Lippincott's Manual of

TOXICOLOGY

Wolters Kluwer | Lippincott Williams & Wilkins
Health

Philadelphia · Baltimore · New York · London
Buenos Aires · Hong Kong · Sydney · Tokyo

Acquisitions Editor: Rebecca Gaertner
Product Manager: Tom Gibbons
Vendor Manager: Alicia Jackson
Senior Manufacturing Manager: Benjamin Rivera
Marketing Manager: Kimberly Schonberger
Design Coordinator: Teresa Mallon
Production Service: Aptara, Inc.

© 2012 by LIPPINCOTT WILLIAMS & WILKINS, a WOLTERS KLUWER business
Two Commerce Square
2001 Market Street
Philadelphia, PA 19103 USA
LWW.com

All rights reserved. This book is protected by copyright. No part of this book may be reproduced in any
form by any means, including photocopying, or utilized by any information storage and retrieval system
without written permission from the copyright owner, except for brief quotations embodied in critical articles
and reviews. Materials appearing in this book prepared by individuals as part of their official duties as U.S.
government employees are not covered by the above-mentioned copyright.

Printed in China

Library of Congress Cataloging-in-Publication Data available upon request.
978-1-4511-7330-7
1-4511-7330-X

Care has been taken to confirm the accuracy of the information presented and to describe generally accepted
practices. However, the authors, editors, and publisher are not responsible for errors or omissions or for any
consequences from application of the information in this book and make no warranty, expressed or implied,
with respect to the currency, completeness, or accuracy of the contents of the publication. Application of the
information in a particular situation remains the professional responsibility of the practitioner.

The authors, editors, and publisher have exerted every effort to ensure that drug selection and dosage set
forth in this text are in accordance with current recommendations and practice at the time of publication.
However, in view of ongoing research, changes in government regulations, and the constant flow of information relating to drug therapy and drug reactions, the reader is urged to check the package insert for each
drug for any change in indications and dosage and for added warnings and precautions. This is particularly
important when the recommended agent is a new or infrequently employed drug.

Some drugs and medical devices presented in the publication have Food and Drug Administration (FDA)
clearance for limited use in restricted research settings. It is the responsibility of the health care provider to
ascertain the FDA status of each drug or device planned for use in their clinical practice.

To purchase additional copies of this book, call our customer service department at (800) 638-3030 or fax
orders to (301) 223-2320. International customers should call (301) 223-2300.

Visit Lippincott Williams & Wilkins on the Internet: at LWW.com. Lippincott Williams & Wilkins
customer service representatives are available from 8:30 am to 6 pm, EST.

10 9 8 7 6 5 4 3 2 1

PREFACE

Why another toxicology handbook for the busy clinician? Many toxicology handbooks provide the reader with generalizations and bullet points but are not specific enough to guide the care of the individual patient who requires immediate emergency management. Other handbooks may be overly prescriptive in their recommendations and fail to adequately consider the nuances of diagnosis and management that vary with each patient and each poisoning.

Those who are familiar with *Harwood-Nuss's Clinical Practice of Emergency Medicine* already know it as a concise and practical, yet comprehensive and accurate, bedside guide to emergency care, as well as a valuable resource for education and reference.

These chapters, extracted from the Harwood-Nuss textbook, are easy to read and easy to use, with critical interventions and common pitfalls specifically highlighted. They are written by an impressive array of board-certified practicing medical toxicologists, who have drawn from their extensive clinical experience and well-established expertise to provide the clinician with the latest practical evidence-based recommendations—on both the common poisonings and the rare and obscure ones.

A world of toxicologic wisdom is packaged in this pocket-sized handbook, ready for use at a moment's notice to guide the critical emergency management of the poisoned patient.

Allan B. Wolfson, MD
Louis J. Ling, MD

ACKNOWLEDGMENTS

Lippincott's Manual of Toxicology has been adapted with permission from *Harwood-Nuss' Clinical Practice of Emergency Medicine*, Fifth Edition, edited by Allan B. Wolfson, Gregory W. Hendey, Louis J. Ling, Carlo L. Rosen, Jeffrey Schaider, and Ghazala Q. Sharieff (Philadelphia: Lippincott Williams & Wilkins, 2010). Additional content is taken from *Rosen & Barkin's 5-Minute Emergency Medicine Consult*, Fourth Edition, edited by Jeffrey J. Schaider, Stephen R. Hayden, Richard E. Wolfe, Roger M. Barkin, and Peter Rosen (Philadelphia: Lippincott Williams & Wilkins, 2007).

We would like to acknowledge the original authors of the chapters:

Joshua G. Schier and Robert S. Hoffman
Chapter 1

Alexander D. Miller and Binh T. Ly
Chapter 2

Mark Su
Chapter 3

Michael Joseph Burns
Chapter 4
Chapter 47

Thomas C. Arnold
Chapter 5

Jeffrey R. Suchard
Chapter 6
Chapter 38
Chapter 56
Chapter 60

Jeffrey Brent and Robert P. Palmer
Chapter 7

Christopher H. Linden and Gerald E. Maloney, Jr.
Chapter 8

Marco L. A. Sivilotti
Chapter 9
Chapter 18

Anna M. Arroyo Plasencia and R. Brent Furbee
Chapter 10

James A. Feldman, Lauren M. Nentwich, and Geoffrey M. Gray
Chapter 11

Carson R. Harris
Chapter 12

Matthew W. Morgan and Carson R. Harris
Chapter 13

Stephen W. Smith
Chapter 14

E. Martin Caravati and Barbara Insley Crouch
Chapter 15

Ejaaz A. Kalimullah and Steven E. Aks
Chapter 16

Allan R. Mottram and Sean M. Bryant
Chapter 17

Jenny J. Lu and Mark B. Mycyk
Chapter 19

Timothy E. Albertson, Kathy A. Marquardt, and Judith A. Alsop
Chapter 20

Christopher H. Linden and William J. Lewander
Chapter 21

Alan D. Woolf
Chapter 22

Jeanmarie Perrone
Chapter 23

William K. Chiang and Richard Y. Wang
Chapter 24

Richard D. Shih and Robert S. Hoffman
Chapter 25

S. Rutherfoord Rose and James E. Cisek
Chapter 26

Susan E. Farrell
Chapter 27

Fermin Barrueto, Jr.
Chapter 28

Matthew D. Sztajnkrycer and G. Randall Bond
Chapter 29

John S. Kashani
Chapter 30

Beth A. Baker
Chapter 31

Kent R. Olson
Chapter 32

Larissa I. Velez and Collin S. Goto
Chapter 33

Heather Long
Chapter 34
Chapter 42

Kennon Heard
Chapter 35

K. Sophia Dyer
Chapter 36

Howard K. Mell and Matthew D. Sztajnkrycer
Chapter 37

Steven M. Marcus
Chapter 39

David A. Tanen and Michael J. Matteucci
Chapter 40

Kenneth D. Katz and Robert D. Cannon
Chapter 41

Michael C. Young, Alexander D. Miller, and Richard F. Clark
Chapter 43

William J. Cimikoski and Keith K. Burkhart
Chapter 44

Michael C. Young, Megan Demott, and Richard F. Clark
Chapter 45

Kenneth W. Kulig
Chapter 46

Claudia L. Barthold, Jennifer A. Oakes, and Andis Graudins
Chapter 48

Andis Graudins
Chapter 49

Richard D. Shih and Judd E. Hollander
Chapter 50

Howard A. Greller
Chapter 51

Pierre Gaudreault
Chapter 52

Cyrus Rangan
Chapter 53

Michael J. Lynch and Anthony F. Pizon
Chapter 54

Milton Tenenbein
Chapter 55

Michael Joseph Burns and Christopher H. Linden
Chapter 57

Paul M. Wax and Richard Barrera
Chapter 58

Adhi Sharma
Chapter 59

Brandon K. Wills and Steven E. Aks
Chapter 61

Judith A. Alsop
Chapter 62

Samara Soghoian and Lewis S. Nelson
Chapter 63

Brenna M. Farmer, Robert B. Dowsett, and Lewis S. Nelson
Chapter 64

We would like to acknowledge the reviewers of these chapters:

Joshua J. Lynch, DO, EMT-P
Clinical Instructor of Emergency Medicine
School of Medicine and Biomedical Science
University at Buffalo
EMS Medical Director
FDR Medical Services
Buffalo, New York

Kevin R. McGee, D.O.
Assistant Clinical Professor of Emergency Medicine
School of Medicine and Biomedical Sciences
University at Buffalo
Buffalo, New York

CONTENTS

General Considerations

General Considerations: Recognition, Initial Approach, and Early Management of the Poisoned Patient

PRE-HOSPITAL CONSIDERATIONS

- Search for clues at the scene:
  - Pills and pill bottles
  - Drug paraphernalia
- Obtain information from witnesses.
- Transport all drugs and pill bottles for identification.
- Restrain uncooperative patients for the protection of the patient and health care personnel.
- Consider comorbid conditions:
  - Trauma
  - Medical illness
  - Environmental exposure
- Consider prehospital administration of activated charcoal, which may optimize decontamination if a prolonged transport time is expected.

Poisoning is a clinical or physiologic state induced by exposure to a xenobiotic (a foreign chemical). The presence and severity of poisoning after exposure to a particular agent is dependent on a number of unalterable factors, including the agent itself, dose of agent, route and duration of exposure, age, weight, and health status (e.g., presence of comorbid conditions) of the patient. However, factors that occur after exposure can be optimized for the best outcome. These include time to emergency department (ED) presentation, whether the history is adequate to diagnose a possible poisoning, and finally, the timely delivery of potentially beneficial therapies. Emergency physicians see acutely poisoned patients first and have the best opportunity to limit the severity of poisoning. This chapter focuses on the most common type of poisonings, which are ingestions and respiratory exposures, and does not discuss dermal or eye exposures.

DIFFERENTIAL DIAGNOSIS

The first challenge in a poisoned patient is to recognize that a chemical exposure has occurred. Frequently, patients or witnesses may suggest an accidental poisoning, a potential suicide, or recreational drug use. At other times, the history is not available. Clinical manifestations of poisoning can often mimic other diseases. For instance, an elderly patient with chronic salicylate toxicity may present solely with altered mental status, and the diagnosis may be delayed while the patient is evaluated and treated for infection. Patients may not be aware that a chemical exposure is the cause of their symptoms, may choose not to share information about it (e.g., intentional drug overdose in a suicidal patient), or may be unable to communicate because of altered mental status. Therefore, it is critical to (a) consider poisoning in the undifferentiated patient presenting to the ED, (b) be familiar with toxidromes, the potential signs and symptoms associated with a variety of toxic poisonings, (c) be familiar with laboratory and diagnostic methodologies and other resources such as poison centers, and (d) know how to effectively manage poisoning-associated conditions.

DIAGNOSTIC APPROACH

The initial approach to the poisoned patient is similar to that used with other undifferentiated patients (Fig. 1.1). Patients should be identified as stable or unstable. Unstable patients with (a) one or more abnormal vital signs, (b) dyspnea, or (c) altered mental status should be treated with aggressive supportive measures and should have cardiac monitoring, continuous pulse oximetry, and IV access. A 12-lead electrocardiogram (ECG) should be evaluated for dysrhythmias and conduction disturbances. If altered mental status is present, a rapid blood glucose test should be done and IV dextrose administered if needed. Toxicologic causes of hypoglycemia are numerous and include insulin, sulfonylureas, ethanol, and beta-blockers. Specific antidotes are available. Thiamine may be of benefit in selected cases, and naloxone is indicated if an opioid toxidrome is present in a patient with an altered mental status. The dyspneic patient should be given oxygen, and airway stabilization measures should be taken. Toxicologic causes of dyspnea and shortness of breath can include carbon monoxide and methemoglobin-inducing agents (e.g., nitrates, dapsone), metabolic poisons (cyanide, sodium monofluoroacetate), irritative or asphyxiant gas inhalation, and atypical agents such as paraquat.

A thorough history and physical examination should be performed in both stable and unstable patients. This should include focused questioning of the emergency medical services personnel and/or family members who brought the patient to the ED. If the patient is able to communicate, the history should include questions about the possibility of a toxic exposure. If the patient is unable or unwilling to cooperate, family members or friends should be contacted for additional information.

Some poisonings may be diagnosed if patients present with a toxidrome that is associated with exposure to a particular agent. Common toxidromes are described in Table 1.1. However, a mixed overdose may not manifest with a clear toxidrome. Potential etiologies stratified by mechanism of action are listed in Table 1.2.

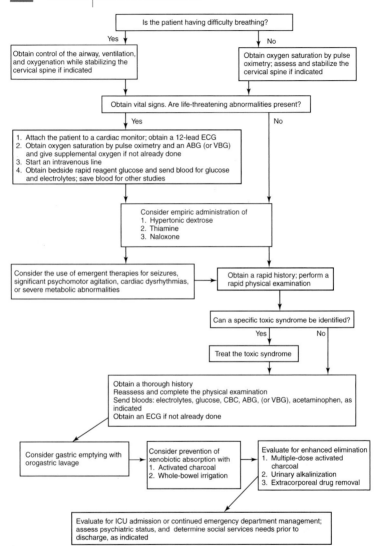

FIGURE 1.1. The algorithm is a basic guide to the management of poisoned patients. A more detailed description of the steps in management may be found in the accompanying text. This algorithm is only a guide to actual management, which must, of course, consider the patient's clinical status.

TABLE 1.1 Recognized Toxidromes with Potential Etiologies

Toxidrome	Signs and Symptoms	Mechanism of Action	Potential Etiologies
Cholinergic	DUMBELS (diarrhea, urination, miosis, bradycardia, bronchorrhea, bronchospasm, emesis, lacrimation, salivation)	Overstimulation of cholinergic receptors by acetylcholine via inhibition of acetylcholinesterase	Organic phosphorous compounds, carbamates
Anticholinergic	Flushed and dry skin, hyperthermia, urinary retention, confusion	Competitive inhibition of acetylcholinesterase receptors	Anticholinergic or antihistaminic compounds, tricyclic antidepressants, disopyramide
Sedative–hypnotic	Coma, hypothermia, sinus bradycardia, bradypnea, hyporeflexia, hypotension or normal BP	Enhanced central nervous system inhibitory tone or alteration of normal glucose homeostasis	Sedative–hypnotics, ethanol and other alcohols, hypoglycemia-inducing agents
Opioid	Coma, miosis, hyporeflexia, hypothermia, decreased bowel sounds, bradycardia, bradypnea, hypotension or normal BP	Overstimulation of opioid receptors	All opioids, agents with capability of stimulating opioid receptors
Sympathomimetic	Hypertension, hyperthermia, tachypnea, tachycardia, agitation, confusion, aggressive behavior	Alterations in normal neurotransmitter production, release or function	Stimulants (e.g., amphetamines, cocaine, phencyclidine), monoamine oxidase inhibitors, antipsychotics (neuroleptic malignant syndrome), serotonin reuptake inhibitors (serotonin syndrome)
Withdrawal syndromes: sedative–hypnotic	Hyperthermia, tachypnea, tachycardia, agitation or confusion; sometimes seizures, tremor and hypertension	Alterations in neurotransmitter production, release or function due to abrupt cessation of a chronically used agent	Ethanol, sedative–hypnotic agents, gamma hydroxybutyrate
Withdrawal syndromes: opioid	Piloerection, vomiting, rhinorrhea, diarrhea, yawning; sometimes tachycardia and tachypnea	Alterations in neurotransmitter production, release or function due to abrupt cessation of a chronically used agent	Opioids

TABLE 1.2 Vital Sign Abnormalities Stratified by Mechanism of Action and Potential Etiology in the Poisoned Patient

Abnormality	Mechanism	Potential Etiologies
Hyperthermia	Interfere with normal neurotransmitter production, release, or function	Stimulant drugs (amphetamines, phencyclidine), antipsychotic drugs (neuroleptic malignant syndrome), serotonin reuptake inhibitors (serotonin syndrome), ethanol withdrawal, anticholinergic drugs
	Inhibitors of oxidative phosphorylation	Dinitrophenol, salicylates
	Hormone-induced changes	Thyroid replacement hormone
Hypothermia	Slow metabolism (typically via interference with normal neurotransmitter production, release or function)	Ethanol and other alcohols, sedative–hypnotic drugs, opioids
	Interfere with normal glucose homeostasis	Insulin, sulfonylureas
Sinus tachycardia	Interfere with normal neurotransmitter production, release, or function	Stimulants (amphetamines, phencyclidine), antipsychotic drugs (neuroleptic malignant syndrome), serotonin reuptake inhibitors (serotonin syndrome), withdrawal syndromes, anticholinergic drugs and cholinergic agents (e.g., organic phosphorous compounds)
	Hypovolemia-inducers	Diuretics
	Respiratory distress-inducers (secondary effect)	Irritant or asphyxiant gases, inducers of abnormal hemoglobin (e.g., nitrites)
	Metabolic poisons	Cyanide, sodium monofluoroacetate, hydrogen sulfide
Sinus bradycardia	Slow normal metabolism (typically via interference with normal neurotransmitter production, release or function)	Opioids, sedative–hypnotic agents, cholinergic agents (e.g., organic phosphorous compounds), baclofen, beta-adrenergic antagonists
	Interfere with voltage-gated ion channel function in the myocardium	Calcium-channel blockers, digoxin and other cardioactive glycosides
	Hypoglycemic-inducing agents	Sulfonylureas, insulin

Tachypnea	Metabolic poisons	Cyanide, sodium monofluoroacetate, hydrogen sulfide
	Interfere with normal neurotransmitter production, release, or function	Stimulants (amphetamines, phencyclidine), antipsychotic drugs (neuroleptic malignant syndrome), serotonin reuptake inhibitors (serotonin syndrome), withdrawal syndromes, anticholinergic drugs and cholinergic agents (e.g., organic phosphorous compounds)
	Hematotoxic agents	Abnormal hemoglobin inducers including carbon monoxide, nitrites, dapsone, and others
	Uncouple oxidative phosphorylation	Dinitrophenol, salicylates
	Inducers of metabolic acidosis	Toxic alcohols and metabolic poisons
	Irritant and asphyxiant gases	Chlorine and other gases
	Selective pulmonary system damage	Paraquat
Bradypnea	Interfere with normal neurotransmitter production, release, or function	Gamma-aminobutyric acid, opioids, sedative-hypnotics, cholinergic agents
	Interfere with glucose homeostasis	Insulin, sulfonylureas
Hypertension	Interfere with normal neurotransmitter production, release, or function	Stimulants (amphetamines, phencyclidine), antipsychotic drugs (neuroleptic malignant syndrome), serotonin reuptake inhibitors (serotonin syndrome), withdrawal syndromes, anticholinergic drugs and cholinergic agents (e.g., organic phosphorous compounds)
Hypotension	Slow metabolism (typically via interference with normal neurotransmitter production, release or function)	Opioids, sedative-hypnotic agents, cholinergic agents (e.g., organic phosphorous compounds), baclofen, beta-adrenergic antagonists
	Interfere with voltage-gated ion channel function in the myocardium	Anti-dysrhythmic agents, digoxin, other cardioactive glycosides
	Hypovolemia and relative hypovolemia	Diuretics, peripheral vasodilating agents

Laboratory and diagnostic testing such as a blood cell count, serum electrolytes, renal function tests, liver function tests, arterial or venous blood gas analysis with co-oximetry testing for dyshemoglobinemia, and ECG can be helpful in determining the etiology and severity of poisoning. In the undifferentiated patient, these routine, readily available laboratory tests are more likely to be of greater benefit than toxicology screening, except in the case of commonly used drugs such as ethanol, phenytoin, and digoxin for which drug levels are readily available.

Acidosis or acidemia, as indicated by serum bicarbonate level or arterial blood gas analysis, suggests toxic alcohols, salicylates, iron, isoniazid, or metabolic poisons such as cyanide and hydrogen sulfide. Acidosis combined with severe hypocalcemia and hyperkalemia strongly suggests exposure to a fluoride-containing compound. Multiple organ toxicity in conjunction with acidosis, hypotension, tachycardia, and gastrointestinal manifestations over several hours is suggestive of heavy metal, ricin, or colchicine toxicity. When these same symptoms develop over the course of minutes or a few hours, however, a metabolic poison (cyanide, hydrogen sulfide, sodium monofluoroacetate) should be suspected. Pulse oximetry can be falsely reassuring in some poisonings. A cyanotic patient with dyspnea, headache, and a normal pulse oximetry reading may suffer from carbon monoxide poisoning whereas a similar patient with pulse oximetry readings that are lower than expected suggests methemoglobinemia.

The ECG can identify toxin-induced cardiac abnormalities such as prolongation of the QRS interval (tricyclic antidepressants, antidysrhythmic agents) and prolongation of the QT interval (antipsychotics, antidysrhythmics, lithium). Many agents produce dysrhythmias either directly or indirectly. Finally, the urine drug screen is typically not helpful in identifying the etiologic agent causing poisoning in most undifferentiated patient. It may be helpful in a patient with a new acute psychosis or may provide a clue in the critical unstable patient of unknown etiology. Because tests vary among institutions and the sensitivity and specificity are also variable, it is important for emergency physicians to be familiar with the urine drug screen available at their own institutions and its applicability in different clinical settings.

A national network of poison centers (PC) provide toxicology consultation for the clinician. (Dialing 1-800-222-1222 automatically connects to the closest PC within the continental United States.) The primary service provided by PCs is to assist with the identification and treatment of poisoned patients and with chemical terrorism preparedness. They also provide public education and assist public health departments. PC-collected data are reviewed for potential chemical terrorism, epidemics, and trends affecting the public health. Physicians are, therefore, strongly urged to report all cases of poisoning, adverse drug events, and therapeutic misadventures to PCs.

IMMEDIATE CRITICAL INTERVENTIONS

As with all emergency patients, stabilization is the first priority. Toxin-induced seizures should be treated with benzodiazepines, barbiturates, and propofol, in that order. Toxin-induced seizures are the result of a systemic metabolic process affecting a large number of neurons. Anticonvulsants such as phenytoin are designed to block impulse *propagation,* as seen in epilepsy, which explains their ineffectiveness in toxin-induced seizures. Seizures associated with a recognizable toxidrome respond best to benzodiazepines, but other appropriate antidotes should be considered (e.g., atropine and pralidoxime for organic phosphorous compound poisoning). True toxin-induced status epilepticus is rare but can result from ingestion of theophylline, isoniazid, hydrazine-associated agents, or monomethylhydrazine-containing mushrooms. The latter three entities should be treated with pyridoxine (vitamin B_6).

After initial evaluation and stabilization, further evaluation and treatment should follow a sign- and symptom-oriented approach focused toward creation of a differential diagnosis of potential etiologies.

Gastrointestinal Decontamination   The severity of poisoning is related directly to the amount of compound absorbed by the patient. If the dose absorbed can be minimized, toxicity may be minimized as well. In some cases, removing a fraction of available drug from the gastrointestinal tract may convert a fatal poisoning to a severe but nonfatal one. The patient's presentation, the type of substance or drug ingested, and the time since ingestion determine the best method of gastrointestinal decontamination (GID) to be utilized: orogastric lavage (OGL), single- or multiple-dose activated charcoal (AC), or whole-bowel irrigation (WBI). Syrup of ipecac is obsolete and is no longer used (2).

Whether to use GID depends on a risk-benefit assessment of the procedure, the likelihood of removing a clinically significant amount of toxin, and the availability of alternative treatments, such as antidotes (4). GID is unnecessary in a patient with a benign overdose who is expected to do very well with minimal treatment, whereas a patient who has just ingested a large number of highly toxic tablets (e.g., extended-release verapamil) is at high risk of severe toxicity and may benefit from a GID. The possibility of removing a clinically significant amount of toxin by GID depends on drug pharmacokinetics and time from ingestion. Generally, there is little likelihood of removing significant amounts of drug from the stomach beyond 1 to 2 hours after ingestion, with the exception of drugs that slow gastrointestinal mobility (e.g., anticholinergics, opioids, or sedative–hypnotics) (1,4,5). Occasionally, concretions of partially digested drug tablets in the stomach may serve as a reservoir for delayed absorption. Drugs that form such concretions or bezoars include salicylates, meprobamate, phenobarbital, and iron (4). The availability of antidotes (e.g., *N*-acetylcysteine for acetaminophen toxicity) also decreases the need for GID.

Orogastric Lavage.   OGL refers to the use of a No. 36 to 40 French tube inserted through the mouth to evacuate the contents of the stomach. Nasal tubes are much smaller (14–18 French) and cannot remove pills, pill fragments, or other particulate matter as easily, although they may be able to remove some ingested liquids still in the stomach. Complications of OGL include aspiration pneumonia, laryngospasm, tension pneumothorax, charcoal empyema, esophageal perforation, atrial and ventricular ectopic beats, and conjunctival hemorrhage.

Gastric lavage is rarely needed but may have a beneficial effect on outcome if performed in the sickest patients within 1 hour of ingestion (9,10), but data neither support nor refute the utility of OGL in other situations. Gastric emptying half-times >120 minutes are seen in almost half of tricyclic antidepressant (TCA), acetaminophen, opioid-acetaminophen, and carbamazepine overdoses, and these patients may benefit from OGL when there has been a serious or life-threatening ingestion (1). In the majority of patients, those who present more than 1 hour after ingestion or who are asymptomatic, OGL is unlikely to add any benefit to AC administration alone (3). OGL should be strongly considered for ingestion of a life-threatening or difficult-to-treat poison (such as the tricyclic antidepressants, calcium channel blockers, and β-adrenergic blockers), and for severely ill patients who present within one hour of ingestion (3,4,9). Other factors that may make gastric emptying appropriate include an ingested amount that exceeds the adsorptive capacity of AC, an ingested agent that is poorly adsorbed to AC, absence of effective antidotal therapy, and the possibility that the ingested agent may form concretions in the stomach (4). OGL should be avoided in nontoxic ingestions, when the procedure entails avoidable risk (e.g., increasing aspiration risk after a hydrocarbon ingestion), when the airway is unprotected, and in general when the risks outweigh the potential benefits (4).

OGL should be performed only if the patient's airway is secure. The length of tube to be inserted should be estimated externally and marked prior to insertion, and the patient should be placed in the left lateral decubitus position. The lubricated tube should be inserted into the mouth, taking care to not force it if significant resistance is encountered. Placement should be confirmed by auscultation of insufflated air over the stomach. Lavage should be conducted with small amounts (adults, 200–300 mL; children, 10 mL/kg) of warm normal saline and with removal of most of the administered fluid before giving more, until the fluid recovered from the stomach no longer has any particulate matter (4). A dose of AC should be administered, after which the tube is removed.

Activated Charcoal. AC decreases the systemic absorption of many drugs, although its efficacy, much like the other GID techniques, decreases with the presence of food, when administration is delayed and depends significantly on the particular drug ingested. Chemicals that are not bound by AC include alcohols, small ions such as caustics, hydrocarbons, and most metals. AC is most effective if administered within 1 hour after ingestion of a toxin. Administration of AC to patients beyond 1 hour of poisoning may be of benefit for controlled-release formulations and anticholinergic drugs, or opiates such as oxycodone, which delay gastrointestinal motility (1,4,6–8).

The risks associated with single-dose AC administration include emesis, nausea, and vomiting, which are common. Of greatest concern is pulmonary aspiration, which may be fatal. Aspiration is often a result of inappropriate administration or inadequate airway control, but even endotracheal intubation does not provide an absolute guarantee against aspiration. Correctly placed nasogastric or orogastric tube in an awake, alert patient does not increase the risk of pulmonary aspiration (4,8).

The dose of AC is theoretically a 10:1 ratio of charcoal to drug or 1 g/kg patient body weight (whichever is larger). The 10:1 ratio is easily achievable when the amount ingested per unit dose is small (e.g., clonidine, 0.2 mg, or levothyroxine, 0.3 mg), but ingestions with very large amounts per unit dose (e.g., aspirin, 325 mg, or theophylline, 300 mg) should be treated with a higher initial dose of AC but not exceeding, 1.5 to 2.0 g/kg. A small nasogastric tube and antiemetics may be needed to facilitate AC administration (4,8). The routine use of cathartics with AC is discouraged (4,8).

Volunteer studies and some clinical studies demonstrate that multiple-dose activated charcoal (MDAC) enhances elimination (although a clinical benefit has not been confirmed in all): carbamazepine, dapsone, phenobarbital, quinine, theophylline, phenylbutazone, digitoxin, digoxin, salicylate, cyclosporine, propoxyphene, nortriptyline, amitriptyline, phenytoin, sotalol, nadolol, piroxicam, and disopyramide. Other ingestions that may benefit from MDAC include controlled-release formulations, agents that form concretions in the stomach (e.g., salicylate), large ingestions wherein a 10:1 ratio of AC to drug cannot be achieved with a single dose, or if the agents undergo enteroenteric or enterohepatic cycling. Reported dosing regimens vary, but a reasonable dosing regimen for most ingestions is 1 g/kg of AC as the initial dose followed with 0.5 g/kg every 3 to 4 hours for a total of three additional doses. Complications of MDAC are similar to those of single-dose AC, with the addition of intestinal obstruction. Contraindications to MDAC administration are also similar, with the addition of patients with decreased peristalsis as a relative contraindication (4,8).

Whole-Bowel Irrigation. The goal of WBI is to prevent absorption by flushing any unabsorbed toxin rapidly through the intestinal tract. Polyethylene glycol electrolyte lavage solution (PEG-ELS, available as Go-Lytely, Colyte and others) causes minimal water and electrolyte shifts (8).

Certain "controlled-release" drug formulations are designed specifically not to dissolve immediately but rather to dissolve at a predesignated rate. Many cardiovascular drugs are available as once- or twice-a-day formulations designed to enhance patient compliance. The controlled-release formulations of β-blockers and calcium channel blockers are good candidates for WBI. "Body packers" who ingest carefully packaged units of illegal drugs for the purpose of transporting them across international borders are also candidates for WBI (4,8). Finally, WBI enhances the elimination of metals such as iron, lead, and arsenic, which are not well adsorbed to activated charcoal (4,8).

WBI should be performed with PEG-ELS and administered orally or through a small nasogastric tube. A recommended dosing regimen is 0.5 L/hours for small children and 1.5 to 2 L/hours for adolescents and adults until all ingested drug has passed or until the rectal effluent is clear. Contraindications to WBI include gastrointestinal disease or dysfunction (ileus, perforation, obstruction, and hemorrhage), an unprotected airway, hemodynamic instability, absent bowel sounds, or intractable vomiting (4,8).

Specific Treatments There are a number of potential antidotes readily available to the emergency physician for the treatment of specific poisonings (Table 1.3). Examples include atropine for cholinergic crisis, dextrose for hypoglycemia, sodium bicarbonate for tricyclic antidepressants and other fast sodium-channel blocking agents, physostigmine for pure anticholinergic compound overdose (e.g., diphenhydramine), intravenous potassium and calcium salt administration for fluoride-containing compounds, hydroxycobalamin for cyanide, and *N*-acetylcysteine for acetaminophen. There are numerous other antidotes that are not as readily available to the emergency physician but that are typically stocked in most hospital pharmacies for selected poisonings. Some examples include deferoxamine for iron poisoning, succimer for lead toxicity, pralidoxime for organic phosphorus compound poisoning, digoxin-specific

TABLE 1.3	Poisonings with Specific Antidotes
Drugs	**Antidotes**
Acetaminophen	N Acetylcysteine (NAC)
Anticholinergics	Pralidoxime/Atropine
Anticoagulants	
Benzodiazepines	Flumazenil
β-Blockers	Glucagon
Calcium channel blockers	Glucagon/Calcium
Carbon monoxide	O2/Hyperbaric O2
Cyanide	Hydroxycobalamin/Lilly Kit
Digitalis	Digoxin immune FAB
Ethylene glycol	Ethanol/fomepizole
Envenomations	Too many to list specific
Fluoride	Calcium gluconate
Heavy metals	EDTA-Calcium
Heparin	Protamine sulfate
Hydrogen sulfide	Nitrites
Hypoglycemics	Sulfonylureas- octreotide
Isoniazid	Pyridoxine (vitamin B6)
Methanol	Fomepizole/Ethanol
Methemoglobinemia	Methylene Blue
Opioids	Naloxone
Pradaxa (dabigatran)	No true antidote
Sympathomimetics	No specific antidote
Vacor	No specific antidote
Warfarin	Vitamin K/FFP

antibody fragments for digoxin and cardioactive glycoside poisoning, and vitamin K for complications of long-acting anticoagulant. These treatments are discussed in detail in the corresponding specific chapters.

CRITICAL INTERVENTIONS

- Always consider the possibility of a toxic exposure in the undifferentiated patient.
- Utilize readily available bedside testing as appropriate, including bedside glucose, 12-lead ECG, and pulse oximetry monitoring.
- Consider the time since ingestion, potential severity of poisoning, and complications before performing GID.
- Assess the patient's ability to protect the airway and the potential for deterioration prior to performing GID.
- Consult a poison center regarding GID in questionable cases.

DISPOSITION

After an appropriate observation period, usually 4 to 6 hours, asymptomatic patients may be discharged from the ED. The disposition of symptomatic patients depends on the actual or predicted severity and the need or potential need for therapeutic interventions. Most patients develop only mild toxicity after exposure and can be observed in the ED until they are asymptomatic or improved. Those with significant physiologic effects, hypoxia, hypercarbia, acid-base disturbances, metabolic abnormalities, extremes of temperature, or cardiac conduction or rhythm abnormalities should be admitted to an intensive care unit. Patients who require close monitoring of antidotal therapy or high-risk elimination procedures, those showing progressive clinical deterioration or long-acting or delayed poisonings, and those with significant underlying medical problems are also candidates for the intensive care unit. Continuous observation of suicidal patients may require a higher level of care than is necessary for the medical consequences of a toxic exposure.

Consultation with a poison center is recommended whenever the treating physician is not familiar with the specific agent or agents involved in a given exposure.

Parents and other caretakers of children should be instructed to store alcoholic beverages; medications; household chemicals; nonedible plants; vitamins; and toiletries above or out of the child's reach or in cabinets with locks or childproof latches. Safety caps are always advisable but are not necessarily sufficient to prevent access by children. Adults with accidental home exposures should be instructed regarding the safe use of drugs and other chemicals, advised to read the instructions on labels carefully, and encouraged to avoid the circumstances that caused the current problem. Notifying the appropriate governmental agency (e.g., Environmental Protection Agency, Occupational Safety and Health Administration, National Institute for Occupational Safety and Health, the local health department) should be considered in cases of environmental or workplace exposure. Unsafe working conditions should also be brought to the attention of the employer. For cases in which confused patients had accidental exposures caused by dosing errors, assistance with the administration of medicines should be arranged.

COMMON PITFALLS

- Failing to consider the possibility of poisoning in the undifferentiated patient
- Relying on urine toxicology screens for a diagnosis
- Failing to appreciate that in select cases GID can be effective beyond an hour or two of ingestion
- Failing to secure the airway prior to GID when there is central nervous system depression
- Failing to appreciate that for most ingestions AC alone is the most appropriate method of GID
- Failing to consider WBI for ingestions of controlled-release formulations or agents that are slowly absorbed

ICD 9

977.8 Poisoning by other specified drugs and medicinal substances
977.9 Poisoning by unspecified drug or medicinal substance
989.9 Toxic effect of unspecified substance, chiefly nonmedicinal as to source

REFERENCES

1. Adams BK, Mann MD, Aboo A, et al. Prolonged gastric-emptying half-time and gastric hypomotility after drug overdose. *Am J Emerg Med* 2004;22(7):548–554.
2. American Academy of Pediatrics, Committee on Injury, Violence, and Poison Prevention. Poison treatment in the home. *Pediatrics* 2003;112:1182–1185.
3. Bond GR. The role of activated charcoal and gastric emptying in gastrointestinal decontamination: a state-of-the-art review. *Ann Emerg Med* 2002;39:273–286.
4. Christophersen ABJ, Hoegberg LCG. Techniques used to prevent gastrointestinal absorption. In: Flomenbaum NE, Goldfrank LR, Hoffman RS, et al., eds. *Goldfrank's Toxicologic Emergencies,* 8th ed. New York: McGraw-Hill, 2006.
5. Comstock EG, Boisaubin EV, Comstock BS, et al. Assessment of the efficacy of activated charcoal following orogastric lavage in acute drug overdose. *J Toxicol Clin Toxicol* 1982;19:149–165.
6. Green R, Sitar DS, Tenebein M. Effect of anticholinergic drugs on the efficacy of activated charcoal. *J Toxicol Clin Toxicol* 2004;42(3):267–272.
7. Halcomb SE, Sivilotti ML, Goklaney A, et al. Pharmacokinetic effects of diphenhydramine or oxycodone in simulated acetaminophen overdose. *Acad Emerg Med* 2005;12(2):169–172.
8. Howland MA. Antidotes in depth: syrup of ipecac, activated charcoal, and whole bowel irrigation and other intestinal evacuants. In: Flomenbaum NE, Goldfrank LR, Hoffman RS, et al., eds. *Goldfrank's Toxicologic Emergencies,* 8th ed. New York: McGraw-Hill, 2006.
9. Kulig K, Bar-Or D, Cantrill SV, et al. Management of acutely poisoned patients without gastric emptying. *Ann Emerg Med* 1985;14:59–64.
10. Pond SM, Lewis-Driver DJ, Williams GM, et al. Gastric emptying in acute overdose: a prospective randomized controlled trial. *Med J Aust* 1995;163:345–349.

SECTION 2

Alcohol-Related Agents and Conditions

CHAPTER 2

Ethanol

PRE-HOSPITAL CONSIDERATIONS
- Administer benzodiazepines for seizures.
- Give naloxone, oxygen, and dextrose to comatose individuals.
- Intubate as necessary for airway protection to prevent aspiration.
- Immobilize cervical spine in cases of suspected trauma.

CLINICAL PRESENTATION

Clinical manifestations following acute ethanol consumption vary considerably, and caution must be employed when trying to attribute clinical manifestations to any specific serum ethanol concentration. At lower dosages, ethanol's depression of inhibitory cortical pathways in the brain may create the appearance of central nervous system (CNS) stimulation through disinhibition. These effects may be most pronounced in mildly to moderately intoxicated individuals who engage in functions requiring higher degrees of cortical integration. Individuals exhibit euphoria, gregariousness, verbosity, or emotional lability. Frequently, disinhibited behavior strongly reflects the individual's basic personality and results in boisterous or aggressive behavior. Other manifestations may include ataxia, nystagmus, and impaired reaction time. With deeper intoxication, disinhibition and impairment of cognitive integration may be progressive. Overt displays of hostility and aggressiveness emerge. Finally, with higher dosages of ethanol and severe intoxication, profound CNS depression, coma, and respiratory depression occur with an increased risk of morbidity as concomitant loss of airway-protective reflexes may ensue.

Because gluconeogenesis is impaired by rising levels of NADH produced during ethanol metabolism, hypoglycemia may develop, particularly in the malnourished adult or the young child. With acute ethanol ingestion, abdominal pain, nausea or vomiting may be present because of either direct gastric irritation by ethanol or secondary processes such as pancreatitis or hepatitis.

Clinical findings suggestive of alcohol abuse are listed in Table 2.1. An alcoholic who is still able to function socially or occupationally may present with chief complaints of memory difficulties, gastrointestinal (GI) dysfunction (including abdominal pain, diarrhea, vomiting, hematemesis, and hepatitis), respiratory complaints, frequent infections, weakness, polysubstance use, withdrawal, or

TABLE 2.1	Clinical Manifestations of Alcohol Abuse
Nervous System	Inebriation Seizures Dementia Coma Wernicke-Korsakoff psychosis Polyneuropathy
Cardiovascular System	Autonomic dysfunction Congestive cardiomyopathy Atrial fibrillation
Gastrointestinal System	Alcoholic hepatitis Alcoholic cirrhosis Peptic ulcer disease Gastrointestinal bleeding Pancreatitis Pancreatic pseudocyst Varices and hemorrhoids Ascites Malabsorption and malnutrition Cancers of the gastrointestinal tract
Genitourinary System	Uric-acid nephropathy Acute tubular necrosis Hepatorenal syndrome
Hematologic	Myelosuppression Coagulopathies Microcytic anemia Megaloblastic anemia Thrombocytopenia
Infectious	Pneumonia Spontaneous bacterial peritonitis
Metabolic	Ketoacidosis Electrolyte abnormalities Vitamin deficiencies Hypothermia
Musculoskeletal	Myopathies Gout Rhabdomyolysis
Pulmonary	Sleep apnea Chronic respiratory insufficiency Tuberculosis
Psychiatric	Anxiety, insomnia Abnormal behaviors Borderline personality Polysubstance abuse

recurrent trauma. Electrolyte imbalances (hypokalemia, hypomagnesemia, and hypocalcemia) are more common in the chronic alcoholic but may occur in the setting of acute intoxication as well (6). Adolescents may present to the emergency department (ED) with a myriad of nonspecific complaints, none of which may directly point to alcohol abuse as a possible underlying etiology. Obtaining a history from family members can be invaluable. The adolescent may have recently undergone significant changes in personality, behavior, peer contacts, or peer relations. College-aged alcoholics, who may use the ED as their only source of health care, can present with vague flu-like symptoms, headache, insomnia, chest palpitations, trauma, GI disturbances, or psychiatric complaints.

Young, otherwise healthy males presenting with chest palpitations, showing paroxysmal atrial fibrillation, atrial tachycardia, or frequent atrial extrasystoles, should be questioned about their ethanol use. Female alcoholics may present with symptoms of anxiety, increased fatigue, insomnia, depression, or irregular menses (7). Geriatric alcoholics may be brought to the department by their families with altered mental status, daytime sleepiness, and irrational behavior.

Occasionally, chronic alcoholics are treated with disulfiram to encourage abstinence. Small amounts of ethanol may induce an adverse reaction in a patient taking disulfiram. Signs and symptoms of the disulfiram-ethanol reaction (DER) include flushing of the face and body, tachycardia, sensations of warmth, urticaria, pruritus, light-headedness, headache, nausea, and vomiting. Complaints of palpitations, chest pain, and shortness of breath are common. In addition, disulfiram may cause inhibition of dopamine-β-hydroxylase, blocking the conversion of dopamine to norepinephrine, which may lead to hypotension. Myocardial ischemia is usually only associated with severe hypotension. In general, deaths attributable to DERs are extremely rare. Manifestations of DER usually begin within 30 minutes of ethanol exposure and may last for several hours. A number of natural and synthetic compounds may induce a disulfiramlike reaction in the presence of ethanol (Table 2.2). Often, the source of ethanol may be elusive because ethanol-containing products in the home are ubiquitous. Similar findings may result from exposure unrelated to ethanol, such as niacin, monosodium glutamate, rifampin, vancomycin, boric acid, and scombroid poisoning.

DIFFERENTIAL DIAGNOSIS

Patients with acute altered mental status in the setting of ethanol use must be carefully evaluated for other causes of altered sensorium unrelated to ethanol intoxication. In the appropriate setting, head injuries, CNS infections, and encephalopathy merit consideration as sources of cognitive impairment. Co-ingestion of other sedating drugs also leads to more pronounced CNS depression. Exposure to other toxic alcohols (see Chapters 4, "Ethylene Glycol" and 5, "Methanol") may create a similar picture of inebriation, but failure to recognize their separate toxicities may have negative consequences for the patient.

TABLE 2.2	Causes of Disulfiram-like Reactions Following Ethanol Exposure
Mushrooms	*Coprinus* sp mushrooms
Chemicals	Carbon disulfide Carbon tetrachloride Tetramethylthiuram (thiram) Trichloroethylene
Medications	Antimicrobials Cephalosporins Cefamandole Cefmenoxime Cefoperazone Cefotetan Metronidazole Trimethoprim-sulfamethoxazole Chloramphenicol Griseofulvin Nitrofurantoin Sulfonylureas Chlorpropamide Tolbutamide Chloral hydrate
Genetic	Aldehyde-dehydrogenase deficiency

An acutely intoxicated patient may present with classic features that include flushed skin, diaphoresis, tachycardia, hypothermia, hypoventilation, vomiting, nystagmus, dysarthria, and incoordination.

However, it is important to recognize signs of coexisting medical illnesses, even in the presence of overt ethanol intoxication. Hypoglycemia can complicate ethanol ingestion in a child or malnourished patient. Abdominal pain in acute alcohol ingestion may simply be related to gastric mucosal irritation, ethanol-induced hepatitis, or pancreatitis, but may be a more serious complication, such as esophageal rupture and perforated gastroduodenal ulcer. Ophthalmoplegia, ataxia, and characteristic mental status alterations suggest Wernicke encephalopathy.

Chronic ethanol use has serious deleterious effects on virtually all organ systems and tissues (2,4,8). The differential diagnosis can include hypoglycemia, sepsis, drug or other toxin exposures, carbon monoxide poisoning, Wernicke-Korsakoff syndrome, tumors, blunt traumatic injury, meningitis, epidural or subdural hematoma, subarachnoid hemorrhage, and dementia, among others (2,7). There is always the danger that an alcoholic may substitute ethanol with potentially lethal intoxicants such as isopropyl alcohol, methanol, ethylene glycol, and sedative drugs, particularly when deprived of access to ethanol.

ED EVALUATION

Obtaining an accurate and thorough history may be impossible when the patient is intoxicated. In the lucid, cooperative patient, information regarding the type, amount, and time of last ethanol use should be obtained, in addition to basic medical history. Clues from friends, family members, or witnesses may be helpful in assessing the risk of trauma or other organ system involvement. Such sources can also be helpful in identifying other substances that might have been co-ingested.

Clinicians should avoid complacency when performing a physical examination, as biased assessments of uncomplicated inebriation may occur with frequent presentations by the same intoxicated individual. The initial evaluation of the acutely intoxicated patient or chronic alcohol abuser is identical to the evaluation of any other potentially ill patient. Patients with altered mental status require an immediate bedside fingerstick blood glucose determination. A complete set of vital signs, including core temperature and oxygen saturation, should be obtained and continuously monitored or frequently reassessed. Subsequently, the patient should be disrobed and carefully examined for signs of trauma or other medical illnesses. Particularly in the patient who is unable to offer a medical history, clinicians must be vigilant when performing a physical examination and consider other diagnostic adjuncts such as computed tomography (CT) of the head or abdomen and laboratory testing to assess for the presence of associated pathology. During initial evaluation, signs of head trauma, pupil size, appropriate response to voice, and hemotympanum should be noted. Signs of trauma or coexistent pathology may become more apparent as the patient becomes less intoxicated. Patients with abnormal vital signs, cardiorespiratory complaints, thoracoabdominal pain, or nonspecific constitutional symptoms should have continuous electrocardiographic monitoring and possibly a 12-lead electrocardiogram (ECG) to evaluate for ischemia and dysrhythmias, particularly atrial fibrillation.

Whether it is necessary to measure ethanol concentrations in the patient who presents with a clinical presentation consistent with uncomplicated acute ethanol intoxication remains controversial. The subjective perception of the presence or absence of ethanol on a patient's breath by care is often an unreliable means of assessing whether an individual has recently used ethanol even under optimum laboratory conditions (5). An initial breath-alcohol level may be helpful in confirming the presence of ethanol, although an accurate level depends on patient compliance. The absence of ethanol or the finding of a low ethanol level should prompt a search for other conditions that may mimic ethanol intoxication. An accurate blood ethanol level may help the clinician estimate a reasonable time for observation while the patient metabolizes. Comatose patients with lower blood ethanol levels than expected for the level of consciousness should be considered for more extensive diagnostic evaluation that may include CT of the head and lumbar puncture, especially if signs of trauma or a fever are present.

In addition to ethanol levels, other blood tests that may be helpful include a complete blood count, serum electrolytes, blood urea nitrogen (BUN), creatinine, ketones, acetone, lipase, transaminases, coagulation profile, ammonia level, cardiac markers, calcium, and magnesium. The decision to initiate these tests will depend upon specific scenarios. An anion gap metabolic acidosis and elevated serum ketones may signify acute alcoholic ketoacidosis and warrants measurement of serum osmolality and calculation of the osmolal gap (the difference between the measured and the calculated osmolality). Ethanol's contribution to the osmolality can be estimated by dividing the serum ethanol level in milligrams per deciliter by 4.6. Ethanol-like intoxication in a patient with an osmolal gap unexplained by the amount of ethanol present should raise suspicion of acetone, isopropanol, methanol, or ethylene glycol ingestion and should prompt measurement of these agents; however, the absence of an osmolal gap cannot exclude the presence of a toxic alcohol.

Although blood-ethanol concentrations may not reliably predict clinical intoxication, it is used legally to define driving while under the influence. In October 2000, the U.S. Congress established a blood-alcohol concentration (BAC) of 0.08 g/dL as the national standard for impaired driving above which it is illegal to drive a motor vehicle, but it is not illegal to have this BAC while not driving. An individual who is not tolerant to ethanol often exhibits impaired driving at blood ethanol concentrations as low as 0.02 g/dL (9). A typical nontolerant adult with a BAC >0.3 to 0.35 g/dL will often be comatose.

The BAC is a measure of ethanol in whole blood and because ethanol more readily distributes into aqueous solutions, serum ethanol concentrations (the standard measurement in most medical institutions) are generally 15% to 20% higher than BAC because of the higher water content in serum compared to whole blood. Because alcohol intoxication can mimic as well as mask disease and injury, a blood- or breath-ethanol level may be obtained to estimate the contribution of alcohol in all patients with systemic complaints. The serum ethanol level can be expected to fall by 0.01 to 0.03 g/dL/h, depending, in part, on individual variables and the timing of the ethanol ingestion (1). In chronic alcoholics, clinical sobriety may occur at blood levels of 0.1 to 0.3 g/dL and may be accompanied by withdrawal in highly tolerant individuals. Once clinical criteria for sobriety are met, the patient may be safely discharged, regardless of the BAC. If the patient fails to improve within a reasonable time or if there is a disparity between the patient's clinical examination and their BAC further investigation is needed to exclude occult head trauma or other life-threatening condition (2,4).

Chronic alcoholism itself can be difficult to diagnose. Laboratory abnormalities have been linked to chronic alcohol intake, but sensitivities and specificities vary from study to study. γ-Glutamyl transferase, the most sensitive indicator of hepatic injury, rises in patients who have had more than five drinks a day for several weeks. Also readily available is an elevated mean red blood cell corpuscular volume. A carbohydrate-deficient transferrin test is highly sensitive and specific for detecting alcohol abuse (3). Table 2.3 summarizes some pertinent aspects of the laboratory and radiologic assessment.

TABLE 2.3	Laboratory and Radiographic Evaluation

Laboratory	**Radiographic**
Complete blood count	Chest radiograph
Cell counts for evaluation of marrow function	Pneumonitis
Indices for folate, iron, pyridoxine, B_{12}	Aspiration
deficiencies	Tuberculosis
Serum chemistries	Pneumothorax
Anion gap	Fractured ribs/trauma
Hypoglycemia or hyperglycemia	Cardiac size
Renal failure	Abdominal radiograph
Electrolyte imbalance (Na, K, Mg, Ca)	Pancreatic calcifications
Hypophosphatemia	Free air
Hyperphosphatemia	Limb radiograph
Arterial blood gas with carbon monoxide oximetry	Fractures
Hypoxemia	Dislocations
Hypercarbia	Osteomyelitis
Metabolic disturbances	Foreign bodies
Carbon monoxide exposure	Computed tomography
Anticonvulsant drug levels	Extra-axial hemorrhage
Urinalysis	Intracerebral hemorrhage
Crystalluria	Intracerebral contusion
Myoglobinuria	Intra-abdominal pathology
Hemoglobinuria	
Liver function tests	
GGT elevation	
AST elevation	
ALT elevation	

GGT, β-glutamyl transferase; AST, aspartate aminotransferase; ALT, alanine aminotransferase.

ED MANAGEMENT

As with all patients with acute mental status changes, rapidly reversible causes such as hyperglycemia and opiate abuse must first be identified and addressed. If occult trauma is suspected, cervical spinal immobilization may be required until the patient is sober and can cooperate with a thorough examination (2). Agitated or combative patients should be restrained with physical and pharmacologic means. Intravenous or intramuscular benzodiazepines or butyrophenones (haloperidol or droperidol) are recommended for pharmacologic sedation. Vigilant and repeated assessments should be performed to monitor for signs of deterioration. Patients who do not respond appropriately as they metabolize the absorbed ethanol should be subjected to further diagnostic examinations and possible therapeutic interventions such as advanced airway management.

Treatment of DERs is also supportive. Intravenous crystalloids should be administered. Antiemetics can be given for nausea and vomiting. Antihistamines such as diphenhydramine (H_1 subtype) may help alleviate cutaneous flushing. Benzodiazepines may be helpful in alleviating associated anxiety and dysphoria. Most DERs can be managed in the ED. Patients can be discharged once they become asymptomatic and vital signs normalize, provided there are no cardiac complications or further evaluation of chest complaints is not indicated. Chronic alcoholics who are malnourished or suspected of Wernicke encephalopathy should receive intravenous thiamine as well as hydration with a balanced electrolyte solution containing dextrose. Significant cost savings may be possible with oral repletion, and those who are frequent ED patients do not need to receive vitamins on every visit. Glucose supplementation remains important, as many alcoholics have inadequate glycogen stores and become hypoglycemic with stress (3). Concomitant medical or surgical problems are treated through standard measures, and treatment of ethanol withdrawal (see Chapter 3) may be required.

CRITICAL INTERVENTIONS

- Perform a fingerstick blood glucose determination to rule out hypoglycemia as a cause of altered mental status in patients with alcohol ingestion.
- Observe patients to assure a clinical course consistent with uncomplicated intoxication.
- In patients whose mental status and level of consciousness are not consistent with the measured ethanol level, obtain a CT scan of the head and rule out infection, metabolic disturbances, and co-ingestants.
- Administer thiamine to alcoholic patients with altered mental status, cerebellar ataxia, or cranial neuropathy.
- Advise or arrange for counseling or detoxification in patients with suspected alcohol abuse or dependence.

DISPOSITION

A patient with uncomplicated intoxication can be discharged after a period of observation when the patient is deemed clinically sober enough to make sound decisions and care for himself. Because clinical sobriety may not correlate with measured ethanol levels, particularly in the tolerant alcoholics, a repeat ethanol level is not necessary before discharge. However, serial assessments of cognitive and neurologic function should be made to avoid prematurely discharging a patient who is still clinically intoxicated. When a safe destination with a responsible adult is available, discharge may be considered for a patient who is still clinically intoxicated but otherwise stable and improving with intact protective reflexes. Such patients should not be discharged until after they have been completely evaluated medically. Prior to discharge, the patient should be offered available social assistance, medical follow-up, and referral to detoxification programs.

Indications for hospitalization include prolonged and inappropriate depressed mental status, metabolic derangements not correctable in a timely manner, persistently abnormal vital signs, associated major trauma, severe withdrawal, mixed overdose, and concomitant medical processes such as GI bleeding, pancreatitis, or severe acute hepatitis. A lower threshold for admission should be applied to those patients who lack social support or who have baseline organic brain syndromes that may be related to chronic ethanol abuse. If the patient is admitted, the potential for ethanol withdrawal needs to be considered, and therapy with benzodiazepines should be instituted.

COMMON PITFALLS

- Failure to appreciate that alcohol intoxication can mask or mimic medical and traumatic conditions
- Failure to obtain a BAC when the history is unclear or inconsistent with clinical findings
- Failure to consider the possibility of a concomitant medical or psychiatric disorder
- Failure to obtain a complete set of vital signs and to fully undress and examine the alcoholic patient
- Failure to re-evaluate the patient frequently and prior to discharge
- Failure to refer intoxicated patients for counseling or detoxification

ICD CODE

980.0 Toxic effect of ethyl alcohol

REFERENCES

1. Enoch M, Goldman D. Problem drinking and alcoholism: diagnosis and treatment. *Am Fam Phys* 2002;65:441–448.
2. Lieber CS. Medical disorders of alcoholism. *N Engl J Med* 1995;333:1058–1065.
3. Lieber CS. Microsomal ethanol-oxidizing system (MEOS): the first 30 years (1968–1998)—a review. *Alcohol Clin Exp Res* 1999;23:991–1007.
4. Martinez R. Alcoholism and society. *Emerg Med Clin North Am* 1990;8:904–909.
5. Moskowitz H, Burns M, Ferguson S. Police officer's detection of breath odors from alcohol ingestion. *Accid Anal Prev* 1999;31:175–180.
6. Ragland G. Electrolyte abnormalities in the alcoholic patient. *Emerg Med Clin North Am* 1990;8:761–773.
7. Ross SM, Chappel JN. Diagnostic dilemmas, part II: substance use disorders—difficulties in diagnoses. *Psychiatr Clin North Am* 1998;21:803–828.
8. Urbano-Marquez A, Estruch R, Navarro-Lopez F, et al. The effects of alcoholism on skeletal and cardiac muscle. *N Engl J Med* 1989;320:409–415.
9. Zador PL. Alcohol-related relative risk and fatal driver injuries in relation to driver age and sex. *J Stud Alcohol* 1991;52:302–310.

CHAPTER 3

Ethanol Withdrawal

PRE-HOSPITAL CONSIDERATIONS
- Assess vital signs.
- Assess capillary glucose.

CLINICAL PRESENTATION

Alcohol withdrawal may present with a wide spectrum of clinical signs and symptoms. For classification purposes, there are four distinct withdrawal syndromes: alcoholic tremulousness, alcoholic hallucinosis, alcoholic withdrawal seizures, and delirium tremens (7). These four clinically distinct entities may occur in isolation or simultaneously in any combination (Fig. 3.1).

Alcoholic tremulousness is characterized by catecholamine excess as a result of abstinence. Patients present to the emergency department (ED) with hypertension, tachycardia, diaphoresis, tremor, fasciculations, mild hyperthermia, agitation, and insomnia (6). The patient appears to be extremely uncomfortable but usually has a normal mental status. Symptoms may begin as early as 6 hours after the last drink, and most patients will be symptomatic within 24 to 48 hours after the last intake of alcohol (7). Symptoms are delayed up to 7 days in a few patients (7).

Alcoholic hallucinosis is characterized by visual or auditory hallucinations that may be persecutory in nature. Formication, the sensation of insects or snakes crawling on the skin, may also occur. The onset is often within a few hours of alcohol cessation and can occur with normal vital signs and without any other manifestations of withdrawal (7).

Alcohol withdrawal seizures, or "rum fits," are the acute onset of a single seizure or a brief flurry of seizures that peak within 24 hours after the last drink. More than 60% of patients have a single seizure characterized by a brief postictal state; status epilepticus is rare (8). As with alcoholic hallucinosis, other signs of alcohol withdrawal may occur either before or after the seizures. About one-third of patients with seizures who are untreated progress to delirium tremens (8).

Delirium tremens is the most severe form of alcohol withdrawal. It includes all of the manifestations of the acute withdrawal syndrome in combination with

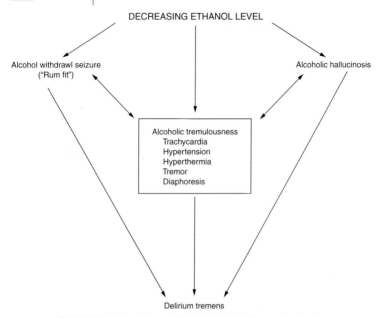

FIGURE 3.1 Adapted from *Goldfrank's Toxicologic Emergencies,* 7th ed.

delirium. Only 5% of patients with alcohol withdrawal progress to delirium tremens. Signs of delirium tremens include extreme autonomic hyperactivity and alteration in sensorium. Delirium tremens usually occurs within 24 to 96 hours after the last drink and has a typical duration of 3 to 7 days (7). In the past, mortality from delirium tremens was 15% to 20% from fluid and electrolyte abnormalities, seizures, and/or infection. Today, the mortality rate is only 5% in properly treated patients (8).

DIFFERENTIAL DIAGNOSIS

The differential diagnosis of alcohol withdrawal is extremely broad because of the many clinical manifestations that occur in isolation or simultaneously and the progression of the condition if left untreated. Furthermore, because patients often suffer from other illnesses, the diagnosis of alcohol withdrawal may be initially overlooked. Consequently, it is crucial to be aware of other etiologies that may mimic the spectrum of alcohol withdrawal (Table 3.1).

TABLE 3.1 Differential Diagnosis of Major Withdrawal Symptoms

Tremor	Seizures	Hallucinations	Delirium
Withdrawal	Withdrawal	Withdrawal	Withdrawal
Ethanol	Ethanol	Ethanol	Ethanol
Sedative–	Sedative–hypnotics	Sedative hypnotics	Sedative–
hypnotics	Intoxications	Intoxications	hypnotics
Intoxications	Cocaine	LSD	Intoxications
Theophylline	Anticholinergics	Mescaline	Cocaine
Caffeine	Phenothiazines	Mushrooms	Amphetamine
Beta agonists	TCAs	Peyote	Phencyclidine
Mercury	Theophylline	Phencyclidine	Anticholinergics
Lithium	Camphor	Anticholinergics	LSD
TCAs	Isoniazid	Ergot	Infectious
Phenytoin	Phencyclidine	Nutmeg	Meningitis
Metabolic	Lidocaine	Infectious	Encephalitis
Hypoglycemia	Organophosphates	Meningitis	Sepsis
Thyrotoxicosis	Infectious	Encephalitis	Thyrotoxicosis
Metabolic	Meningitis	Sepsis	Hypoglycemia
Structural	Encephalitis	Metabolic	Hyperglycemia
Cerebellar	Metabolic	Hypoglycemia	Hypocalcemia
disease	Hypoglycemia	Hypoxia	Hypoxia
Other	Hypoxia	Structural	Thiamine
Parkinsonism	Hypothyroidism	CNS hemorrhage	deficiency
	Thyrotoxicosis	Tumor	Structural
	Hypocalcemia	Psychiatric	Head trauma
	Hyperosmolar state	Schizophrenia	CNS
	Hepatic failure	Bipolar disorder	hemorrhage
	Uremia	Other	Tumor
	Structural	Seizures	Psychiatric
	Head trauma	Heat-related	Other
	CNS hemorrhage	illness	Seizures
	Tumor		Heat-related
	CVA		illness
	Other		
	Idiopathic epilepsy		
	Posttraumatic		
	epilepsy		
	Degenerative		
	disease		

Reproduced from *Withdrawal Syndromes in Emergency Medical Clinical Care,* 3rd ed.

ED EVALUATION

The clinical presentation of alcohol withdrawal may be extremely unpredictable and depends on the particular patient. Most alcohol-dependent patients do not intentionally stop drinking without a new medical illness or social barrier that prevents continued consumption. Therefore, when patients are identified in alcohol withdrawal, it is crucial to determine the underlying reason for alcohol abstinence.

All patients should have a fingerstick glucose, and oxygen saturation measured. A complete history includes substance abuse, previous withdrawal episodes, and all current and former medications. If possible, family, friends, and pre-hospital personnel are interviewed to gain additional information. Vital signs, including rectal temperature, are recorded and closely monitored. Examination of the skin, abdomen, eyes, and pulse rate may help to distinguish a distinct toxidrome (e.g., anticholinergic, sympathomimetic). Attention should be paid to any signs of chronic liver disease or intravenous drug use.

As substance abusers are at high risk for concomitant trauma, traumatic injury should always be considered, especially in patients with an altered sensorium. These patients should also be evaluated for other complications of ethanol and drug abuse, such as pneumonia, skin abscesses, bacterial endocarditis, acquired immunodeficiency syndrome, pancreatitis, liver disease, and gastrointestinal bleeding.

Laboratory studies may include a complete blood count; electrolytes, glucose, blood urea nitrogen, and serum creatinine; aminotransferases; coagulation studies; and ethanol concentration. Ethanol concentrations are likely to be negligible or low in most patients in withdrawal; however, measurable serum ethanol concentrations in patients experiencing alcohol withdrawal correlate with the severity of symptoms. Patients with delirium tremens may need computed tomography of the brain and, if negative, a subsequent lumbar puncture to rule out organic central nervous system (CNS) pathology as the cause of their altered mental status.

ED MANAGEMENT

In any patient with an altered sensorium, a toxin-related condition is always a possibility. Intravenous dextrose is indicated if the patient has hypoglycemia (usually <60 mg/dL). Chronic alcohol use is commonly associated with hypoglycemia for several reasons. Alcoholics are often nutritionally depleted and may have insufficient glycogen stores from liver dysfunction. Chronic ethanol use also leads to an impaired redox potential owing to the accumulation of NADH and subsequent depletion of pyruvate, one of the major precursors of gluconeogenesis.

Thiamine (vitamin B_1) is also indicated for patients with an altered sensorium and patients with a history of alcohol abuse because of the possibility of Wernicke's encephalopathy (triad of ataxia, dementia or confusion, and ophthalmoplegia). This condition is rare but may occur as a result of nutritional deficiency. The standard initial dose of thiamine is 100 mg intravenously (higher dose of thiamine (up to 500mg) is needed for the treatment of Wernicke's). For patients who are known alcoholics, other multivitamin preparations and magnesium sulfate may also be administered, but their benefit is unproven.

Intravenous fluids are often necessary and important for the treatment of alcohol withdrawal, because alcohol induces a diuresis and leads to volume depletion.

Alcohol withdrawal is often due to an underlying medical condition (e.g., pneumonia, pancreatitis, head trauma) that prevents the usual alcohol intake. These patients may require aggressive volume resuscitation for the treatment of this concurrent condition.

Agitated patients may need soft restraints to prevent injury, facilitate intravenous access, and enhance sedation. Prolonged use of restraints with continued struggling may lead to rhabdomyolysis, hyperthermia, and metabolic acidosis.

The goal of therapy for the agitated alcohol withdrawal patient is sedation. Benzodiazepines, the cornerstone of therapy (2) are sedative-hypnotics, like ethanol, and exert their pharmacologic effect via the gamma-aminobutyric acid (GABA) receptor. Benzodiazepines are effective in the treatment of alcohol withdrawal because they often restore inhibitory tone owing to their *cross-tolerance* with alcohol. Nevertheless, some patients require massive doses of intravenous benzodiazepines for treatment. Patients "refractory" to benzodiazepines should be treated with a different GABA agonist, such as a barbiturate. "Anesthetic" barbiturates (e.g., thiopental, methohexital) have direct effects on the GABA receptor and exert a synergistic effect with benzodiazepines. Patients with severe refractory alcohol withdrawal, unresponsive to benzodiazepines, may respond to a propofol infusion. Propofol is both a GABA agonist and an NMDA antagonist and has been effective in several case reports as a treatment of alcohol withdrawal. Patients who receive barbiturates or propofol often require airway protection, because of the potential respiratory depression.

Symptom-triggered therapy refers to the administration of intravenous benzodiazepines when the patient's symptoms exceed a threshold of severity and is given until the patient's symptoms are adequately controlled. This is in contrast to a fixed-dose regimen of a set amount of benzodiazepine at regular intervals with a subsequent taper after the patient's symptoms are under control. The symptom-triggered method is a better technique and decreases the total amount of benzodiazepines administered, the duration of treatment and the incidence of delirium tremens, as compared to the fixed-dose method (3,5).

Diazepam (Valium), chlordiazepoxide (Librium), and lorazepam (Ativan) are the most commonly used agents for alcohol withdrawal and can also be used for sedative–hypnotic withdrawal. These agents are preferred over benzodiazepines with shorter half-lives, because they require less frequent dosing and allow gradual elimination of the drug over several days.

Long-acting agents may be more effective than short-acting agents in preventing withdrawal seizures and can contribute to smoother withdrawal with fewer rebound symptoms (4). The active metabolites of diazepam and chlordiazepoxide prolong their therapeutic effect. In elderly patients and those with hepatic dysfunction, lorazepam may be preferred because it has no active metabolites. In other cases, lorazepam does not appear to offer any distinct advantage over diazepam or chlordiazepoxide (1). See Table 3.2 for dosing recommendations for various benzodiazepines.

TABLE 3.2 Pharmaceutical Management of Ethanol and Drug Withdrawal

Ethanol or Sedative-Hypnotic Withdrawal

1st choice: diazepam
    5 mg IV bolus every 5–15 min until sedated
    May increase dose to 20 mg every 5–15 min in refractory cases
    Total over 24-hr period may exceed 1,000 mg
    If >300 mg given, may consider adding another GABA agent (e.g., barbiturate, propofol)
    Do not exceed 5 mg/min

2nd choice: lorazepam
    1–2 mg IV bolus every 5–15 min until sedated
    Not as long-acting as diazepam
    Preferable in cases of hepatic failure or recurrent seizures

3rd choice: pentobarbital
    100-mg IV bolus
    Continue titration to sedation or 600 mg total.
    Potential for more respiratory depression than benzodiazepines
    Do not exceed 50 mg/min.
    Alternatives
    Chlordiazepoxide, secobarbital, phenobarbital

Reproduced from *Withdrawal Syndromes in Emergency Medical Clinical Care,* 3rd ed.

Intravenous dosing of benzodiazepines is preferred in all but the mildest cases of ethanol withdrawal. Agitation may preclude oral administration, and gastritis may impair drug absorption. Intramuscular lorazepam (but not diazepam or chlordiazepoxide) is absorbed predictably and is recommended when intravenous access is not readily obtained.

Patients who have abstinence seizures should be given standard supportive therapy and benzodiazepines to stop seizure activity. Phenytoin is not useful for the treatment of alcohol withdrawal seizures and should not be given unless the patient has a known seizure focus and was previously taking this drug prior to presentation. Carbamazepine and valproic acid are mildly efficacious in certain settings but have not been studied in an ED setting or in patients with delirium tremens. Consequently, these anticonvulsants are not recommended for patients with significant signs and symptoms of alcohol withdrawal.

Historically, beta-adrenergic antagonists, clonidine, and antipsychotics (phenothiazines and butyrophenones) have been used for the treatment of alcohol withdrawal, but none of these agents exerts its primary effects through GABA. Though they may appear to control symptoms, their efficacy in improving alcohol withdrawal outcomes has not been demonstrated, and their routine use is discouraged.

CRITICAL INTERVENTIONS

- Identify and treat alcohol withdrawal early with IV fluids and IV benzodiazepines. Treatment becomes increasingly more difficult as the disease progresses.
- Identify any precipitating illness. Concurrent infection is often the precipitant for ethanol abstinence and subsequent withdrawal.

DISPOSITION

Depending on the particular withdrawal syndrome, the reason for cessation of alcohol, and the severity of alcohol withdrawal signs and symptoms, the disposition of patients with alcohol withdrawal is extremely variable. As long as there are no critical medical conditions that will prevent the patient with mild alcohol tremulousness from resuming normal activities, patients may be safely discharged with treatment and referral to a detoxification program.

Patients with more severe signs and symptoms of alcohol withdrawal, including alcohol withdrawal seizures and alcoholic hallucinosis, will require hospital admission. Patients with delirium tremens will require admission to an intensive care unit for close cardiac and hemodynamic monitoring. Patients who are not adequately sedated with conventional doses of benzodiazepines may require propofol, necessitating intensive care unit admission for respiratory monitoring and subsequent endotracheal intubation, if necessary.

COMMON PITFALLS

- Overlooking alcohol withdrawal as a potential cause of altered sensorium and autonomic instability
- Failing to perform computed tomography of the brain and a lumbar puncture to exclude organic CNS pathology in patients with delirium tremens
- Using a fixed-dose schedule of benzodiazepines to treat ethanol withdrawal rather than escalating doses or symptom-triggered therapy

ICD 9

291.0 Alcohol withdrawal delirium
291.81 Alcohol withdrawal

REFERENCES

1. Bird RD, Makela EH. Alcohol withdrawal: what is the benzodiazepine of choice? *Ann Pharmacother* 1994;28:67–71.
2. Holbrook AM, Crowther R, Lotter A, Cheng C, King D. Meta-analysis of benzodiazepine use in the treatment of acute alcohol withdrawal. *CMAJ (Ottowa)* 1999;160:649–655.
3. Jaeger TM, Lohr RH, Pankratz VS. Symptom-triggered therapy for alcohol withdrawal syndrome in medical inpatients. *Mayo Clin Proc* 2001;76:695–701.

4. Mayo-Smith MF. Pharmacological management of alcohol withdrawal. A meta-analysis and evidence-based practice guideline. American Society of Addiction Medicine Working Group on Pharmacological Management of Alcohol Withdrawal. *JAMA* 1997;278:144–151.

5. Saitz R, Mayo-Smith MF, Roberts MS, et al. Individualized treatment for alcohol withdrawal. Arandomized double-blind controlled trial. *JAMA* 1994;272:519–523.

6. Trevisan LA, Boutros N, Petrakis IL, Krystal JH. Complications of alcohol withdrawal. Pathophysiological insights. *Alcohol Health Res World* 1998;22:61–66.

7. Victor M, Adams, RD. The effect of alcohol on the nervous system. *Res Public Assoc Res Nerv Ment Dis* 1953;32:526–573.

8. Victor M, Brausch C. The role of abstinence in the genesis of alcoholic epilepsy. *Epilepsia* 1967;8:1–20.

Ethylene Glycol

PRE-HOSPITAL CONSIDERATIONS

- Bring containers of all possible ingestants.
- Monitor airway and central nervous system (CNS) depression.
- After an ethylene glycol spill, decontaminate the skin by removing clothing and jewelry and irrigating with soap and water.

CLINICAL PRESENTATION

With ethylene glycol (EG) poisoning, there are three distinct stages of CNS, cardiopulmonary, and renal organ system involvement, but the onset, progression, and confluence of these stages vary widely (1,6,7). Thirty minutes to 12 hours after ingestion, CNS signs and symptoms predominate. Initially, slurred speech, ataxia, nystagmus, and lethargy occur. The patient may appear drunk but lacks the breath odor of ethanol; instead, a faint, sweet, or aromatic odor may be detected. Nausea, vomiting, and abdominal pain may also be present.

During this early stage, an elevated osmolal gap may provide a clue to the diagnosis of EG poisoning (5,6,8). Because of its low molecular weight (62 g/mol), only high concentrations of EG increase the serum osmolality appreciably. This results in an increase in the osmolal gap, the difference between the serum osmolality measured by the freezing-point depression (but not the vapor pressure method) and the calculated osmolarity ([2 $\times$ sodium] + [glucose/18] + [blood urea nitrogen/2.8] + [serum ethanol concentration/4.6]). Normally, serum osmolality ranges from 280 to 300 mOsmol/kg H_2O, with a normal osmolal gap of -2 ± 6 mOsmol/kg. The osmolal gap is not precise enough to make a diagnosis, but a very large osmolal gap is strongly suggestive. Measurement of EG in serum or urine will confirm the diagnosis.

A decreased serum bicarbonate and an increased anion gap metabolic acidosis may be seen as early as 3 hours after EG ingestion (1,2). The normal anion gap (serum sodium minus chloride and bicarbonate) is 12 $\pm$ 2 mEq/L and represents unmeasured anions in the serum. In EG poisoning, glycolic acid accounts for a large part of the unmeasured anions The absence of metabolic acidosis is consistent with an early presentation, an insignificant ingestion, or the coingestion of ethanol, which blocks the metabolism of EG.

After a latent period of 3 to 12 hours, signs and symptoms develop from accumulated toxic metabolites. CNS depression progresses to stupor and coma.

Hyperreflexia, tremor, tetany, cranial nerve abnormalities, and seizures (both focal and generalized) may occur. Severe CNS disturbances may reflect the development of cerebral edema and meningoencephalitis (5,6). In the late stages of poisoning, when most or all EG has been metabolized, measuring the serum glycolic acid level may be the only way to confirm the diagnosis.

Cardiopulmonary signs such as hypertension, tachycardia, dysrhythmias, and pulmonary edema develop 12 to 36 hours after the ingestion of EG. During this stage, compensatory tachypnea and Kussmaul respirations reflect a progressively worsening anion gap metabolic acidosis.

Urinalysis may provide additional evidence of EG poisoning. Proteinuria and microscopic hematuria are seen in more than 60% of cases (2,5,6,8). The presence of hematuria and oxaluria is not predictive of acute renal failure (8). Calcium oxalate crystalluria, although nonspecific, is present on admission in more than 40% of patients; this percentage increases with serial urinalysis and delayed presentation (2,6,8). Calcium oxalate is often excreted as needle-shaped monohydrate crystals that may be misidentified as hippuric or uric acid crystals (6). At higher urinary concentrations, calcium oxalate is also excreted in an envelope-shaped dihydrate form (5,6). The binding of calcium to oxalate may result in hypocalcemia, causing myoclonic jerks or tetanic contractions (1,5,6). Because fluorescein is added to many commercial antifreeze preparations, fluorescence of urine or gastric contents with a Wood lamp supports EG poisoning early after ingestion. Fluorescence is insensitive and nonspecific, however, and should not be relied on to make or exclude the diagnosis of EG poisoning.

EG plasma concentrations do not correlate with mortality (8). Death results from cerebral edema and infarction, multiple organ failure, and irreversible shock (1,5,6). The time delay between ingestion and treatment and the degree of metabolic acidosis at the initiation of treatment are the factors that correlate most with survival (6). Rapid diagnosis and treatment prevents EG bioactivation and lethality, regardless of the initial plasma EG concentration (6). Even with treatment there is a 5% to 17% mortality rate (2).

Renal dysfunction is seen in nearly 70% of cases and is characterized by oliguria, proteinuria, and urine with a low specific gravity and sodium content (acute tubular necrosis). Patients may complain of severe flank pain (1,5,6). Renal dysfunction may be noted as early as 9 hours after ingestion (2). The high frequency of renal injury reflects delayed presentation and delayed diagnosis and treatment (8). The degree of metabolic acidosis or glycolic acid accumulation at the initiation of treatment, rather than EG plasma concentration, correlates closely with the subsequent development of renal injury (2,6,8). In one retrospective study, an initial glycolic acid level of >8 mmol/L, anion gap of >20 mmol/L, or arterial pH of <7.30 were highly predictive of acute renal failure (8).

Conversely, patients who have an initial glycolic acid level of <8 to 10 mmol/L, arterial pH of >7.30, or normal renal function upon initiation of appropriate treatment are unlikely to develop acute renal insufficiency (2,8). Although most treated patients have a complete recovery, some may have protracted renal insufficiency that requires months of hemodialysis. Cranial neuropathies and bilateral basal ganglia and brainstem infarction may rarely develop 2 to 18 days after acute poisoning (1,5,6).

DIFFERENTIAL DIAGNOSIS

EG intoxication can mimic a large variety of poisonings or disease states, depending on the amount of EG ingested and the degree of EG metabolism at presentation. Diagnostic clues include drunkenness without the odor of ethanol, a delay between ingestion and significant illness, hyperventilation on physical examination, increased osmolal or anion gaps, metabolic acidosis, calcium oxalate crystalluria, and hypocalcemia. The differential diagnosis includes alcoholic, diabetic, and starvation ketoacidosis; lactic acidosis; renal failure; methanol poisoning; and advanced, untreated acetaminophen or salicylate poisoning. If the history is not suggestive of lactic acidosis or ketoacidosis, a high osmolal gap with anion gap metabolic acidosis strongly points toward EG or methanol poisoning (5,6). In methanol intoxication, crystalluria is absent, and visual complaints and an abnormal eye examination may be present. Although a large osmolal gap (particularly if >25) is suggestive of toxic alcohol poisoning, a small gap (<10), cannot be used to exclude significant EG poisoning, particularly in the later stages of poisoning, when significant metabolism has already occurred (1,5,6,8). The presence of glycolate can cause artifactual elevation of the plasma lactate level with lactate analyzers that use the reagent L-lactate oxidase and lead to a misdiagnosis of lactic acidosis (3). Previously unrecognized disorders of inborn organic acid metabolism should be considered in the differential diagnosis of young children with an increased anion gap metabolic acidosis.

ED EVALUATION

The history should include the time of ingestion, the volume and concentration of the ingested product, and the onset, nature, and progression of symptoms. The ingestion of other substances, particularly ethanol, should be documented. Patients should be asked specifically about ethanol-like intoxication, shortness of breath, flank pain, and urinary dysfunction.

The physical examination should focus on the neurologic status, cardiopulmonary function, and any abdominal and back tenderness. In symptomatic patients, evaluation should include a complete blood count; serum electrolytes, blood urea nitrogen, creatinine, glucose, amylase, calcium, ketones, and lactate; serum osmolality; arterial blood gas; toxicologic screen; urinalysis; electrocardiogram; and a chest radiograph.

A quantitative serum EG concentration should be obtained in all patients, preferably by gas chromatography and mass spectrometry (GC/MS). Semiquantitative alcohol oxidase reagents (enzymatic assays) are too insensitive and nonspecific to confirm or exclude the presence of EG (3). Patients with intentional ingestion often drink ethanol, and a serum ethanol concentration can help in planning treatment. In addition, as many antifreeze products also contain methanol or propylene glycol, serum concentrations of these agents should be ordered if the identity of the ingested substance cannot be confirmed. Occasionally, propylene glycol or propionic acid may be misinterpreted as EG by GC/MS. Occasionally, glycolic acid quantification by special GC/MS techniques may be necessary for those patients who present very late (e.g., renal failure and no detectable EG) (2,8).

If EG analysis is not readily available, the serum level (milligrams per deciliter) can be roughly estimated by multiplying the osmolal gap by 6.2 (mg/dL per mOsm of EG). When interpreting the osmolal gap and using it in calculations, the contribution of ethanol (1 mOsm for each 4.6 mg/dL of serum ethanol) must first be subtracted (5,6,8).

ED MANAGEMENT

Airway protection and respiratory and circulatory support with cardiac and hemodynamic monitoring, should be instituted as necessary. Intravenous (IV) fluids should be liberally administered initially to maintain an adequate urine output; a large urine flow increases the urinary excretion of EG in those without renal failure (5,6). If the patient has ingested EG only shortly before presentation, gastric aspiration via a nasogastric tube should be performed immediately. Activated charcoal adsorbs EG but may be clinically ineffective because EG is rapidly absorbed and the capacity of charcoal to bind EG is exceeded when moderate amounts of EG are ingested. Activated charcoal is recommended if a co-ingestant is suspected.

Specific treatment for EG poisoning consists of sodium bicarbonate to correct metabolic acidosis, calcium to correct symptomatic hypocalcemia, ethanol or fomepizole to inhibit production of toxic metabolites, hemodialysis to remove EG and its toxic metabolites, and cofactors (e.g., magnesium, pyridoxine, and thiamine) to theoretically enhance endogenous clearance of toxic metabolites (1).

Correction of metabolic acidosis may require large amounts of IV sodium bicarbonate ($NaHCO_3$):

$$0.7 \times kg \times (24 - actual[HCO_3^-]),$$

where 0.7 is the volume of distribution of bicarbonate in acidemia, 24 is the desired $[HCO_3^-]$, and kg is the lean body weight.

$NaHCO_3$ should be given in 1 mEq/kg increments (1,5,6). Increasing the serum pH increases the fraction of ionized acid metabolites, thereby minimizing their tissue redistribution and maximizing their renal clearance through ion trapping. The acid-base status should be frequently re-evaluated to assess the response to therapy. Hypocalcemia may be worsened by sodium bicarbonate administration (1,5,6).

Serum calcium levels should be monitored frequently. Symptomatic hypocalcemia (e.g., cardiac dysrhythmias, tetany, and seizures) should be treated with IV calcium chloride or gluconate (7 to 14 mEq for adults and 1 to 7 mEq for children). The

10% calcium chloride solution contains 1.4 mEq of calcium per milliliter, and 10% calcium gluconate solution contains 0.46 mEq/mL. Calcium is not recommended for those with asymptomatic hypocalcemia, as its administration could theoretically increase calcium oxalate tissue precipitation and overall EG toxicity. Seizures should otherwise be treated with standard drugs (diazepam, lorazepam, or a barbiturate).

Traditionally, ethanol has been used to inhibit the alcohol dehydrogenase–mediated metabolism of EG. Fomepizole (4-methylpyrazole, 4-MP; Antizol) is a potent, long-acting, competitive alcohol dehydrogenase inhibitor that is a safe, easy, and effective alternative to ethanol (1,2,6,7,9). Unlike ethanol, fomepizole is approved by the U.S. Food and Drug Administration for the treatment of EG and methanol poisoning. Fomepizole attenuates and prevents metabolic acidosis and renal failure in humans and animals poisoned by EG by halting the accumulation of glycolic and oxalic acids, respectively (1,2,7,8). Fomepizole has higher potency, longer duration of action, more predictable kinetics, an easier dosing regimen than ethanol (1,2,5,8), and does not require frequent monitoring and adjustment of plasma concentrations. In addition, fomepizole does not produce the CNS depression, hypoglycemia, gastritis, pancreatitis, fluid overload, and habituation commonly associated with ethanol therapy (1,2,5,7).

A disadvantage of fomepizole is its high acquisition cost (~$1,000 U.S. per 1.5-g vial). Although it has been associated with dizziness, eosinophilia, headache, nausea, rash, transient hepatic transaminase elevation, phlebitis, and seizures, it is generally safe in humans (1,2,5,7). The higher acquisition cost of fomepizole is balanced by greater patient safety and decreased cost of monitoring patients, and fomepizole has become preferred to ethanol in the United States (5,7). Fomepizole is contraindicated in pregnant patients and in those with a known previous allergy to pyrazole derivatives (7).

Regardless of which antidote is used, both ethanol and fomepizole preferentially bind alcohol dehydrogenase, which prevents further EG metabolism to the toxic metabolites. EG can then be eliminated by urinary excretion or hemodialysis. Indications for treatment with ethanol or fomepizole include a measured serum EG concentration >20 mg/dL; a documented history of significant recent EG ingestion when a serum EG concentration is not immediately available, particularly if the osmol gap is elevated; or strong suspicion of EG ingestion based on abnormal clinical or laboratory findings (e.g., unexplained anion gap metabolic acidosis, elevated corrected osmolar gap, or both, or oxalate crystalluria) (1,2,5–7).

For fomepizole, a loading dose of 15 mg/kg IV should be administered, followed by doses of 10 mg/kg IV every 12 hours thereafter (2,7). All doses are diluted in 100 mL of 5% dextrose in water or normal saline and are administered by slow IV infusion over 30 minutes (2,7). Like ethanol, fomepizole is also effective after oral administration (1,7). Antidotal therapy is continued until EG concentrations fall below 20 mg/dL (2,7).

For ethanol therapy, the therapeutic goal is a serum ethanol concentration of at least 100 mg/dL (5,6), which is theoretically sufficient to prevent metabolism of EG at a serum concentration of 546 mg/dL (6). IV administration is preferred as it provides a more rapid and constant serum concentration (1,5,6). An IV loading dose of 10 mL/kg of 10% ethanol (preferably in a glucose-containing solution, such as D5W to avoid hypoglycemia) over 30 to 60 minutes, followed by a maintenance infusion of 1.5 mL/kg/h, generally produces a serum ethanol concentration of slightly >100 mg/dL (5,6). Alternatively, 5 mL/kg of 20% (40 proof) ethanol may be administered orally or via nasogastric tube to achieve the desired loading dose; the hourly maintenance oral dose is similar to that for IV administration (1.5 mL/kg/h of 10% ethanol) (1,5,6). Serum ethanol and glucose concentrations should be monitored and the dose of ethanol adjusted, as necessary, to maintain a therapeutic ethanol concentration.

Hemodialysis rapidly removes both EG and glycolic acid (5–7). Elimination half-lives are reduced to approximately 3 hours for each, as compared with 19 and 10 hours, respectively, with alcohol dehydrogenase inhibitor therapy alone (1,2,7,9). Indications for hemodialysis include significant metabolic acidosis (arterial pH <7.30), renal insufficiency (serum creatinine >1.2 mg/dL), or deterioration in these parameters or clinical status despite conventional treatment (1,2,5–8).

Traditionally, hemodialysis has been recommended for a serum EG concentration of 50 mg/dL or greater (5–7). However, this concentration does not define toxicity, predict prolonged elimination, or correlate with patient outcome. Recent evidence suggests that patients who present before the development of metabolic acidosis and renal impairment can be effectively and safely managed with fomepizole monotherapy (i.e., without hemodialysis) regardless of the initial EG concentration (1,2,7,8). In these patients, EG is excreted by the kidneys, with an approximate half-life of 18 hours (1,2,7–9). For patients who present with elevated serum creatinine, however, EG elimination half-life is prolonged to approximately 49 hours, and hemodialysis is recommended (2,7,9). These patients will also likely require hemodialysis based on the presence of a significant metabolic acidosis. Hemodialysis should be continued until acid-base and metabolic abnormalities are corrected and serum EG concentrations are below 50 mg/dL (2,5–7).

The infusion rate of ethanol should be increased to 3 mL/kg/h during hemodialysis to compensate for increased clearance (1,5,6). Because fomepizole is also dialyzable, it should be administered by a continuous IV infusion of 1 to 1.5 mg/kg/h or its dosing frequency increased to every 4 hours during hemodialysis (2,7). If hemodialysis is unavailable or technically difficult (e.g., in infants), peritoneal dialysis can be used, although this method is considerably less effective than hemodialysis.

Pyridoxine, thiamine, and magnesium are cofactors in the metabolism of EG to less toxic products (Fig. 4.1). Their administration may preferentially shunt metabolism of glyoxylic acid away from oxalic acid.

Both pyridoxine and thiamine are given intravenously in doses of 100 mg four times daily (5,6).

Treatment of cultured human proximal renal tubular cells with ethylenediaminetetraacetic acid to solubilize calcium oxalate crystals, or with aluminum citrate to prevent crystal precipitation, significantly reduces cytotoxicity associated with calcium oxalate (4). These may prove in the future to be useful treatments.

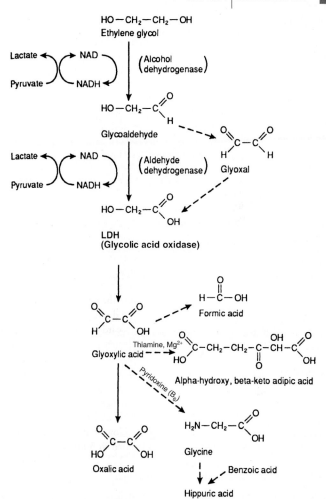

FIGURE 4.1 Metabolism of ethylene glycol. *Solid lines,* known pathways of metabolism; *dashed lines,* postulated pathways of metabolism.

CRITICAL INTERVENTIONS

- Administer fomepizole or ethanol to patients with signs, symptoms, or laboratory evidence of EG poisoning.
- Administer IV sodium bicarbonate to patients with acidemia.
- Arrange hemodialysis for patients with EG poisoning that is severe or refractory to other treatment.

DISPOSITION

Patients with EG poisoning almost always require admission to an intensive care unit. The need for hemodialysis should always be anticipated, and the patient should be transferred if such treatment is unavailable. Patients who accidentally ingest a small volume and who do not develop acidosis or have toxic levels of EG can be discharged.

COMMON PITFALLS

- Failure to consider EG as a cause of ethanol-like intoxication and increased anion gap metabolic acidosis
- Failure to appreciate that a normal osmolal or anion gap does not exclude the presence of potentially toxic amounts of EG
- Failure to observe and monitor all patients with known or suspected ethylene EG ingestion until an EG level can be obtained or until the time of expected toxicity has passed without incident
- Failure to appreciate the importance of fully correcting acidemia
- Failure to appreciate that ethanol and fomepizole are removed by hemodialysis and to increase their dosing accordingly during this procedure

ICD 9

982.8 Toxic effect of other nonpetroleum-based solvents

REFERENCES

1. Barceloux DG, Krenzelok EP, Olsen K, et al. American Academy of Clinical Toxicology practice guidelines on the treatment of ethylene glycol poisoning. *J Toxicol Clin Toxicol* 1999;37:537–560.
2. Brent J, McMartin K, Phillips S, et al. Fomepizole for the treatment of ethylene glycol poisoning. *N Engl J Med* 1999;340:832–838.
3. Brindley PG, Butler MS, Cembrowski G, Brindley DN. Falsely elevated point-of-care lactate measurement after ingestion of ethylene glycol. *CMAJ (Ottawa)* 2007;176:1097–1099.
4. Guo C, Cenac TA, Li Y, et al. Calcium oxalate, and not other metabolites, is responsible for the renal toxicity of ethylene glycol. *Toxicol Lett* 2007;173:8–16.
5. Jacobsen D, McMartin KE. Antidotes for methanol and ethylene glycol poisoning. *J Toxicol Clin Toxicol* 1997;35:127–143.
6. Jacobsen D, McMartin KE. Methanol and ethylene glycol poisonings: mechanisms of toxicity, clinical course, diagnosis and treatment. *Med Toxicol* 1986;1:309–334.
7. Megarbane B, Borron SW, Baud FJ. Current recommendations for treatment of severe toxic alcohol poisonings. *Intensive Care Med* 2005;31:189–195.
8. Porter WH, Rutter PW, Bush BA, et al. Ethylene glycol toxicity: the role of serum glycolic acid in hemodialysis. *J Toxicol Clin Toxicol* 2001;39:607–615.
9. Sivilotti M, Burns M, McMartin K, et al. Toxicokinetics of ethylene glycol during fomepizole therapy: implications for management. *Ann Emerg Med* 2000;36:114–125.

CHAPTER 5

Methanol

PRE-HOSPITAL CONSIDERATIONS

- Transport all possibly ingested substances.
- After a methanol spill, decontaminate the skin by removing clothing and jewelry and irrigating with soap and water.
- Monitor airway and central nervous system depression.

CLINICAL PRESENTATION

Usually 6 to 24 hours elapse from the time of methanol ingestion to the occurrence of symptoms. This period of time is required for sufficient amounts of formic acid to be produced by methanol metabolism. A latent period up to 90 hours has been reported when ethanol is coingested (2) because ethanol competitively inhibits methanol metabolism by alcohol dehydrogenase.

Methanol itself has few direct effects. Mild ethanol-like central nervous system (CNS) depression has been reported (7). Methanol is about half as potent as ethanol in this regard. With concentrated methanol solutions, nausea, vomiting, and abdominal pain may develop shortly after ingestion. During the early stages of poisoning, the diagnosis is confirmed by measuring the serum methanol level, but levels are often not readily available or rapidly obtainable. Because of its low molecular weight (32 g/mol), high concentrations of methanol (and other low-molecular-weight solutes—see Chapter 1, "General Considerations: Recognition, Initial Approach, and Early Management of the Poisoned Patient") increase the serum osmolality. The diagnosis may therefore be suggested by an increased osmolal gap, the difference between the measured osmolality and the calculated osmolality (2 × sodium [mEq/L] + blood urea nitrogen [mg/dL]/2.8 + glucose [mg/dL]/18 + ethanol [mg/dL]/3.7) (9). The "normal" range for the osmolal gap has been debated extensively and has been reported to vary from −10 to 20 mOsm (1). Although an osmolal gap above 20 indicates exogenous osmoles of some kind, an osmolal gap within the normal range does not exclude the possibility of a toxic methanol ingestion. The serum methanol level can be estimated (in mg/dL) by multiplying the excess osmolal gap by 2.6, the amount of methanol that increases the osmolality by 1 mOsm/kg H_2O. Shortly after ingestion, when the highest methanol levels and osmolal gap are present, metabolic acidosis can be absent as significant conversion to formate has not yet occurred.

Clinical features during the intermediate stage of poisoning include anorexia, headache, nausea, and vomiting, accompanied or followed by increasing hyperventilation as a result of progressive anion gap metabolic acidosis (7). The "normal" range for the anion gap ($[Na + K] - [Cl + HCO_3]$) is 13 ± 4 mEq/L (mean $\pm$ SD) (1). Visual symptoms (blurred vision, decreased acuity, halo vision, tunnel vision, photophobia, and "snowfields") may precede or accompany the aforementioned symptoms. Objective signs, such as dilated pupils that are partially reactive or nonreactive to light and funduscopy showing optic disk hyperemia with blurring of the margins, occur later. During this stage, the diagnosis is confirmed by detecting methanol or formate in the serum, and an elevated osmolal gap may or may not be present. Occasionally, patients may present with abdominal pain from an associated acute pancreatitis (7,8).

Without treatment, coma and respiratory and circulatory failure may ensue. A few patients may develop methemoglobinemia from an interaction between formate and the ferric part of hemoglobin. In the late stages of methanol poisoning, when most or all of the methanol has been metabolized to formate, the anion gap is elevated, but the osmolal gap is normal, and methanol may not be detectable. In this situation of undetectable methanol, measurement of the serum formate may be the only way to confirm the diagnosis. Toxic effects on the basal ganglia do not immediately produce detectable signs and symptoms as they are masked by the pronounced CNS depression. Survivors may later manifest a Parkinson-like syndrome with basal ganglion necrosis seen on computed tomography (CT) scan or magnetic resonance imaging (MRI) (3).

DIFFERENTIAL DIAGNOSIS

Other causes of metabolic acidosis and increased serum osmolality should be considered in the differential diagnosis (Fig. 5.1), particularly when the history is unclear and quantitative methanol and formate levels are not readily available. Increased anion and osmolal gaps also occur in ethylene glycol poisoning. Differentiating the two may be difficult, but the treatments are essentially the same. Visual complaints suggest methanol poisoning, whereas hypocalcemia, seizures, and urine oxalate crystals indicate ethylene glycol poisoning (7).

ED EVALUATION

Important aspects of the history include the amount, concentration, and time of methanol ingestion, the nature and onset of symptoms, and whether ethanol was coingested. Patients should be questioned carefully about the presence or absence of visual complaints, gastrointestinal (GI) symptoms, and a feeling of intoxication. The physical examination should focus on vital signs (especially respiratory rate) and the neurologic, visual, and cardiopulmonary status. Visual acuity and funduscopic examinations should be documented. Laboratory evaluation should include arterial blood gas analysis, measurement of electrolytes, blood urea nitrogen, creatinine, glucose, lipase, urinalysis, and quantitative serum methanol or formic

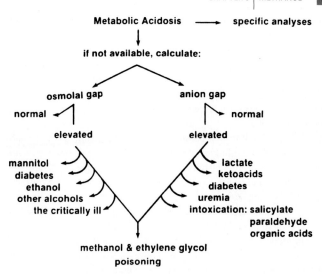

FIGURE 5.1 Causes of increased anion and osmolal gaps.

acid levels. A chest radiograph and an electrocardiogram should be obtained if clinical toxicity is pronounced.

If the diagnosis is based on the osmolal and anion gaps, osmometry must be performed by the freezing-point depression technique and not by the vapor pressure technique, as the latter does not detect the increased osmolality caused by volatile alcohols. A CT scan or MRI of the brain should be performed on patients with coma or persistent neurologic dysfunction.

ED MANAGEMENT

General treatment measures include supportive care and GI decontamination. Immediate gastric aspiration via nasogastric tube may be helpful if performed within 1 hour of ingestion. Activated charcoal is probably of limited value because of limited binding (2).

Specific treatment of methanol poisoning includes intravenous (IV) sodium bicarbonate for metabolic acidosis, antidotal therapy with ethanol or fomepizole to inhibit methanol metabolism to formate, and hemodialysis to remove methanol and formate. Folinic acid (leucovorin), 1 mg/kg IV up to 50 mg every 4 hours, may be of value to increase the metabolism of formate (2). If folinic acid is unavailable, folic acid in the same dose may be used.

Metabolic acidosis should be aggressively treated with enough sodium bicarbonate ($NaHCO_3$) to fully correct acidemia:

$$NaHCO_3 \text{ dose} = 0.7 \times \text{kg} \times 24 - \text{actual } [HCO_3],$$

where 0.7 is the volume of distribution of bicarbonate, 24 is the desired [HCO_3^-] and kg is the lean body weight.

$NaHCO_3$ should be given in 1-mEq/kg increments. As much as 400 to 600 mEq of $NaHCO_3$ may be required during the first few hours. Bicarbonate therapy decreases the amount of undissociated formic acid, and decreases CNS toxicity (7). Hence, metabolic acidosis from methanol poisoning should *always* be treated with bicarbonate. Frequent reassessment of acid-base and electrolyte status is prudent during treatment.

Alkali treatment must be accompanied by administration of ethanol or fomepizole to block further production of formic acid. If methanol poisoning is suspected and a level cannot readily be obtained, ethanol or fomepizole therapy should be started in any patient with an increased osmolal gap, acidosis, symptoms, or a potentially toxic ingestion by history. Antidotal treatment may be discontinued when the methanol level drops below 20 mg/dL, provided the acid-base status is normal and there are no complications.

For antidotal treatment, a therapeutic blood ethanol level of at least 100 mg/dL is recommended by most authors. However, the ethanol level necessary to block methanol metabolism varies with the blood level of methanol, because of competition for alcohol dehydrogenase The molar ethanol concentration should be at least one fourth of the molar methanol concentration (7).

A blood ethanol level of 100 mg/dL may be achieved by giving a bolus dose of 0.6 mg/kg, followed by 66 to 154 mg/kg/hr intravenously or orally, with the higher maintenance dose for heavy drinkers. Mixing 50 mL of absolute ethanol with 500 mL isotonic glucose yields a 10% ethanol solution. With this solution, a bolus of 10 mL/kg (>0.5 hour), followed by 1.5 mL/kg/hr, will produce the desired blood level. The maintenance infusion should be adjusted according to frequently measured ethanol levels. As a rule of thumb, the maintenance dose of ethanol should be doubled during hemodialysis. If this is not done, as ethanol is removed, methanol metabolism can resume, resulting in worsening toxicity despite hemodialysis.

Fomepizole (4-methylpyrazole; Antizol) is an alternative to ethanol (4,5). The loading dose of 15 mg/kg IV is followed by doses of 10 mg/kg IV every 12 hours. During hemodialysis, dosing frequency should be increased to every 4 hours. Fomepizole is superior to ethanol as an antidote, without the risk of respiratory depression, the need to monitor blood ethanol, or requiring an intensive care unit (ICU) setting for an IV infusion, with only the expense being a negative consideration.

Hemodialysis efficiently removes methanol and formate and helps to correct the metabolic acidosis (5,7). The one absolute indication for hemodialysis is any visual impairment in a patient with metabolic acidosis or a detectable methanol level. Other indications include severe acidemia (particularly if unresponsive to bicarbonate and ethanol therapy), a blood methanol level above 50 mg/dL (because of the very slow elimination of methanol during antidotal therapy), renal insufficiency, or ingestion of more than 1 g/kg of methanol. With the use of fomepizole, most patients need dialysis only to shorten the duration of fomepizole treatment by removing unmetabolized methanol. However, in the severe poisoning with pronounced acidemia and visual disturbances, hemodialysis should be performed to remove formate and methanol. Hemodialysis should be continued until the blood methanol level is below 20 mg/dL and acidemia is corrected. If methanol analyses are unavailable, hemodialysis should be continued for at least 8 hours or until the osmolal gap is normal (5,6). Peritoneal dialysis is not effective enough to be clinically useful.

CRITICAL INTERVENTIONS

- Administer ethanol or fomepizole to patients with signs, symptoms, or laboratory evidence of methanol poisoning.
- Administer intravenous sodium bicarbonate to patients with acidemia.
- Arrange hemodialysis for patients with methanol poisoning that is severe or refractory to other treatment.

DISPOSITION

When the diagnosis of methanol poisoning is made or suspected, a nephrologist should be consulted, as many of these patients will require hemodialysis, especially when admitted in a late stage. If hemodialysis is likely to be needed, the patient should be transferred to a facility with this capability. Bicarbonate and antidotal therapy should be given prior to and during transport.

If a methanol level is not immediately available, asymptomatic patients with known or suspected methanol ingestion and a normal anion and osmolar gap should be observed and be re-evaluated for clinical and acid-base status until the methanol level becomes known. Patients with signs, symptoms, or laboratory evidence of methanol intoxication should be admitted, usually to an ICU because of the frequency of monitoring required. They should also have an ophthalmologic evaluation for detection and management of ocular injury.

COMMON PITFALLS

- Failure to consider methanol poisoning in the differential diagnosis of metabolic acidosis of unknown origin
- Failure to consider the possibility of multiple victims when the source of methanol is unknown or is known to be contaminated ethanol
- Failure to appreciate that the absence of early symptoms, a normal anion gap, or a normal osmolal gap does not exclude a potentially serious methanol intoxication
- Failure to observe and monitor patients with known or suspected methanol ingestion until a methanol level can be obtained or until the time of expected toxicity has passed without incident
- Failure to fully correct the acidemia

- Failure to appreciate that ethanol and fomepizole are removed by hemodialysis and to adjust their dosing during this procedure accordingly
- Failure to have the visual function of patients with poisoning formally assessed by an ophthalmologist

ICD 9

980.1 Toxic effect of methyl alcohol

REFERENCES

1. Aabakken L, Johansen KS, Rydningen EB, et al. Osmolal and anion gaps in patients admitted to an emergency medical department. *Hum Exp Toxicol* 1994;13:131.
2. Barceloux DG, Bond GR, Krenzelok EP, et al. American Academy of Clinical Toxicology practice guidelines on the treatment of methanol poisoning. *J Toxicol Clin Toxicol* 2002;40:415.
3. Bessell-Browne RJ, Bynevelt M. Two cases of methanol poisoning: CT and MRI features. *Australasian Radiol* 2007;51:175.
4. Brent J, McMartin KE, Phillips S, et al. Fomepizole for the treatment of methanol poisoning. *N Engl J Med* 2001;344:424.
5. Hovda KE, Froyshov S, Urdal P, Jacobsen. Severe methanol poisoning treated with fomepizole and hemodialysis. *J Toxicol Clin Toxicol* 2003;41:473.
6. Hunderi OH, Hovda KE, Jacobsen D. Use of the osmolal gap to guide the start and duration of dialysis in methanol poisoning. *Scand J Urol Nephrol* 2006;40:70.
7. Jacobsen D, McMartin KE. Methanol and ethylene glycol poisonings: mechanism of toxicity, clinical course, diagnosis and treatment. *Med Toxicol* 1986;1:309.
8. Jacobsen D, Webb R, Collins TD, et al. Methanol and formate kinetics in late diagnosed methanol intoxication. *Med Toxicol* 1988;3:418.
9. Purssell RA, Pudek M, Brubacher J, et al. Derivation and validation of a formula to calculate the contribution of ethanol to the osmolal gap. *Ann Emerg Med* 2001;38:653.

CHAPTER 6

Isopropanol, Acetone, and Other Glycols

PRE-HOSPITAL CONSIDERATIONS

- Search for and transport all medications, including medication containers, that may have been ingested by the patient.

CLINICAL PRESENTATION

Isopropanol poisoning is characterized by central nervous system (CNS) depression, gastrointestinal effects, ketosis, and an elevated osmolal gap without metabolic acidosis. Two common scenarios are (a) chronic alcoholics seeking an alternative when deprived of ethanol and (b) exploratory ingestions by children. It is difficult to correlate the degree of intoxication with serum isopropanol levels, probably because of cross-tolerance to isopropanol in alcoholics or to lack of previous exposure to intoxicants among children. Complicating the issue is the ubiquitous presence of acetone, an isopropanol metabolite that is also a CNS intoxicant.

With a few exceptions, signs and symptoms of isopropanol and acetone intoxication are very similar to those of ethanol. The disinhibited phase that may be seen with early ethanol intoxication has not been reported with isopropanol, but the CNS depressant effects are otherwise the same. Patients ingesting isopropanol often have higher levels of acetone than isopropanol by the time of presentation. The duration of isopropanol intoxication is longer than that with ethanol because of the slower metabolism of the former and the fact that the acetone metabolite is itself a CNS depressant. Gastrointestinal effects are common and include nausea, vomiting, abdominal pain, and hemorrhagic gastritis.

Acetone produces a characteristic fruity or ether-like odor in the breath. Serum acetone levels after isopropanol or acetone ingestion often greatly exceed those found in diabetic ketoacidosis, so this olfactory clue may be even more obvious than usual. Ketonemia and ketonuria occur rapidly after isopropanol or acetone poisoning (3).

Most cases of propylene glycol (PG) toxicity occur iatrogenically in hospitalized patients, particularly with high doses of intravenous benzodiazepines (5,6), but it can also result from ingestion of PG-containing household products such as cosmetics and automotive antifreezes (sold as safer alternatives to ethylene glycol). Signs and symptoms include CNS depression, hyperosmolality, lactic acidosis, and renal insufficiency.

Diethylene glycol (DG) and glycol ether poisoning may result in CNS depression, metabolic acidosis, renal failure, hepatitis, and pancreatitis. Glycol ethers can also cause hemolysis, hypotension, hypoglycemia, hematuria, and acute respiratory distress syndrome (1).

DIFFERENTIAL DIAGNOSIS

The differential diagnosis of isopropanol and acetone exposure includes any of the other CNS depressants, and other medical or surgical conditions that alter mental status, including intracranial trauma, CNS infection or tumors, hypoglycemia and other severe metabolic derangements.

The primary exogenous substances in the differential diagnosis are other alcohols. Patients ingesting any of the short-chain alcohols typically present with a similar clinical picture of CNS depression and an elevated osmolal gap. Differentiating the early stages of intoxication with any of these agents may be difficult. Fortunately, the most commonly ingested alcohol is ethanol, which can be rapidly quantified by most clinical laboratories. Late-presenting patients might be differentiated by an anion-gap metabolic acidosis (methanol and ethylene glycol), renal insufficiency (ethylene glycol), visual symptoms (methanol), hyperlactatemia (PG), and the smell of acetone on the breath (isopropyl alcohol or acetone). Patients with ethanol-like CNS effects, an elevated osmolal gap, and a normal anion gap and who smell like acetone may presumptively be diagnosed with isopropanol or acetone toxicity pending laboratory confirmation. Concurrent ingestion of isopropanol and ethanol or another "toxic alcohol" is not uncommon (4).

Ketones from isopropanol or acetone ingestion may falsely elevate measurements of serum creatinine (2), and an elevated creatinine with a normal blood urea nitrogen (BUN) suggests this diagnosis. Renal insufficiency from ethylene glycol should occur in conjunction with an increased BUN and a significant anion-gap metabolic acidosis. Other causes of ketosis to consider include diabetic ketoacidosis and alcoholic ketoacidosis, both of which also elevate the osmolal gap, and starvation ketosis. Elevated serum acetone levels are found in patients with ketoacidosis, although these levels are usually lower than those seen with isopropanol or acetone ingestion.

Although fingernail-care product ingestion is a common and usually benign source of acetone exposure, care should be taken to confirm the history and product ingredients in such cases. The ingestion of artificial nail remover (as opposed to nail polish remover) containing acetonitrile, rather than acetone, has resulted in fatal cyanide toxicity.

PG-induced lactic acidosis, especially among hospitalized patients, may be confused with many other serious causes of lactic acidosis, including hypoxia, hypotension, and sepsis that need to be excluded before ascribing the lactic acidosis to PG toxicity.

ED EVALUATION

The history should include identification of the substance(s) involved, concentration, route(s) of exposure, estimated volume ingested, and time elapsed since exposure. Any history of potential co-ingestants or trauma should be elicited. Early definitive product identification can help rule out potential disasters, such as acetonitrile-containing nail-care products in children or methanol and ethylene glycol ingestion by chronic alcoholics deprived of ethanol. Physical examination should focus on the patient's mental status, airway, and vital signs.

A rapid serum glucose determination to rule out hypoglycemia is essential. With serious intoxication, laboratory tests should include a quantitative level of the substance involved (if available). Routine serum chemistries (to rule out anion gap metabolic acidosis), an ethanol level, arterial blood gas, and measurement of serum and urinary ketones may also be helpful where the diagnosis is not clear by history. The close chemical structural relationship between ethanol, isopropanol, and acetone can cause analytical interference when employing breath ethanol tests and enzymatic ethanol assays using ADH.

The serum osmolal gap (OG) can be helpful as a screening tool for detecting exogenous low-molecular-weight alcohols or glycols. A serum osmolality measured by freezing-point depression exceeding the calculated osmolality (2[Na] + [BUN]/2.8 + [Glucose]/18 + [Ethanol]/4.2) suggests the presence of isopropanol, acetone, methanol, ethylene glycol, or PG. If the identity of the substance is known, its serum concentration in milligrams per deciliter can be roughly estimated by multiplying the OG by the substance's molecular weight and dividing by 10. The molecular weight of isopropanol is 60 g/mol, acetone is 58 g/mol, and PG is 76 g/mol. For example, if a patient with an acetone ingestion has an OG of 20, the estimated serum acetone concentration is (20 × 58)/10 = 116 mg/dL. Because the molecular weights of glycol ethers are higher than those of the other alcohols, toxic levels of glycol ethers often do not significantly elevate the osmolal gap.

ED MANAGEMENT

Treatment of isopropanol or acetone toxicity is supportive, with most patients requiring only observation. Early-presenting patients should be observed for deterioration, as toxicity should manifest within the first few hours. Activated charcoal does not bind these toxins well, unless given in very large doses, which is not recommended. Patients not adequately protecting their airway should be endotracheally intubated. Hypotension, if present, should be treated with intravenous saline and, if necessary, vasopressor agents.

Hemodialysis can greatly enhance isopropanol and acetone elimination. Hypotension refractory to treatment with intravenous saline is the primary indication for hemodialysis. Because acetone is not substantially more toxic than isopropanol, treatment with ethanol or fomepizole to inhibit alcohol dehydrogenase is not recommended. Patients with abdominal pain or heme-positive emesis may have a hemorrhagic gastritis and should be evaluated for gastrointestinal bleeding and anemia.

The treatment of severe toxicity from DG, PG, or glycol ethers should include ethanol or fomepizole and hemodialysis, with similar doses and protocols as used with ethylene glycol (see Chapter 4) or methanol (see Chapter 5) toxicity (1,5).

CRITICAL INTERVENTIONS

- Support the airway and respiratory function in patients with CNS depression.
- Administer intravenous fluids and pressors for hypotension.
- Consider hemodialysis for profound CNS depression, refractory hypotension, metabolic acidosis, or renal failure.
- Administer ethanol or fomepizole to patients with severe DG, PG, and glycol ether poisoning.

DISPOSITION

Patients with minor exposures to isopropanol or acetone, as often occurs with pediatric nonintentional ingestions, will need only 2 or 3 hours of observation to ensure they do not develop CNS depression. Patients with mild symptoms can be observed as with ethanol intoxication. Patients with coma, hypotension, metabolic disturbances, or end-organ toxicity should be admitted to an intensive care unit with poison center, toxicologist, and nephrologist consultation as needed.

COMMON PITFALLS

- Assuming that all isopropanol and acetone exposures are benign
- Failure to monitor and re-evaluate both asymptomatic and intoxicated patients
- Failure to appreciate that acetone and isopropanol affect breathalyzer measurement
- Failure to appreciate that acetone causes falsely elevated serum creatinine levels and diagnosing renal failure when the BUN is normal
- Failure to appreciate that DG, PG, and glycol ethers can cause toxicity similar to ethylene glycol

ICD 9

980.2 Toxic effect of isopropyl alcohol

REFERENCES

1. Gualtieri JF, DeBoer L, Harris CR, Corley R. Repeated ingestion of 2-butoxyethanol: case report and literature review. *J Toxicol Clin Toxicol* 2003;41:57–62.
2. Hawley PC, Falko JM. "Pseudo" renal failure after isopropyl alcohol intoxication. *South Med J* 1982;75:630–631.

3. Lacouture PG, Heldreth DD, Shannon M, Lovejoy FH. The generation of acetonemia/acetonuria following ingestion of a subtoxic dose of isopropyl alcohol. *Am J Emerg Med* 1989;7:38–40.
4. Pappas AA, Ackerman BH, Olsen KM, Taylor EH. Isopropanol ingestion: a report of six episodes with isopropanol and acetone serum concentration time data. *J Toxicol Clin Toxicol* 1991;29:11–21.
5. Parker MG, Fraser GL, Watson DM, Riker RR. Removal of propylene glycol and correction of increased osmolar gap by hemodialysis in a patient on high dose lorazepam infusion therapy. *Intensive Care Med* 2002;28:81–84.
6. Yorgin PD, Theodorou AA, Al-Uzri A, et al. Propylene glycol-induced proximal renal tubular cell injury. *Am J Kidney Dis* 1997;30:134–139.

Analgesics and Related Conditions

CHAPTER 7

Acetaminophen

PRE-HOSPITAL CONSIDERATIONS
- Transport all pills and pill bottles involved in overdose for identification in the emergency department.
- Keep in mind that over-the-counter cold remedies often contain acetaminophen.

CLINICAL PRESENTATION

Acetaminophen (*N*-acetyl-p-aminophenol, or APAP) toxicity can be divided into four stages (Table 7.1). The first stage of APAP poisoning is a relatively subtle period characterized by nausea, vomiting, and general malaise. In this phase, APAP is being absorbed and metabolized, and glutathione stores are being consumed. Although hepatotoxicity is beginning, it is often not apparent clinically or in laboratory results. Phase I typically lasts <24 hours. The antidote *N*-acetylcysteine (NAC) is most effective during this early phase and is virtually 100% effective in preventing hepatotoxicity if initiated within 8 hours of ingestion.

During phase II, which usually starts late on the day of the ingestion, the gastrointestinal effects of phase I resolve, and plasma concentrations of APAP are low or nondetectable. The hepatotoxic effects of the *N*-acetyl-p-benzoquinoneimine (NAPQI), which has not been inactivated by glutathione, begins to cause hepatocellular destruction. The predominant clinical picture is of hepatotoxicity but, as toxicity evolves, cholestatic features may occur. However, primary cholestatic injury is not caused by APAP.

Phase III of acetaminophen toxicity is the time of maximum hepatotoxicity. During this phase, transaminases will peak and then decline, but effects on coagulation may continue to increase. Patients who present in stage II or III may have right upper quadrant pain, nausea, vomiting, jaundice, bleeding, and encephalopathy. Associated with this is a progressive increase in bilirubin, alanine aminotransferase (ALT), and aspartate aminotransferase (AST) levels, as well as prothrombin time (PT)/international normalized ratio (INR). The magnitude of these liver function abnormalities can be dramatic, with ALT and AST levels of 10,000 to 20,000 IU/L frequent. In most cases, these abnormalities peak in 48 to 96 hours (stage III) and gradually resolve.

TABLE 7.1   Stages in the Clinical Course of Acetaminophen Toxicity

Stage	Time after Ingestion	Characteristics
I	0.5–24 h	Anorexia, nausea, vomiting, malaise, pallor
II	24–48 h	Right upper quadrant abdominal pain and tenderness; elevated bilirubin, prothrombin time, hepatic enzymes; oliguria
III	72–96 h	Peak liver function abnormalities; anorexia, nausea, vomiting, malaise may reappear
IV	4 d–2 wk	Resolution of hepatic dysfunction or fulminant hepatic failure

Modified from Linden CH, Rumack BH. Acetaminophen overdose. *Emerg Med Clin North Am* 1984;2:103.

In the final phase (IV), there will be either recovery or fulminant hepatic failure. Patients with severe untreated APAP toxicity exhibit a pattern of continued rising PT, bilirubin, and ammonia levels as the AST and ALT decline. This pattern signifies fulminant hepatic failure. However, most patients, even those with severe hepatotoxicity, eventually recover, with normal livers. It is not expected that patients who recover from APAP hepatotoxicity will suffer any residual liver abnormalities, and there is no reason for concern regarding future therapeutic APAP use.

The relationship between the plasma concentration of APAP, the time after acute ingestion, and the potential for toxicity is described by the nomogram developed by Rumack and Matthew (Fig. 7.1) (14). The nomogram stratifies patients into risk categories of "probable" or "possible" hepatotoxicity. Toxicity has not occurred in the "possible risk" area, which represents a 25% margin of safety to account for possible errors in establishing the time of ingestion, and is traditionally considered an indication for antidotal therapy in the United States. In most other countries, treatment is initiated only when the APAP level is in the probable toxicity area. The practice of treating patients with "possibly toxic" APAP levels has been questioned (2), and some toxicologists and poison centers in the United States are now treating otherwise healthy patients only if the measured plasma acetaminophen concentration falls in the "probable toxicity" area of the nomogram.

The nomogram begins at 4 hours after ingestion and extends to 24 hours. Plasma APAP concentrations obtained before this time—during the absorption and distribution phases—are difficult to interpret. However, early APAP concentrations of <100 μg/mL suggest a lack of toxicity risk (8). The nomogram cannot be used to assess potential toxicity of plasma concentrations obtained beyond 24 hours from the ingestion. Both nomogram lines have a slope equivalent to a 4-hour half-life so by remembering that the nomograms begin at plasma concentrations of 150 and 200 μg/mL, the level at each subsequent 4-hour time can be calculated by halving the previous level.

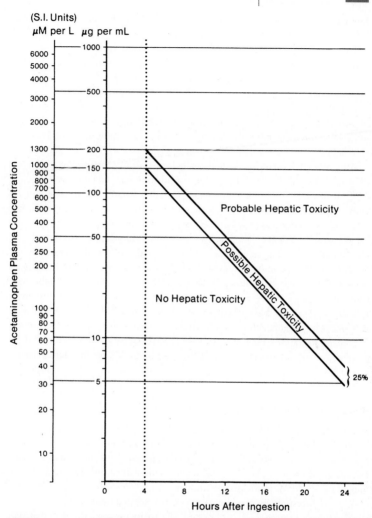

FIGURE 7.1 Rumack-Matthew nomogram for acetaminophen poisoning. Relation between plasma APAP levels and toxicity correlated with time after exposure. (Reproduced with permission from Rumack BH. *Pediatr Clin North Am* 1986;33:691–701.)

The APAP nomogram is based on initial plasma concentrations. Repeat levels offer no further useful information and should not be routinely obtained. Although this has been recommended for delayed release APAP overdose (e.g., Tylenol Extended-Relief, Tylenol Arthritis Pain), the value of this practice for determining risk of hepatotoxicity has been studied only in a very small case series (6). Based on the known volume of distribution of APAP of 0.9 to 1.0 L/kg, an ingestion of 10.5 g APAP in a 70-kg adult, or 150 mg/kg in a child, may produce plasma concentrations in the possible toxicity range. The current nomogram is derived solely from adult cases. Children with toxic plasma levels appear to be less susceptible to APAP toxicity than adults (13). Because there have been no reported cases of APAP-induced hepatotoxicity in infants after a single overdose, the utility of the nomogram in this population is unknown, and some clinical toxicologists and poison centers do not routinely treat infants.

Patients who have ingested a potentially toxic dose of APAP and have a history of alcoholism, chronic liver disease, or malnutrition may be more susceptible to APAP hepatotoxicity because of decreased glutathione stores. Conversely, patients with cirrhotic liver disease and, consequently, poorly functioning cytochrome P450 enzyme systems may be relatively protected owing to the inability to generate the toxic metabolite. Nonetheless, in acute overdose, these patients should also be evaluated using the standard nomogram. Ethanol is a inducer of the 2E1 isozyme of the hepatic P450 system (CYP2E1), the enzyme responsible for generation of the toxic metabolite. Alcoholics without liver disease and who have both induced CYP2E1 systems and depressed hepatic glutathione stores are theoretically more susceptible to the hepatotoxic effects of APAP. The same situation may occur in patients with acute illnesses associated with poor oral food intake (e.g., acute starvation). However, given the large therapeutic index for APAP, these populations are not expected to be at risk for hepatotoxicity with normal therapeutic doses (10).

DIFFERENTIAL DIAGNOSIS

In the earliest stage of APAP poisoning, the presumptive diagnosis is made by a history suggestive of overdose. Because there is no consistently reliable or pathognomonic signs or symptoms the possibility of occult APAP poisoning must be considered when one is confronted with any overdose or chronic pain patient. The finding of any APAP in the plasma must alert the clinician to the possibility of a toxic APAP ingestion, especially in the setting of elevated transaminases.

The patient in stage II, III, or IV of APAP toxicity present a different diagnostic challenge. By this time, there may be little or no detectable APAP in the serum, so the diagnosis depends heavily on the history and clinical suspicion.

The differential diagnosis of hepatic injury includes most commonly viral, autoimmune, ischemic, or chemical etiologies. Virtually any drug can cause hepatotoxicity as an idiosyncratic reaction. The correct diagnosis requires an astute history supplemented by laboratory studies. One particularly difficult diagnostic quandary is distinguishing between Reye's syndrome and APAP toxicity in the child given acetaminophen for an antecedent viral syndrome. The chemistry profiles typically seen with the different types of hepatitis are shown in Table 7.2. As

Hepatotoxin	Acute Viral Studies	AST (IU/L)	ALT (IU/L)
TABLE 7.2	**Laboratory Values in the Common Acute Hepatitides: Viral, Alcoholic, Acetaminophen**		
Viral	Usually positive	Hundreds to low thousands	Variable but less than AST
Alcohol	Negative	Usually <300 or 10× normal	Usually 100 and ALT/AST >2
APAP	Negative	May be very high	Much less than AST

AST, aspartate aminotransferase; ALT, alanine aminotransferase.

shown in Figure 7.2, liver function test (LFT) results may not rise dramatically until a day after the ingestion, although LFT elevations are often seen within the first day (17).

ED EVALUATION

The amount, formulation, and time(s) of APAP or other drug ingestion should be noted. Because of the myriad over-the-counter medications containing APAP, the patient may not even be aware of the danger. The history should address risk

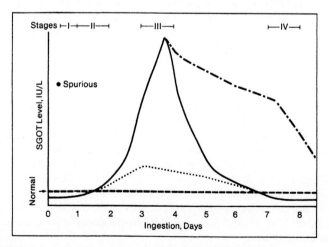

FIGURE 7.2 *Dotted line:* the course of those who received acetylcysteine. *Solid line:* those with natural a course. *Dotted–dashed line:* those with a severe course. (Reproduced with permission from Smilkstein MJ, Knapp GL, Kulig KW, Rumack BH. Efficacy of oral N-acetylcysteine in the treatment of acetaminophen overdose. Analysis of the national multicenter study (1976 to 1985). *N Engl J Med* 1988;319:1557–1562.)

factors such as acute or chronic alcohol use, pre-existing liver disease, and chronic malnutrition or acute starvation. The physical examination should focus on the vital signs and assessment of cardiovascular, gastrointestinal, and neurologic function and hydration status. An APAP level should be obtained and compared to the nomogram. If the level is potentially toxic or the time of ingestion is unknown and APAP is present, baseline liver function tests (AST, ALT, and total bilirubin levels and PT time), renal function tests (plasma urea nitrogen and creatinine concentrations), and urinalysis should be obtained.

ED MANAGEMENT

Advanced life-support measures should be provided if necessary (e.g., for coingested agents). Intravenous fluids may be required for patients with vomiting and dehydration. Treatment of acute APAP overdose is directed toward preventing absorption and administering NAC when indicated. Although the use of activated charcoal (AC) is common, the efficacy of this intervention for altering clinical course or outcome has not been firmly established. There is evidence that early administration of a single dose of AC given within 2 hours after ingestion may decrease measured plasma APAP concentrations, the single metric relied on for the determination of the need for therapy (4).

Although charcoal binds NAC, charcoal therapy does not have a clinically significant effect on plasma NAC concentrations. Therefore, it is unnecessary to increase the NAC dose when the patient is receiving both of these therapies (3). However, charcoal and NAC should not be mixed together before administration. Gastric emptying, by syrup of ipecac or lavage, has significant associated risk and no demonstrable benefit and should be avoided.

The most effective treatment for patients with a potentially toxic APAP level is NAC (4,12,15,18,19). NAC is metabolized by hepatocytes to the amino acid cysteine, a precursor of glutathione. NAC also enhances APAP sulfation, potentially leaving less APAP available to the hepatic P450 system (Fig. 7.3). NAC therapy is essentially 100% effective in preventing APAP toxicity if it is started within 8 hours of the ingestion, regardless of the plasma APAP concentration (19). Delay in starting therapy beyond this time results in a progressive diminution of its effectiveness (15,19). If a plasma APAP concentration is unavailable within 8 hours after ingestion, a history (or suspicion) of APAP overdose is sufficient to warrant the initiation of NAC therapy until the plasma APAP levels are known. If APAP is present and the time of ingestion is unknown or liver function tests are abnormal as a possible result of APAP poisoning, NAC therapy should be instituted regardless of the APAP level.

Two protocols are now used for the treatment of APAP overdose (Table 7.3). For both, it is best to treat patients with NAC until plasma APAP concentrations are undetectable and to discontinue therapy at that time if transaminase levels and PT remain normal or are falling and approaching normal values (7). The duration of NAC therapy using these criteria is frequently <24 hours. A

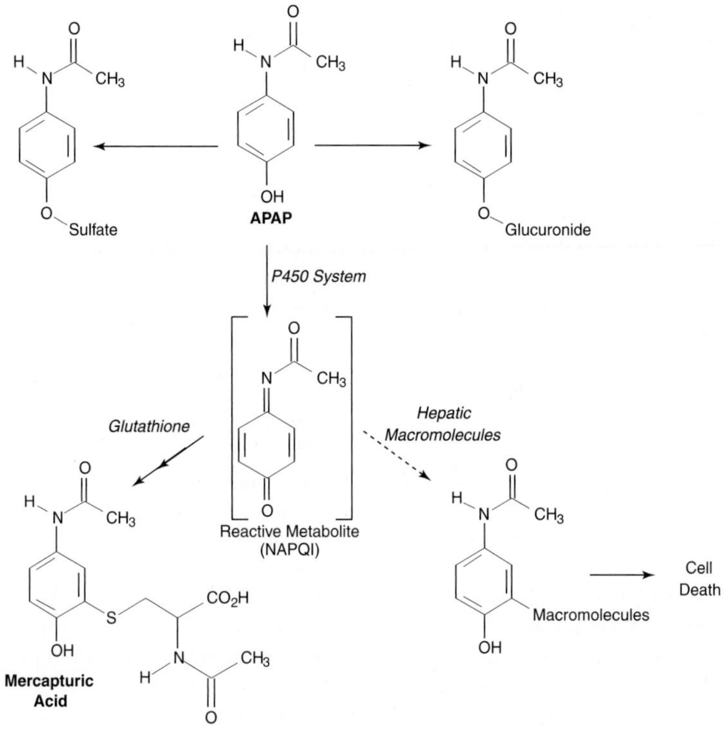

FIGURE 7.3 Metabolic pathways for acetaminophen metabolism.

prospective evaluation demonstrated that a shortened 20- to 48-hour course of oral NAC is an effective treatment option for patients meeting specific laboratory criteria of normal serum APAP <10 $\mu g/mL$ and liver function tests (serum aminotransferase and INR) and receiving a minimum of 20 hours of oral NAC therapy (1).

TABLE 7.3	**Protocols for *N*-Acetylcysteine Administration**	
Route of Administration	**Loading Dose**	**Subsequent Doses**
Oral	140 mg/kg	70 mg/kg q4h
Intravenous	150 mg/kg over 30 min	50 mg/kg over 4 h, followed by 100 mg/kg over 16 h

Giving oral NAC can be challenging. Because it tastes and smells like "rotten eggs," it is poorly tolerated. NAC is available as the mucolytic agent Mucomyst in a 10% or 20% solution. Before administration, it should be diluted to 5% in a soft drink to increase its palatability. It is also helpful to have the patient drink it through a straw from a closed container to prevent the unpleasant odor from causing emesis. Adding ice is helpful as it decreases the vapor pressure, and therefore the odor, of NAC. Emesis after NAC ingestion is common; and the dose should be repeated in full if emesis occurs within an hour of the dose. Standard antiemetics such as metoclopramide (Reglan; 0.1–1.0 mg/kg), promethazine (Phenergan; 12.5–25 mg IV), ondansetron (Zofran, 0.15 mg/kg IV), or another 5HT3 antagonist (e.g., granisetron, dolasetron) may be given and repeated as necessary. Rarely, an increase in hepatic transaminases may occur with ondansetron, which can obscure the assessment of APAP hepatotoxicity. If emesis continues, it is best to switch to IV NAC administration to assure adequate and timely therapy.

Intravenous NAC was approved for use in the United States in 2004 but has long been the standard therapy outside the United States. Even before formal approval, many clinical toxicologists and poison centers were giving oral NAC intravenously with an in-line filter and considered it to be first-line therapy (11). Although NAC given intravenously is easier to administer than oral NAC, IV administration may be associated with anaphylactoid reactions (primary itching and rash but also bronchospasm and hypotension). These may be related to the rate of NAC infusion. Debate continues regarding which route and dosing protocol are the most effective, cost-effective, and favorable in terms of risk-benefit profile (5). The major practical pitfall in using IV NAC occurs when a patient receives the loading dose in the emergency department but the maintenance infusion is neglected for some period, often because the patient is being transferred to the ward. Though there is inadequate literature addressing this specific circumstance, the authors recommend that the entire IV loading dose be readministered prior to starting the maintenance infusion.

APAP crosses the placenta, so when a pregnant patient overdoses on APAP, fetal hepatotoxicity is possible. However, NAC also appears to cross the placenta. If spontaneous delivery occurs while the mother is being treated, NAC may be given to the newborn. However, the necessity for NAC administration to neonates has not been established because their immature P450 system may not produce significant quantities of NAPQI.

A particularly perplexing group of patients are those who have taken a potentially toxic cumulative amount of APAP but have done so by ingesting multiple excessive doses over a period of time (16). If a patient has ingested more than 10.5 g or 150 mg/kg during the preceding 24 hours and has elevated transaminases, he or she should be treated with NAC. If the transaminases are normal, the plasma APAP concentration should be assessed. However, there is no consensus or controlled study that can provide guidance in the interpretation of these plasma levels. Non-validated recommendations range from treating patients with plasma APAP concentrations at least 10 μg/mL to treating patients with a potentially

TABLE 7.4	Transplantation Criteria for Patients with APAP-Induced Fulminant Hepatic Failure

Arterial pH <7.25–7.30 after adequate fluid resuscitation OR all of the following:
  Prothrombin time of >100–180 sec, AND
  Serum creatinine >3.4 mg/dL, AND
  Grade III–IV encephalopathy

toxic plasma APAP level based on the time since the last dose on the Rumack-Matthew nomogram.

The management of patients with APAP-induced hepatic or renal failure consists of NAC and supportive care (9). Patients who appear to have fulminant hepatic failure may be candidates for transplantation. However, transplantation should not be done simply on the basis of elevated transaminases, because this does not necessarily portend a poor prognosis. The most commonly used transplantation criteria are given in Table 7.4.

CRITICAL INTERVENTIONS

- Obtain a serum APAP level on all patients with a known or suspected drug overdose or hepatotoxicity of unknown cause.
- Administer NAC if the APAP level is potentially toxic by the nomogram, if APAP is present and the time of an acute overdose is unknown, or if the APAP level is elevated or liver function tests are abnormal after chronic excessive dosing.
- Administer the initial dose of NAC within 8 hours of ingestion.

DISPOSITION

Any patient who has a potentially toxic APAP level by the nomogram requires admission and continued treatment. Patients who present more than 24 hours after acute APAP ingestion or who have taken repeated supratherapeutic doses and have abnormal liver function test results should receive NAC therapy until the hepatotoxicity resolves (9). All intentional overdose patients should undergo a psychiatric evaluation before discharge.

COMMON PITFALLS

- Failing to consider an occult APAP overdose in all patients with intentional overdose, chronic pain, or unexplained hepatitis
- Withholding AC because of concern about its effect on NAC therapy
- Delaying NAC treatment beyond 8 to 10 hours while waiting for APAP levels or not starting NAC therapy in the emergency department when indicated
- Failing to appreciate that NAC has beneficial effects in patients with established hepatotoxicity

ICD 9

965.4 Poisoning by aromatic analgesics, not elsewhere classified

REFERENCES

1. Betten DP, Cantrell FL, Thomas SC, Williams SR, Clark RF. A prospective evaluation of shortened course oral *N*-acetylcysteine for the treatment of acute acetaminophen poisoning. *Ann Emerg Med* 2007;50:272–279.
2. Brandwene EL, Williams SR, Tunget-Johnson C, et al. Refining the level for anticipated hepatotoxicity in acetaminophen poisoning. *J Emerg Med* 1996;14:691–695.
3. Brent J. Are activated charcoal-N-acetylcysteine interactions of clinical significance? *Ann Emerg Med* 1993;22:1860–1862.
4. Buckley NA, Whyte IM, O'Connell DL, Dawson AH. Activated charcoal reduces the need for *N*-acetylcysteine treatment after acetaminophen (paracetamol) overdose. *J Toxicol Clin Toxicol* 1999; 37:753–757.
5. Buckley NA, Whyte IM, O'Connell DL, Dawson AH. Oral or intravenous N-acetylcysteine: which is the treatment of choice for acetaminophen (paracetamol) poisoning? *J Toxicol Clin Toxicol* 1999;37:759–767.
6. Cetaruk EW, Dart RC, Hurlbut KM, Horowitz RS, Shih R. Tylenol Extended Relief overdose. *Ann Emerg Med* 1997;30:104–108.
7. Clark D, Ruck B, Jennis T, Marcus S. Compliance with PCC recommendations: discontinuation of NAC [abstract]. *J Toxicol Clin Toxicol* 2001;39:485.
8. Douglas DR, Smilkstein MJ, Rumack BH. APAP levels within 4 hours: are they useful? *Vet Hum Toxicol* [abstract]. 1994;36:350.
9. Keays R, Harrison PM, Wendon JA, et al. Intravenous acetylcysteine in paracetamol induced fulminant hepatic failure: a prospective controlled trial. *BMJ* 1991;303:1026–1029.
10. Kuffner EK, Green JL, Bogdan GM, et al. The effect of acetaminophen (four grams a day for three consecutive days) on hepatic tests in alcoholic patients—a multicenter randomized study. *BMC Med* 2007;5:13.
11. Perry HE, Shannon MW. Efficacy of oral versus intravenous N-acetylcysteine in acetaminophen overdose: results of an open-label, clinical trial. *J Pediatr* 1998;132:149–152.
12. Prescott LF, Illingworth RN, Critchley JA, et al. Intravenous N-acetylcysteine: the treatment of choice for paracetamol poisoning. *Br Med J* 1979;2:1097–1100.
13. Rumack BH. Acetaminophen overdose in young children. Treatment and effects of alcohol and other additional ingestants in 417 cases. *Am J Dis Child* 1984;138:428–433.
14. Rumack BH, Matthew H. Acetaminophen poisoning and toxicity. *Pediatrics* 1975;55:871–876.
15. Rumack BH, Peterson RC, Koch GG, Amara IA. Acetaminophen overdose. 662 cases with evaluation of oral acetylcysteine treatment. *Arch Intern Med* 1981;141:380–385.
16. Schiodt FV, Rochling FA, Casey DL, Lee WM. Acetaminophen toxicity in an urban county hospital. *N Engl J Med* 1997;337:1112–1117.
17. Singer AJ, Carracio TR, Mofenson HC. The temporal profile of increased transaminase levels in patients with acetaminophen-induced liver dysfunction. *Ann Emerg Med* 1995;26:49–53.
18. Smilkstein MJ, Bronstein AC, Linden C, et al. Acetaminophen overdose: a 48-hour intravenous N-acetylcysteine treatment protocol. *Ann Emerg Med* 1991;20:1058–1063.
19. Smilkstein MJ, Knapp GL, Kulig KW, Rumack BH. Efficacy of oral N-acetylcysteine in the treatment of acetaminophen overdose. Analysis of the national multicenter study (1976 to 1985). *N Engl J Med* 1988;319:1557–1562.

CHAPTER 8

Salicylates

PRE-HOSPITAL CONSIDERATIONS

- Transport pills and pill bottles to the emergency department for review.

CLINICAL PRESENTATION

Mild or early salicylate poisoning is characterized by respiratory alkalosis with alkalemia and alkaluria (urine pH >6) (Table 8.1). It typically develops 3 to 8 hours after acute overdose but can occur days after chronic overdose. Signs and symptoms include nausea, vomiting, abdominal pain, headache, hearing loss, tinnitus (may occur at therapeutic levels), tachypnea or hyperpnea, ataxia, dizziness, agitation, and lethargy. Mild to moderate dehydration is invariably present. Tachypnea and hyperpnea can be subtle. Hearing loss is typically mild and symmetrical. Tinnitus is often described as a continuous high-pitched sound. Functional hypocalcemia (a decrease in ionized calcium) and tetany may result from respiratory alkalosis. Minor increases or decreases in serum glucose, potassium, and sodium levels are common, but blood urea nitrogen (BUN), creatinine, sodium, and potassium levels often remain normal despite total body fluid and electrolyte deficits.

Moderate poisoning is characterized by metabolic acidosis with respiratory alkalosis, alkalemia, and "paradoxical" aciduria (see Table 8.1). It occurs 6 to 18 hours after an acute overdose and days after chronic overdose. The anion gap may be elevated or normal. Gastrointestinal (GI) effects persist, and dehydration and neurologic symptoms become more pronounced. Fever, asterixis, diaphoresis, deafness, pallor, confusion, slurred speech, disorientation, hallucinations, tachycardia, tachypnea, and mild or orthostatic hypotension may be present. Leukocytosis, thrombocytopenia, increased or decreased glucose and sodium levels, hypokalemia, hypocalcemia, and increased BUN, creatinine, ketone, and lactate levels may be seen on laboratory evaluation.

Severe or late salicylate poisoning is characterized by an increased anion gap metabolic acidosis, acidemia, and aciduria (see Table 8.1) (6). It usually develops 12 to 24 hours after acute overdose and longer after chronic overdose. Hyperventilation (respiratory alkalosis) or hypoventilation (respiratory acidosis) and hypoxemia may be present. Other manifestations include coma, seizures, cerebral edema, papilledema, respiratory depression, hypothermia or hyperthermia, hypotension,

TABLE 8.1	Stages of Salicylate Poisoning	
Stage/Severity	**Plasma pH**	**Urine pH**
Early/mild	>7.4	>6
Intermediate/moderate	≥7.4	<6
Late/severe	<7.4	<6

pulmonary edema, congestive heart failure, dysrhythmias, and profound dehydration with oliguria. The chest radiograph may show pulmonary edema with a normal-sized heart, and brain computed tomography (CT) scan may reveal cerebral edema and hemorrhage. Electrocardiographic (ECG) abnormalities may result from direct cardiotoxicity, electrolyte abnormalities, or coingestants. Sinus tachycardia is common and can be extreme. Other dysrhythmias occur primarily as a terminal event. Asystole is the most common cause of cardiac arrest, but ventricular tachycardia and ventricular fibrillation can also occur (6). When cardiac arrest occurs, death appears to be inevitable. Successful resuscitation in this situation has yet to be reported.

GI bleeding, hepatic toxicity, pancreatitis, proteinuria, abnormal urinary sediment, an increased prothrombin time, and a low serum uric acid level (as a result of salicylate's uricosuric effect) may be present with therapeutic and toxic doses. Clinically significant bleeding, GI perforation, blindness, and inappropriate antidiuretic hormone secretion are rare complications of acute poisoning. Intrauterine fetal demise from poisoning during pregnancy has been described. The ingestion of methyl salicylate (oil of wintergreen, and a variety of Chinese propriety medicines) or salicylic acid (e.g., Compound W) may cause corrosive injury to the GI tract (3). Magnesium and bismuth (Pepto-Bismol) salts and enteric-coated or sustained-release formulations of salicylate may be radiopaque on abdominal radiographs.

Poisoning as a result of acute methyl salicylate ingestion can progress more rapidly, presumably because of liquid nature and higher lipid solubility of this formulation. Poisoning in children tends to progress faster than in adults, whereas adults appear to be more prone to pulmonary complications (3,4,7,10). The onset and progression of toxicity may be delayed, with peak drug levels occurring up to 5 days after overdose, with enteric-coated or sustained-release formulation ingestions (10).

Morbidity is higher in chronic than acute poisoning, and when the diagnosis is delayed (3,6,10). Although the overall mortality is <0.01%, fatality rates of 15% to 50% occur with severe poisoning (1,6). Persistent neurologic dysfunction occurs in those who recover from severe poisoning (1).

DIFFERENTIAL DIAGNOSIS

The pathognomonic increased anion gap metabolic acidosis is seen in only 15% to 20% of adults with such poisoning (1,3). Metabolic acidosis with respiratory alkalosis is the most common acid base abnormality, occurring in 50% to 61%

of poisoned adults. Respiratory alkalosis is the sole acid-base disturbance in 20% to 25%, and a combined respiratory and metabolic acidosis is seen in 5%. Metabolic acidosis is more common and respiratory alkalosis is less common (and often absent) in children, in patients with large acute ingestions, chronic intoxication, and delayed presentation or treatment. The anion gap is rarely above 20 mEq/L, even in advanced poisoning (3).

Salicylate poisoning should be considered in any patient with an unexplained acid-base disturbance. The diagnosis is initially missed in 25% to 60% of patients, particularly those chronically taking the drug (3,6,7,10). These patients are often elderly, take nonaspirin salicylates, and have underlying medical problems. Signs and symptoms of salicylate poisoning have been mistakenly attributed to anxiety, cardiopulmonary disease, cerebrovascular disease, chronic obstructive pulmonary disease, dementia, encephalopathy, alcohol intoxication, ketoacidosis and withdrawal, viral encephalitis and meningitis, pancreatitis, psychiatric disorders, and sepsis. Salicylate poisoning in children may be indistinguishable from Reye's syndrome. A low (subtherapeutic) cerebrospinal fluid salicylate level, high serum alanine, glutamine, and lysine levels, and fatty infiltration of the liver (by CT, ultrasound, or biopsy) indicate Reye's syndrome rather than salicylate poisoning. In infants and children, salicylate poisoning may also be confused with inborn errors of metabolism.

Other causes of anion gap metabolic acidosis include methanol and ethylene glycol, and lactic acidosis may occur in any poisoning that is complicated by hypoxia, seizures, or shock. A persistently normal arterial blood gas and serum electrolytes in a patient who remains symptomatic many hours after an unknown overdose rules out salicylate poisoning.

ED EVALUATION

The history should include the time(s), amount(s), and formulation of salicylate ingested. The physical examination should focus on vital signs, neurologic status, and cardiorespiratory function, especially to accurately measure the respiratory rate, temperature (e.g., rectal), and the degree of dehydration with orthostatic pulse and blood pressure, if possible. Papilledema, peritoneal signs, and occult blood in vomitus and stool should be identified.

With intentional ingestion and when the history is uncertain, a serum salicylate level should be obtained. Aspirin products are frequently misidentified as acetaminophen and vice versa. Unless the product (or its container) is available for positive identification or the history can be confirmed by a third party, serum levels of both drugs should be obtained when the ingestion of either is reported, particularly in those with intentional overdose. Unlike with acetaminophen, routine salicylate levels in all ingestions is unnecessary given that most severe salicylate intoxications present with obvious clinical signs (11).

Because of delayed and prolonged absorption, repeat salicylate levels should be obtained until levels are noted to be declining. A nontoxic salicylate level soon after ingestion does not rule out a significant overdose, particularly with enteric-coated or sustained-release formulations. If the patient is symptomatic or the salicylate level is elevated, an arterial blood gas (ABG), serum electrolytes, glucose, BUN, and creatinine, and a urinalysis should be obtained. If acid-base abnormalities are present, further evaluation should include serum calcium, magnesium, ketone, and lactate levels, liver function tests, complete blood count, coagulation profile, ECG, and chest radiograph. If levels continue to rise, repeated metabolic evaluation is necessary. A CT scan can assess for cerebral edema in comatose patients.

The ferric chloride spot test rapidly detects aspirin in the urine. Several drops of 10% ferric chloride added to 1 mL of urine turns purple if acetylsalicylic acid is present but positive results are also seen with therapeutic doses of aspirin. False-positive reactions may be caused by acetoacetic acid, phenylpyruvic acid, phenothiazines, and phenylbutazone.

ED MANAGEMENT

Advanced life-support measures should be instituted as needed. In patients who require endotracheal intubation, maintaining hyperventilation before, during, and after this procedure is critical because worsening acidemia (as a result of an increase in the pCO_2) enhances toxicity by increasing the fraction of nonionized salicylic acid available for tissue distribution. Failure to adequately hyperventilate intubated patients can result in rapid deterioration and death (7,10). Because artificial ventilation is accompanied by increased airway resistance and dead space, mechanical hyperventilation is unlikely to be as effective as spontaneous hyperventilation, and an increase in the pCO_2 (and decrease in serum pH) after intubation is inevitable in patients with a pCO_2 <20 mm Hg. Therefore, particularly with acidemia, a prophylactic dose of sodium bicarbonate ($NaHCO_3$) should be given at the time of induction. An empiric dose of $NaHCO_3$ of 1 to 2 mEq/kg given over 5 minutes is suggested for patients with acidemia or a pCO_2 less than 20 mm Hg. ABGs should be checked after intubation and after bicarbonate therapy.

Because central nervous system (CNS) hypoglycemia may occur despite a normal serum glucose in patients with salicylate poisoning, 50 mL of 50% dextrose in water (D50W) should be given to those with altered mental status (unless the glucose level is known to be elevated) (4). Anticonvulsants (e.g., benzodiazepines and barbiturates) and supplemental glucose should be given to patients with seizures. It is also advisable to administer $NaHCO_3$ (0.5 mEq/kg IV over 2–5 minutes) and calcium (0.1–0.2 mL/kg of 10% calcium chloride or gluconate IV over 2–5 minutes) as acidemia is likely to pre-exist and worsen after a seizure, and seizures can be as a result of hypocalcemia. This dose of calcium can be safely given even if the serum calcium level is normal (e.g., in functional hypocalcemia) and is the preferred treatment for tetany as a result of hyperventilation (respiratory alkalosis). Paper-bag breathing or sedatives for the treatment of agitation is not recommended because an increase in the pCO_2 can worsen concomitant acidemia. Similarly, an antiemetic should be nonsedating agent such as ondansetron.

Patients who are unresponsive or becomes so after a seizure should be assumed to have cerebral edema and should be treated with head elevation, hyperventilation, and possibly mannitol, furosemide, and dexamethasone. Diuretics should be used cautiously in patients with hypovolemia.

The degree of dehydration is often unappreciated. Volume deficits of 1 to 2, 3 to 4, and 5 to 6 liters (20, 40, and 60 mL/kg in children) are typical with mild, moderate, and severe poisoning, respectively. Fluid should be administered intravenously as 5% dextrose in normal saline or 5% dextrose in one-half normal saline with one 50-ml ampule of $NaHCO_3$ (44 or 50 mEq for the 7.5 and 8.4% solution, respectively) added to each liter of IV fluid and infused over the first few hours. With hypernatremia, a more hypotonic solution should be used. The use of a dextrose-containing solution is important because of the potential for occult CNS hypoglycemia. Such therapy is contraindicated in patients with cerebral or pulmonary edema and should be monitored closely in those with renal dysfunction. Urine output monitoring is helpful for assessing the efficacy of rehydration.

Central venous monitoring may guide treatment of patients with hypotension or oliguria, especially if there is evidence of heart failure or pulmonary edema. Congestive heart failure can be treated by standard measures, but patients with noncardiac pulmonary edema should be treated with positive end-expiratory pressure rather than diuretics. Preventing increased acidemia by maintaining hyperventilation is critical in patients with compromised pulmonary function.

Acidemia should be treated aggressively to slow salicylate tissue distribution. Treatment includes artificial ventilation for respiratory acidosis and IV $NaHCO_3$ for metabolic acidosis. Calculating the dose of $NaHCO_3$ for metabolic acidosis in salicylate poisoning is more complicated than for other causes of metabolic acidosis because respiratory alkalosis is usually present and, in salicylate poisoning, it is a concomitant primary acid-base disturbance, not just a compensatory response to academia. Hence, bicarbonate is unlikely to blunt the respiratory drive (increase the pCO_2), which would otherwise limit the increase in serum pH. The goal of therapy is to limit the tissue distribution of salicylates by increasing the pH to 7.45, not to correct the base deficit, which can result in a dangerous alkalemia.

Empirically: 1 to 2 mEq/kg $NaHCO_3$ is given intravenously either as a slow intravenous bolus (e.g., in aliquots of 0.5–1 mEq/kg given over 2–5 minutes every 10 minutes) or by rapidly infusing a similar dose mixed 5% dextrose (e.g., 3 ampules of $NaHCO_3$ per liter) over the first hour, reassessing the ABG, and repeating the process until the desired result is achieved (2,7,10). This approach, however, is less precise than calculating the dose of bicarbonate.

Potassium supplementation is necessary because patients are typically potassium–depleted, especially the presence of acidemia, wherein hypokalemia is more severe than indicated by the serum potassium level (by approximately 0.6 mEq/L for each 0.1-unit decrease in pH). As a general guideline, 10 to 20 mEq of potassium will be necessary for each 50 mEq of $NaHCO_3$ administered.

Complications of $NaHCO_3$ administration include excessive alkalemia, hypocalcemia, hypokalemia, hypernatremia, and fluid overload with cerebral and pulmonary edema, particularly in the elderly and with severe poisoning. Hence, regardless of the method used, cardiac monitoring, frequent evaluation of vital signs, mental status, cardiorespiratory function, urine output, and laboratory parameters (ABG analysis, serum calcium, and electrolytes) should be performed during and after such therapy. Relative contraindications for NaHCO$_3$ include oliguric renal failure, congestive heart failure, and cerebral or pulmonary edema.

Hyperthermia should be treated with cooling blankets, ice packs, and evaporative methods. Acetaminophen is unlikely to be effective, and nonsteroidal anti-inflammatory drugs should be avoided. The presence of peritoneal signs necessitates evaluation for surgical complications. Vitamin K should be given for coagulation abnormalities. Those with overt bleeding should also receive fresh-frozen plasma. Underlying metabolic derangements should be corrected. Insulin is unnecessary for nondiabetics with hyperglycemia and may be dangerous, particularly if there is coexisting hypokalemia. Hyperkalemia does not usually require specific therapy and can be expected to resolve with fluid administration and correction of acidosis.

GI decontamination with activated charcoal is recommended for patients with accidental ingestions of more than 150 mg/kg and in all patients with intentional overdoses (2,7,10). Because charcoal binds neutral agents better than ionized ones, salicylate may desorb from charcoal in the alkaline milieu of the small intestine. Multiple doses of charcoal may prevent this. Gastric lavage should be considered for large ingestions (500 mg/kg). Even in patients with spontaneous vomiting, large amounts of salicylate have been recovered as long as 18 hours after ingestion, hence the adage, "It's never too late to aspirate with salicylate." Optimal decontamination for large overdoses may include a dose of charcoal before and after gastric lavage. Whole-bowel irrigation should be considered in patients with large ingestions of enteric-coated or sustained-release preparations. Serial salicylate levels should be obtained to assess the efficacy of GI decontamination. Levels that continue to rise despite decontamination measures therapy suggest gastric drug concretion or bezoar, and endoscopy should be considered if clinical toxicity is severe or progressive.

Salicylate elimination can be enhanced by repeated oral doses of activated charcoal, alkaline diuresis, and extracorporeal removal (2,5,7,10). The administration of glycine (or N-glycylglycine), a cofactor for one of the salicylic acid pathways subject to saturation (Table 8.2), can also enhance the elimination of salicylate, but clinical experience with this therapy is limited. Multiple-dose activated charcoal, though not associated with a mortality benefit, has shortened the salicylate half-life to 2 to 4 hours after acute overdose (5) and is recommended for patients with clinical or laboratory evidence of salicylate poisoning or a salicylate level >30 mg/dL after an acute overdose. The optimal dosing and frequency for multiple-dose activated charcoal administration is controversial, though a reasonable approach is to use 25 g orally every 2 to 3 hours after the initial oral dose (12).

Alkaline diuresis can shorten the salicylate half-life to 6 to 12 hours in acute overdose with salicylate levels <70 mg/dL (8). Urinary alkalinization is more effective than either diuresis alone or alkaline diuresis. Indications for alkaline diuresis are the same as for multiple-dose charcoal. Contraindications include

TABLE 8.2   Elimination of a Single Dose of Salicylic Acid

Pathway	Product(s)	Percentage
Conjugation with glycine	Salicyluric acid	75*
Conjugation with glucuronic acid	Salicyl phenolic glucuronide	10*
	Salicylacyl glucuronide	5
Oxidation (hydroxylation)	Gentisic acid	1
Urinary excretion	Salicylic acid	10

*Saturable pathways.

cerebral and pulmonary edema, oliguric renal failure, and a serum pH >7.55. It should be performed with caution in patients with a history of cardiac failure.

The goal of alkaline diuresis is a urine pH ≥7.5 and a brisk (3–6 mL/kg/h) urine output. Once acidemia has been corrected, alkaline diuresis can usually be accomplished by administering the same solution as used for rehydration at a rate equal to the desired urine output. Alternatively, the empiric fluid therapy as described for the correction of acidemia can initially be used. Although counter-intuitive, alkaline diuresis is still indicated during early or mild intoxication, when the serum and urine pH are both alkaline, because respiratory alkalosis with com-pensatory renal bicarbonate and fluid excretion account for these findings. If left untreated, this can lead to dehydration and more severe metabolic acidosis later. Carbonic anhydrase inhibitors (e.g., acetazolamide) should not be used because they can cause acidemia, which increases ionized drug fraction and increased CNS salicylate levels (10). Because bicarbonate reabsorption and hydrogen ion excretion accompany potassium reabsorption, alkalinization of the urine may be ineffective until potassium deficits are corrected but whether this is true or is not is contro-versial (10). In the absence of hyperkalemia, initiation of potassium-containing maintenance fluids at the time of initiation of alkaline diuresis is a reasonable approach. Patients treated with alkaline diuresis should have hourly monitoring of fluid intake, urinary output, and urine pH. If intake persistently exceeds output, diuresis may be enhanced with furosemide.

Hemodialysis can shorten the salicylate half-life to 2 to 3 hours (2,7,9,10,). Peritoneal dialysis (with 5% albumin added to compete with serum proteins for salicylate binding) and exchange transfusion are less effective and should be used only if hemodialysis is unavailable, contraindicated, or technically impossible (e.g., in infants or in patients with active or recent bleeding complications).

Specific indications for hemodialysis include confusion, disorientation, coma, seizures, cerebral or pulmonary edema, renal failure, and clinical or metabolic dete-rioration (or failure to improve) despite other therapies (2,7,10). As acidemia and body temperature >38°C are associated with high mortality (1), their presence should also prompt consideration for hemodialysis, particularly if they persist despite other treatment. Patients with moderate poisoning who have liver dysfunction and hence impaired ability to eliminate salicylate may also benefit from hemodialysis. Although hemodialysis is often recommended if the salicylate level is >100 mg/dL after an acute ingestion, it may not be necessary if an early presentation and aggressive treatment is successful in preventing severe or progressive clinical and metabolic toxicity. Conversely, patients with moderate toxicity that progresses or fails to improve with other treatment (e.g., those with underlying cardiopulmonary disease or limited reserves because of advanced age or coexisting illness) should be considered for hemodialysis even if the salicylate level is not markedly elevated.

In contrast to the usual dialysis patient with chronic renal failure who is fluid-overloaded and hypertensive, those with salicylate poisoning are often hemodynamically compromised or tenuously stable because of underestimated or under-treated dehydration and cardiac dysfunction. As such, they are prone to cardiovascular decompensation on initiation of hemodialysis. Hypotension is common, and dysrhythmias can occur. Priming the dialysis circuit with normal saline and administering a fluid bolus prior to and during dialysis are recommended as prophylactic measures, along with correction of volume deficits and metabolic abnormalities, if possible. The dialysate bath should contain a high concentration of bicarbonate (32 mEq/L) to facilitate the treatment and prevention of acidemia and also to enhance the trapping and removal of salicylate.

Because of reported cases of significant toxicity from dermal absorption of salicylate, external decontamination to remove any further salicylate-containing substance from the skin should be considered if a dermal exposure is suspected.

Clinical improvement and decreasing salicylate levels are the endpoints of therapy. Once the salicylate level has reached 30 mg/dL, first-order kinetics resume. In patients with significantly elevated levels or ongoing absorption from a gastric bezoar, levels may rise again after an initial decline, so repeat levels assure that toxicity does not reappear once treatment is discontinued.

CRITICAL INTERVENTIONS

- Maintain hyperventilation during and after endotracheal intubation and administer $NaHCO_3$ prior to this procedure in patients with acidemia.
- Replace volume deficits with intravenous fluids containing dextrose and saline, and administer intravenous $NaHCO_3$ to correct acidemia and to alkalinize the urine.
- Perform frequent clinical and laboratory re-evaluation and obtain serial salicylate levels to assess the progression and severity of poisoning and the efficacy of decontamination and enhanced drug elimination therapies.
- Consider hemodialysis for patients with severe clinical or metabolic manifestations of salicylate poisoning or progressive deterioration despite other treatments.
- Give activated charcoal in large acute overdose.

DISPOSITION

Patients with mild or absent clinical and laboratory toxicity after acute overdose can often be treated in the emergency department if the peak salicylate level is

<60 mg/dL after aggressive treatment and the level is decreasing. Patients with chronic poisoning, higher levels, underlying medical problems, and moderate or severe toxicity should be admitted to an intensive care unit. A nephrologist should be consulted if poisoning is severe. Patients with severe poisoning or moderate poisoning with very high (or rising) salicylate levels should be transferred to a facility in which such hemodialysis is available. Unless the patient has oliguria, alkaline diuresis should be continued during dialysis.

COMMON PITFALLS

- Failure to ask about salicylate ingestion and to obtain a serum salicylate level on patients with unexplained acid-base disturbances, particularly with altered mental status
- Failure to obtain levels of both aspirin and acetaminophen in patients who report an overdose of either
- Failure to obtain repeat salicylate levels to rule out delayed absorption
- Failure to suspect chronic salicylate poisoning in ill patients
- Failure to monitor for complications of salicylate poisoning and its treatment
- Basing treatment on drug levels instead of clinical and laboratory findings

ICD 9

965.1 Poisoning by salicylates

REFERENCES

1. Chapman BJ, Proudfoot AT. Adult salicylate poisoning: deaths and outcome in patients with high plasma salicylate concentrations. *Q J Med* 1989;72:699.
2. Dargan PI, Wallace CI, Jones AL. An evidence based flowchart to guide the management of acute salicylate (aspirin) overdose. *Emerg Med J* 2002;19(3):206–209.
3. Gabow PA, Anderson RJ, Potts DE, et al. Acid–base disturbances in the salicylate-intoxicated adult. *Arch Intern Med* 1978;138:1481.
4. Gaudrealt P, Temple AR, Lovejoy FH. The relative severity of acute vs. chronic salicylate poisonings in children: a clinical comparison. *Pediatrics* 1982;70:566.
5. Hillman RJ, Prescott LF. Treatment of salicylate poisoning with repeated activated charcoal. *BMJ* 1985;291:1472.
6. Kirshenbaum AL, Mathews SC, Sitar DS, Tenebein M. Does multiple-dose activated charcoal therapy enhance salicylate excretion? *Arch Intern Med* 1990;150:1281–1283.
7. McGuigan MA. A 2-year review of salicylate deaths in Ontario. *Arch Intern Med* 1987;147:510.
8. O'Malley GF. Emergency department management of the salicylate-poisoned patient. *Emerg Med Clin North Am* 2007;25:333.
9. Prescott LF, Balali-Mood M, Critchley JAJH, et al. Diuresis or urinary alkalinization for salicylate poisoning? *Br Med J (Clin Res Ed)* 1982;285:1383–1386.
10. Thisted B, Krantz T, Strom J, et al. Acute salicylate poisoning in 177 consecutive patients treated in ICU. *Acta Anaesthesiol Scand* 1987;31:312.
11. Yip L, Dart RC, Gabow PA. Concepts and controversies in salicylate toxicity. *Emerg Med Clin North Am* 1994;12:351.
12. Wood DM, Dargan PI, Jones AL. Measuring plasma salicylate concentrations in all patients with drug overdose or altered consciousness: is it necessary? *Emerg Med J* 2005;22:401–403.

Nonsteroidal Anti-Inflammatory Drugs

PRE-HOSPITAL CONSIDERATIONS

- Collect pills and pill bottles for identification in the emergency department.

CLINICAL PRESENTATION

Most patients remain asymptomatic or develop only mild gastrointestinal (GI) or neurologic symptoms following acute overdose with nonsteroidal anti-inflammatory drugs (NSAIDs). Specific signs and symptoms are summarized in Table 9.1. Death is rare and usually results from secondary complications such as aspiration or sepsis. In the absence of acute renal failure or secondary complications, full recovery can be expected within 6 to 24 hours. The elderly are more likely to develop adverse effects with therapeutic doses and toxicity with overdoses. The acute toxicity of the selective cyclooxygenase-2 (COX-2) inhibitors appears to resemble the nonselective agents in overdose.

In contrast, the pyrazolones and fenamic acids can cause severe toxicity. Phenylbutazone and its active metabolite oxyphenbutazone can cause coma, seizures, dysrhythmias, cardiogenic shock, respiratory alkalosis, and metabolic acidosis. Tinnitus, deafness, and a rash may be present. Hepatic necrosis, without other symptoms, may develop 24 hours after overdosage. A red discoloration of the urine caused by the metabolite rubazonic acid may be observed. Mefenamic acid can cause muscle twitching and tonic–clonic seizures within 12 hours of ingestion. Both respiratory and cardiac arrest may follow seizures.

Propionic and acetic acid derivatives are associated with relatively low toxicity. Of these agents, fenoprofen appears to be the most toxic. Metabolic acidosis after ibuprofen overdose is probably related to high levels of acidic drug and metabolites. Indomethacin frequently causes headaches and tinnitus, even at therapeutic doses.

After piroxicam overdose, dizziness with blurred vision and brief coma are reported. Because of the long elimination half-life of piroxicam, overdose symptoms can be prolonged. Multisystem toxicity (with GI, neurologic, renal, hepatic, and hematopoietic effects) was noted in a 2-year-old who ingested 100 mg of piroxicam. Prolonged toxicity should be anticipated after overdose of oxaprozin and nabumetone, which also have long half-lives. NSAID plasma levels are not routinely available and are not necessary for the treatment of acute ingestion, despite a rough correlation between ibuprofen plasma levels and clinical toxicity.

TABLE 9.1	**Signs and Symptoms of Nonsteroidal Anti-Inflammatory Drug Overdose**

Gastrointestinal: nausea, vomiting, anorexia, abdominal pain, diarrhea, gastritis, gastrointestinal bleeding, occasional hepatocellular injury, rare cholestasis

Neurologic: dizziness, nystagmus, diplopia, blurred vision, headache, tinnitus, restlessness, lethargy, ataxia, confusion, coma, muscle fasciculations, seizures

Respiratory: hyperventilation, respiratory depression with cyanosis, apnea, diaphoresis

Cardiovascular: hypotension, bradycardia, occasional tachycardia, rare cardiac arrest

Renal: sodium retention and edema, proteinuria, hematuria, acute oliguric or nonoliguric renal failure

Hematologic: decreased platelet aggregation, prolongation of prothrombin time and partial thromboplastin time

Other: occasional metabolic acidosis, rare electrolyte imbalance

DIFFERENTIAL DIAGNOSIS

The diagnosis of NSAID overdose is made primarily on the basis of history and the exclusion of other etiologies. The possibility of acetaminophen, colchicine, and salicylate ingestion should be considered in patients with overdose of an unknown arthritis medication.

The central nervous system (CNS) depression that occurs with NSAID overdose is usually mild; coma unresponsive to stimulation is uncommon. Deep coma, marked hypotension, and severe respiratory depression suggest the presence of other drugs. The metabolic acidosis caused by ibuprofen is relatively mild and short-lived compared with that caused by salicylates, isoniazid, ethylene glycol, and methanol.

ED EVALUATION

A detailed history including available medications should be obtained and may provide the only clue to NSAID overdose. The amount and time of ingestion and the onset, nature, and progression of symptoms should be noted. The physical examination should include complete vital signs, oxygen saturation measurement, and assessment of mental status and cardiorespiratory function. Evaluation for occult GI bleeding should be considered for patients with abdominal pain.

A complete blood count (CBC), electrolytes, blood urea nitrogen (BUN), creatinine, glucose, and urinalysis should be obtained in all symptomatic patients, those with underlying kidney dysfunction, and the elderly. Etodolac may cause a false-positive urine bilirubin and a false-positive urine ketone test on dipstick. Although the time of onset of renal failure is poorly defined, urinalysis, serum BUN, and creatinine may be useful in adults who ingest >6 g of ibuprofen. Arterial or venous blood gases should be monitored in patients with significant mental status changes or respiratory depression. After pyrazolone overdose, liver function tests should be obtained. Toxicology screens of urine and blood rarely detect or correctly identify most NSAIDs other than salicylates.

ED MANAGEMENT

Initial management consists of supportive care. Mechanical ventilation may be necessary in severe poisonings especially if respiratory acidosis is present. Hypotension can be managed with intravenous crystalloids. Vasopressors are seldom necessary. Benzodiazepines should be given for seizures. Sodium bicarbonate should be given to patients with significant metabolic acidosis. GI bleeding should be treated by standard measures. Coagulopathy can be corrected by administering fresh-frozen plasma and vitamin K_1.

Activated charcoal should be considered in all patients with recent intentional overdose of more than 10 therapeutic doses, and children who present within 4 hours of accidentally ingesting more than five adult doses. Fenamic acids or pyrazolones may cause serious toxicity with even a twofold overdose, and decontamination is appropriate for all these patients. Multiple-dose activated charcoal (MDAC) therapy has not been studied with most NSAIDs. Although the elimination half-life of therapeutic doses of phenylbutazone was decreased by 30% using MDAC, the effectiveness of this treatment is likely to be minimal, even for NSAIDs that undergo enterohepatic recirculation. Because most NSAIDs are highly protein-bound and rapidly metabolized, diuresis or dialysis is not expected to remove a significant amount of active drug. Charcoal hemoperfusion may benefit patients with severe phenylbutazone poisoning, but few centers offer this modality.

CRITICAL INTERVENTIONS

- Establish intravenous access, initiate cardiac monitoring, and provide supportive care as clinically indicated.
- Obtain a CBC, electrolytes, BUN, creatinine, glucose, and urinalysis in symptomatic patients, those with underlying kidney dysfunction, and the elderly.
- Exclude the possibility of occult acetaminophen and salicylate ingestion in patients with intentional ingestions.

DISPOSITION

Most patients will be observed for 4 to 6 hours after ingestion or until minor symptoms resolve and then are discharged. After the ingestion of fenamic acids or pyrazolones, symptomatic patients should be monitored for at least 12 hours.

Patients with coma, respiratory depression, seizures, or renal failure should be admitted to a medical intensive care unit. Patients with an abnormal urinalysis or underlying renal dysfunction should have follow-up kidney function tests. A CBC and kidney and liver function tests should be repeated 24 to 48 hours after pyrazolone overdose. Follow-up liver function tests should be obtained in symptomatic piroxicam overdose patients.

Transfer should rarely be necessary. If acute renal failure develops, a nephrologist should be consulted. All intentional ingestions should be evaluated for ongoing suicidal risk.

COMMON PITFALLS

- Failure to consider other ingestions in patients with significant CNS depression, metabolic acidosis, or vital sign abnormalities
- Failure to consider acetaminophen, salicylate, or colchicine ingestion in patients who overdose on an unknown arthritis medicine
- Failure to appreciate that phenylbutazone and mefenamic acid can cause serious toxicity after overdose

ICD 9

965.9 Poisoning by unspecified analgesic and antipyretic

CHAPTER 10

Opioids

PRE-HOSPITAL CONSIDERATIONS

- Transport all pills and pill bottles for identification in the emergency department.
- Provide respiratory support.
- Administer naloxone.

CLINICAL PRESENTATION

Opioid poisoning may occur after intravenous, intramuscular, intranasal, inhalational, oral, subcutaneous, intradermal, or transdermal exposure. Unintentional poisoning in addicts or recreational users and intentional use in suicide attempts is frequently encountered. In the setting of injection, inhalational, and intranasal drug use, poisoning typically occurs in novice users, during binging, or when an experienced user obtains an unfamiliar supply of heroin and accidentally miscalculates the dose owing to differences in purity. The possibility of an intentional self-overdose or attempted homicide must also be considered. Unintentional exposure is most common in children, although iatrogenic poisonings do occur. Children may ingest pills or apply/ingest transdermal patches (that sometimes become stuck on the roof of the mouth). Elderly patients, particularly those on chronic opioid therapy for pain control of chronic illnesses, also represent a high-risk group for unintentional poisoning.

The onset of symptoms is nearly immediate after injection, inhalation, and nasal insufflation. Although effects are usually noted within 30 minutes of ingestion, absorption can be erratic and delayed, particularly in children and with sustained-release formulations. Lomotil (diphenoxylate and atropine) is notorious for causing delayed toxicity, perhaps because both constituents can inhibit gastrointestinal motility. The effects of transdermal medications also begin about 30 minutes after application. They can, however, develop or progress after the patch is removed. Intravenous injection and oral ingestion of fentanyl patches deliver the entire drug content of the patch at one time rather than the ongoing absorption of small aliquots of fentanyl.

Respiratory depression is the common denominator of opioid toxicity. In the overdose setting, it may lead to hypoxia and death. Opioid-induced respiratory depression results from diminished sensitivity to hypercapnia and depressed ventilatory response to hypoxia. The risk of respiratory depression increases after 60 years of age with therapeutic use of opioids. Heroin-related noncardiogenic pulmonary edema (NCPE) appears to be a neurogenic process initiated by central nervous system (CNS) hypoxia. Patients who have not been comatose and apneic do not appear to be at risk for this complication (7). NCPE can occur with any route of exposure. Although historically NCPE was described at a rate of 48% to 80%, recent case studies indicate that NCPE is an infrequent (0.8%–2.4%) complication of acute heroin overdose (7). Respiratory decompensation from NCPE typically develops within minutes to several hours after respiratory depression, but radiographic evidence may be delayed up to 24 hours. The decrease of NCPE in patients with nonfatal overdose may be related to better prehospital care and to regular administration of naloxone.

Another complication of opioid abuse is interstitial lung disease associated with talcosis from the injection of insoluble binding agents in oral opioid preparations such as talc, cornstarch, or cellulose. The result is microscopic pulmonary emboli and inflammation progressing to interstitial fibrosis and pulmonary hypertension. Clinically, this results in emphysema and chronic respiratory failure. Historically, the oral opioid most frequently cited in pulmonary talcosis is pentazocine (often used in conjunction with methylphenidate) and with methadone, meperidine, codeine, and oxycodone (4). Similarly, retinopathy may develop from the injection of oral medications (3).

Opioids have limited effects on the cardiovascular system, specific to a few agents. Opioids increase venous capacitance that may cause a slight decrease in both systolic and diastolic pressures. Opioids may cause bradycardia secondary to decreased CNS stimulation. Nonspecific histamine release can lead to hypotension. Methadone and propoxyphene may produce hypotension and bradycardia through calcium channel blockade (6). Propoxyphene may also produce sodium channel blockade in cardiac myocytes, producing QRS prolongation, ventricular dysrhythmias, hypotension, and decreased contractility. Other electrocardiographic (ECG) abnormalities include right bundle-branch block, left bundle-branch block, first-degree atrioventricular block, ventricular bigeminy, and ventricular fibrillation.

Methadone and its derivative L-α-acetylmethadol (LAAM) represent a unique situation. Both inhibit delayed potassium rectifier currents, increasing the QT interval and the subsequent risk for developing torsades de pointes. Prolonged QT syndrome and torsade de pointes appear to be dose-dependent and are more likely with high-dose methadone.

All opioids can cause CNS depression. Other CNS complications are associated with specific drugs. The mechanisms for seizures with propoxyphene, tramadol, and meperidine are not completely elucidated. Propoxyphene causes seizures in animals although its metabolite, norpropoxyphene does not (2). Inhibition of the reuptake of serotonin and norepinephrine is postulated as the etiology for tramadol associated seizures. Meperidine's metabolite normeperidine may cause excitatory neurotoxicity and serotonin syndrome as it blocks the reuptake of serotonin. Seizures with opioid overdose may also result from hypoxia.

Illicit use of a meperidine analogue synthesized in a clandestine laboratory has caused severe, acute parkinsonism as a result of a metabolite of the contaminant 1-methyl-4-phenyl-1,2,3,6-tetrahydropyridine (MPTP). Affected individuals are known as "frozen addicts."

Gastrointestinal side effects include nausea and vomiting, decreased bowel sounds, and abdominal distention. Urinary retention due to increased sphincter tone may also develop as a complication of opioid use. Other complications include pressure necrosis, compartment syndrome with rhabdomyolysis, hypoglycemia, and hypothermia in patients who have been comatose. Intravenous drug abusers are also at risk for endocarditis, lung and skin abscesses, viral hepatitis, and human immunodeficiency virus (HIV).

CNS depression, miosis, and respiratory depression are suggestive of opioid poisoning, although atypical presentations can occur (Table 10.1). CNS effects range from drowsiness to deep coma. In some cases, however, paradoxic excitation may be seen. Seizures can occur in a pure opioid overdose, particularly in children, but are most common with propoxyphene, tramadol, and meperidine (1) poisoning.

Increased muscle tone, tremors, and twitching may be seen with meperidine, and chest wall or muscle rigidity has been associated with fentanyl. Miosis is present in most cases of opioid poisoning. Mydriasis or midrange pupils do not rule out this diagnosis, however, as they can be seen with diphenoxylate, meperidine, hypoxic injury, hypoglycemia, a postictal state, or co-intoxicant. Initially, the rate (but not the depth) of respirations is decreased. With increasing severity, cyanosis and extreme bradypnea are noted. Rapid, shallow respirations may be noted in

TABLE 10.1	**Atypical Presentations of Opioid Poisoning**
Agent	**Prominent/Atypical Feature**
Propoxyphene (Darvon)	Rapid, sudden onset of opioid effects Seizures, psychosis (unresponsive to naloxone) Hypotension Prolongation of PR, QRS, and ventricular tachycardia Delayed onset of membrane depressant effects Low dose is life-threatening (11 mg/kg) Higher doses of naloxone needed to antagonize narcotic effects
Diphenoxylate (Lomotil)	Initial anticholinergic features Delayed onset of opioid effects Children at high risk for toxicity
Meperidine (Demerol)	Mydriasis Prolonged half-life of metabolite Seizures Increased muscle tone; serotonin syndrome
Pentazocine (Talwin)	Higher doses of naloxone needed to antagonize effects
Tramadol (Ultram)	Seizures unresponsive to naloxone Serotonin syndrome

patients with NCPE. These patients will also demonstrate hypoxemia, hypercarbia, and a respiratory acidosis and copious pink, frothy sputum and rhonchi, rales, or wheezes. Central venous pressure is normal or low, leading to the absence of jugular venous distention and the lack of an S3 gallop. Chest radiograph findings include a normal-sized heart and a variable pattern of pulmonary edema ranging from unilateral localized infiltrates to classic hilar-based bilateral infiltrates. Owing to the CNS depressant effects of opioids, aspiration pneumonia should be considered as a possible cause of abnormal pulmonary findings on examination and chest radiograph.

Opioids may cause a slight decrease in both systolic and diastolic pressures, which is often unnoticed in the supine patient. With the exception of propoxyphene, meperidine, pentazocine, and methadone, opioids have no direct inotropic or chronotropic effects (5). Although significant hypotension can occur as a consequence of nonspecific histamine release, it is usually secondary to hypoxia, a co-intoxicant, or shock from other etiologies. Though rhythm disturbances can occur with propoxyphene, methadone, and LAAM exposure, they otherwise suggest hypoxia or a co-ingestant (5). A murmur in an intravenous drug abuser should raise the possibility of endocarditis. Pulmonary hypertension with cor pulmonale may result from the injection of adulterants or contaminants.

DIFFERENTIAL DIAGNOSIS

Opioid poisoning should be considered in any patient with altered mental status (including seizures), miosis, and respiratory depression. Anticonvulsant, antidepressant, antihistamine, ethanol, muscle relaxant, neuroleptic, and sedative–hypnotic intoxication should also be considered. Pontine hemorrhage, cholinergic agents, clonidine and other imidazolines, phencyclidine, and phenothiazines may also cause miosis. With pontine hemorrhage, the patient exhibits tachypnea (central neurogenic hyperventilation) and hypertension. Cholinergic agents (e.g., organophosphate insecticides) may cause a diagnostic dilemma initially, as the patient may appear to have pulmonary edema (profuse oral secretions, wheezing, and rales). However, the gastrointestinal tract is stimulated rather than depressed, resulting in hyperactive bowel sounds, recurrent vomiting, and diarrhea. An overdose of clonidine or other imidazolines (e.g., tetrahydrozoline, guanabenz) may result in bradycardia, hypotonia, and bradypnea. Phencyclidine intoxication is usually accompanied by tachycardia, hypertension, and muscle rigidity or tremor. In phenothiazine poisoning, hypotension and tachycardia occur in conjunction with coma. Hypothermia, encephalopathy, postictal state, CNS trauma or infection, cerebral vascular accident, and metabolic or electrolyte abnormalities, including hypoglycemia, hypercalcemia, hyponatremia, and hypernatremia, should also be considered in the differential diagnosis.

ED EVALUATION

The history should include the identity of the opioid, co-intoxicants, and the amount, time, intent, and route of exposure. The physical examination should initially focus on assessing the patency of the airway and the adequacy of ventilation.

Patients should be placed on a cardiac monitor and have continuous oxygen saturation monitoring. Intravenous access and bedside glucose for patients with altered mental status should be provided. Electrolytes, creatinine kinase, and urine myoglobin should also be checked in patients who are combative, agitated, or seizing. A chest radiograph and ECG, appropriate in any overdose patient, should be obtained particularly in patients with unstable vital signs, hypoxia, or an abnormal cardiopulmonary examination. An ECG should also be performed on patients with propoxyphene or methadone ingestions and in patients with abnormal rhythm or conduction intervals on cardiac monitoring. Toxicology testing is appropriate to exclude acetaminophen and aspirin, which can be found in combination with opioids in many oral prescription medications. Urine screening and comprehensive toxicology testing for drugs of abuse detect some, but not all, opioids. Hence, a negative toxicology screen does not rule out opioid poisoning. A positive toxicology screen suggests exposure but not toxicity from opioids and should be confirmed by a second method. In contrast, a lack of response to adequate doses of opioid antagonists virtually excludes this diagnosis. A positive response to opioid antagonists is usually diagnostic, but poisoning with clonidine and valproate (and rarely benzodiazepines, ethanol, and chlorpromazine) have been reported to occasionally respond.

ED MANAGEMENT

Supplemental oxygen and assisted ventilation should be provided, as necessary. With the expeditious use of opioid antagonists and temporary ventilation via a bag-valve-mask, endotracheal intubation can often be avoided. The application of four-point restraints should be considered before antagonist administration, as the patient may become uncooperative and combative with reversal of opioid intoxication. Suction equipment should be set up in advance, because vomiting may occur after naloxone administration.

Opioid antagonists are indicated primarily for the treatment of respiratory depression. They may also be effective for opioid-induced seizures and can be used for diagnostic purposes in patients with altered mental status of unknown etiology. In suspected addicts, a low initial dose of naloxone (0.1–0.4 mg intravenously) should be administered to avoid precipitating a severe withdrawal reaction. This dose may be repeated every minute until a total of 2 mg has been given or respiratory depression is reversed and the patient awakens. Because some opioid overdoses (e.g., propoxyphene and methadone) are relatively resistant to naloxone, increments of 2 mg up to a total of 10 mg should be given if there is little or no response to the initial 2-mg bolus. If the patient is not a suspected addict, 0.4 to 2 mg of naloxone can be given as the initial bolus. The dose of nalmefene is essentially the same as for naloxone. Although longer acting than naloxone (4–8 hours vs. 30–100 minutes), this antagonist is more expensive. Naltrexone, an oral opioid antagonist, is used only for abstinence maintenance.

If intravenous access cannot be obtained, naloxone may be administered intramuscularly, subcutaneously, or endotracheally. The time to response after intramuscular administration is about the same as the time required to place an intravenous line and administer the drug. However, intramuscular administration decreases the risk of needlestick injury, reducing the potential for transmission of infections such as hepatitis and HIV to health care workers, especially in an uncooperative patient or in one with veins sclerosed from injection drug use.

Because naloxone has a shorter duration of action than most opioid agents, opioid toxicity can recur, primarily after oral overdose and particularly with diphenoxylate and methadone. Repeat doses may be necessary, and a continuous naloxone drip should be considered when frequent naloxone dosing is required. An infusion of two thirds of the initial dose of naloxone needed to reverse respiratory depression, given every hour, should maintain arousal. It may be necessary to give one-half of the original dose as an additional bolus 15 to 20 minutes after initiation of the drip. Health care providers must be diligent in monitoring patients placed on a naloxone drip.

A partial response to naloxone requires a careful search for other accompanying illnesses, injury, or intoxicants. Endotracheal intubation is necessary in patients with hypercarbia, hypoxia, or an inability to protect their airway. A neuromuscular blocking agent (e.g., succinylcholine) may be needed to perform an atraumatic intubation in some patients. Fluid restriction and positive end-expiratory pressure are also useful in the treatment of noncardiac pulmonary edema, but diuresis is inappropriate. Seizures unresponsive to naloxone should be treated with intravenous benzodiazepines (diazepam or lorazepam) or phenobarbital. Ongoing seizures suggest a cause other than pure opiate poisoning.

Hypotension is usually not a prominent feature of pure opioid overdose, and its presence should be managed with a crystalloid fluid bolus and an aggressive search for another cause. Propoxyphene, however, may necessitate aggressive use of vasopressors such as dopamine. Dysrhythmias due to propoxyphene are similar to those of the tricyclic antidepressants and may require sodium bicarbonate therapy (see Chapter 44, "Cyclic Antidepressants"). Naloxone will not reverse propoxyphene cardiotoxicity. Although naloxone only partially inhibits tramadol-mediated analgesia, it reverses respiratory depression and coma due to this agent. Magnesium with potassium replacement may be required to treat methadone-poisoned patients, especially those who develop a prolonged QTc or torsade de pointes.

CRITICAL INTERVENTIONS

- Administer naloxone to patients with altered mental status and respiratory depression.
- Begin with small doses of naloxone in opioid addicts with unintentional poisoning to avoid withdrawal.
- Give large doses of naloxone to those with intentional overdose and to children with accidental ingestions.
- Admit all patients who require naloxone after oral overdose and all children with possible opioid ingestions.

DISPOSITION

Careful observation is required for any patient who has demonstrated clinical evidence of opioid poisoning requiring naloxone administration. Although it is often recommended that patients with intravenous overdose be observed for 6 hours for evidence of relapse or the development of noncardiac pulmonary edema, this may not be necessary. Such patients usually have taken only slightly more heroin than necessary to achieve the desired effect. In addition, complications, if they develop, are usually evident soon after presentation. In contrast, all patients requiring naloxone after an oral overdose should be admitted to an intensive care unit with cardiac and respiratory monitoring (and suicide precautions, as needed). They should not be discharged until they are symptom-free for 12 hours. Adults who are or become asymptomatic during a 6-hour observation period after an oral overdose may be discharged, whereas all children with an oral overdose should be admitted to the hospital for observation and monitoring for 12 to 24 hours. Psychiatric or social work follow-up must be arranged for all intentional or pediatric poisonings. Asymptomatic patients who have been treated with narcotic antagonists should be monitored.

COMMON PITFALLS

- Failure to consider opioid overdose in patients who present with altered mental status, including seizures or combativeness, and CNS depression
- Failure to apply restraints, thereby risking injury to staff, before giving naloxone to suspected addicts
- Failure to evaluate for pulmonary complications, aspiration, and concomitant traumatic and medical illness
- Failure to examine thoroughly for medication patches (e.g., fentanyl)

ICD 9

965.00 Poisoning by opium (alkaloids), unspecified

REFERENCES

1. Kaiko RF, Foley KM, et al. Central nervous system excitatory effects of meperidine in cancer patients. *Ann Neurol* 1983;13(2):180–185.
2. Lund-Jacobsen H. Cardio-respiratory toxicity of propoxyphene and norpropoxyphene in conscious rabbits. *Acta Pharmacol Toxicol* 1978;42(3):171–178.
3. O'Brien RJ, Schroedl BL. Talc retinopathy. *Optom Vision Sci* 1991;68(1):54–57.
4. Padley SP, Adler BD, et al. Pulmonary talcosis: CT findings in three cases. *Radiology* 1993;186(1):125–127.
5. Routhier DD, Katz KD, et al. QTc prolongation and torsades de pointes associated with methadone therapy. *J Emerg Med* 2007;32(3):275–278.
6. Seyler DE, Borowitz JL, et al. Calcium channel blockade by certain opioids. *Fundam Appl Toxicol* 1983;3:536–542.
7. Sporer KA, Dorn E. Heroin-related noncardiogenic pulmonary edema: a case series. *Chest* 2001;120(5):1628–1632.

CHAPTER 11

Complications of Injection Drug Use

CLINICAL PRESENTATION

Patients with superficial abscesses often complain of localized pain, redness, and swelling at a previous injection site. Associated fever, cellulitis, and systemic complaints may also be present. Potential infection with methicillin-resistant *Staphylococcus aureus* (MRSA) should be considered in all patients presenting with abscesses and particularly in patients presenting with a furuncle or a cellulitis that does not resolve with conventional antibiotics (3).

Tetanus presents as increased muscle tone, spasm, or trismus. Patients with wound botulism usually present with neurologic complaints such as cranial palsies or descending symmetric paralysis. Atypical signs, including asymmetric or unilateral cranial nerve weakness and peripheral motor weakness, may be present. Atypical presentations and false-positive edrophonium tests have caused patients to be misdiagnosed with Eaton-Lambert syndrome or myasthenia gravis, resulting in prolonged delays in appropriate therapy.

Deep soft-tissue infections can have a subtle initial presentation but can rapidly progress to limb- and life-threatening illness. Myositis and pyomyositis may present initially with only mild erythema of the overlying skin but rapidly develop pain, significant edema, and crepitus. Sometimes a brown discoloration of the skin or purplish blebs develop. When the infection has progressed enough to cause marked cutaneous changes, the patient will frequently develop septic shock.

Broken needle fragments at injection sites may be asymptomatic or patients may have localized complaints of pain, as a result of the needle itself or of infectious complications. Patients may present with concerns about the risks of a retained needle fragment. They may also be unaware of its presence or fail to mention it unless asked.

Inadvertent intra-arterial injection causes immediate severe pain, hyperemia, numbness, weakness, distal swelling, cyanosis, and motor deficit and, often, sensory abnormalities. Distal ischemia may progress to gangrene, myonecrosis, and associated complications. The use of crushed oral medications and the lower extremity as a site of injection appear to be associated with more severe complications.

Venous pseudoaneurysms are most commonly noted in the groin and may present bilaterally. Pain, swelling, and purulent drainage may be noted. Some patients may appear clinically septic, with minimal localized complaints. In these patients, either pulmonary complaints or symptoms referable to sites of metastatic septic involvement may be more prominent.

Any mass over a vascular territory may actually be a pseudoaneurysm and should be approached with caution. Arterial mycotic aneurysms usually present as an indurated mass with local pain, and swelling. The mass may not be pulsatile, but a bruit is often heard over the swelling. Fever and leukocytosis are common, but bleeding, although occasionally massive, is usually intermittent, minor, or absent. Claudication, paresthesias, or compression neuropathy can occur. Signs and symptoms of distal embolic phenomenon, including cutaneous purpura, may be present and may precede systemic manifestations.

Injection drug use (IDU) patients with infective endocarditis usually have fever, but a new heart murmur, Roth's spots, Osler's nodes, Janeway lesions, splinter hemorrhages, or embolic phenomena are rare. The history and physical examination have a poor sensitivity and specificity for detecting infective endocarditis (12). The mortality rate in patients with IDU, human immunodeficiency virus (HIV) infection, and endocarditis is associated with the degree of immunosuppression as reflected by CD4 counts.

Patients with pneumothorax typically present with a history of recent neck injection, dyspnea, and pleuritic chest pain. Particulate-induced pulmonary dysfunction frequently presents as progressive dyspnea. Chest radiography can show a micronodular pattern; over time, the pattern changes to show large homogenous opacities, usually in the perihilar regions and upper lobes (8). Chest computed tomography (CT) scans have demonstrated fine micronodular changes, perihilar conglomerate masses, ground glass attenuation, and emphysema, especially of the lower lobes, among patients who inject solubilized oral medications. Retinoscopy can show talc deposits (small, whitish, glistening dots) and may have a higher diagnostic yield than either routine chest x-ray or pulmonary function tests.

Skeletal infections often present as localized pain and tenderness. IDU patients commonly develop septic arthritis and osteomyelitis at sites rarely seen in the general population, including the sternum, sacroiliac joints, and pubic symphysis. Almost 20% of patients with vertebral osteomyelitis related to IDU have had pain for more than 3 months at the time of diagnosis. Fever is usually absent or low-grade. Neurologic signs and symptoms occur infrequently (<15%) and are usually transient. Patients with septic arthritis associated with IDU are similar in presentation to other patients with septic arthritis, except for the prominence of fibrocartilaginous joint involvement. Local signs of inflammation and fever, leukocytosis, and elevated erythrocyte sedimentation rate (ESR) are usually noted. Asymptomatic HIV infection has been reported in one third of IDU patients with septic arthritis (1).

A patient with fungal endophthalmitis usually presents with decreased vision, photophobia, and ocular pain, which develop slowly. The infection may occur in one or both eyes. White vitreal exudates may be seen on funduscopic examination. Bacterial endophthalmitis has a similar but more rapidly progressing presentation.

Patients with cerebral mucormycosis usually have headache, fever, and rapidly developing cranial nerve and motor deficits. Basal ganglia lesions on CT scan should suggest this diagnosis. Cotton fever may cause dyspnea, palpitations, headache, and rigors.

Patients who inject drugs are also at risk for systemic drug or drug-contaminant toxicity (see Chapters 10, "Opioids"; Chapter 15, "Muscle Relaxants and Other Sedative–Hypnotic Agents"; Chapter 50, "Cocaine"; and Chapter 54, "Sympathomimetics"), withdrawal syndromes (see Chapter 58, "Drug Withdrawal"), and central nervous system (CNS) infections.

DIFFERENTIAL DIAGNOSIS

The most important requirement for developing an appropriate differential diagnosis is obtaining the history of IDU. Biases can easily enter into the physician's decision to obtain this information. It may be necessary to consider the possibility of IDU, even if denied by the patient. In such cases, a urine screening test for drugs of abuse may be helpful.

Unless the history of IDU is routinely obtained or considered, conditions such as vertebral osteomyelitis and epidural abscess may not be considered in the differential diagnosis of complaints such as back pain. Consider botulism, endocarditis, or intracranial abscesses and mycotic aneurysms in the IDU patient presenting with stroke symptoms. What appears to be an abscess in an IDU may actually be a pseudoaneurysm, and a simple incision and drainage might have disastrous consequences. The IDU patient who develops a fever or flulike symptoms is much more likely to have an infection requiring hospital admission than is a non-IDU patient who presents with similar complaints. Infective endocarditis should be in the differential diagnosis of all IDU patients with fever, even if another source of fever is found.

ED EVALUATION

The possibility of IDU, recent or remote, should be included in the standard "screening history." A nonthreatening question such as, "Do you smoke cigarettes, or use alcohol or other drugs?" should be routinely asked of all patients. Patients with IDU should be asked about the specifics of drug type, amount, needle sharing, skin preparation (alcohol wipes), and whether they have a history of hepatitis, endocarditis, HIV, pain at injection sites, recent fever, and nonprescribed antibiotic self-treatment. Because many IDU patients will not reveal their drug use, track marks or a positive urine toxicology screen may be the only clue to the diagnosis.

The physical examination of a patient with recognized IDU should include a careful review of vital signs, particularly an accurate temperature. Examination of the skin for signs of endocarditis, jaundice, infection at injection sites, and markers of HIV infection, such as oral thrush, should be performed in addition to a complaint-oriented examination. Evidence of opiate withdrawal, such as diaphoresis, lacrimation, yawning, pupillary dilation, and piloerection, should also be sought.

Routine laboratory tests are of limited use. Drug screens provide little information that will affect decisions, except possibly to suggest drug use when it is denied. Although the complete blood count and ESR lack sufficient sensitivity and specificity to guide disposition decisions, if infection is suspected or diagnosed, a very high or low white blood cell count might prompt admission, even for a simple abscess.

Ultrasonography may identify occult abscesses that require drainage that otherwise would have been missed on physical examination alone. Cutaneous abscesses with associated systemic complaints should be cultured. A radiograph should be routinely considered in patients with cutaneous complaints of pain and tenderness at injection sites to exclude retained needle foreign bodies and to identify gas-forming infections. Surgical consultation is necessary for abscesses that could involve deeper tissue based upon their location or appearance. A retrospective review of IDU patients seeking ED care for soft-tissue infections found that deltoid abscesses were five times more likely to be drained and explored in the operating room as compared to abscesses in other locations, given that the deltoid area has increased potential for deeper and more serious infections (11). Suspected deep soft-tissue infections such as myositis, pyomyositis, or necrotizing fasciitis can be evaluated with magnetic resonance imaging (MRI). However, given the rapid progression of these conditions, MRI should not delay surgical exploration for a definitive diagnosis in cases where there is high clinical suspicion (10). Ultrasound may identify a perivascular abscess but is not very sensitive for detecting pseudoaneurysms. Although digital subtraction angiography may be a useful diagnostic modality, color-flow duplex scans may be the diagnostic study of choice (13). Arteriography may be necessary to confirm the diagnosis.

Patients in whom endocarditis is suspected should have three sets of blood cultures, a chest radiograph, and cardiac ultrasonography. Pocket shooters and those with respiratory complaints should have a chest radiograph and measurement of oxygen saturation.

Patients with joint pain and effusion should have two sets of blood cultures and aspiration, Gram stain, and culture of affected joints. Septic synchondroses may be safely aspirated in the emergency department and should be evaluated similarly. Diagnostic criteria for prosthetic joints infection differ. Two sets of blood cultures and an MRI should be obtained for suspected vertebral osteomyelitis or epidural abscess. An elevated ESR and C-reactive protein (CRP) are not specific for osteomyelitis or septic arthritis and have limited utility for risk stratification or as triage tools (7). MRI is the modality of choice for detection of vertebral osteomyelitis and can be diagnostic for infected joints involving the axial skeleton and pelvis in uncertain cases.

Given that history, physical examination, and all other diagnostic testing lack significant sensitivity and specificity, an MRI should be considered on all IDU patients presenting with back pain.

Patients with complaints that suggest a CNS process (headache, weakness, ataxia) require a detailed neurologic examination, CNS imaging with CT scan or MRI, and a lumbar puncture to identify cerebrovascular complications of IDU use, opportunistic CNS infections, or malignancy (whether related or unrelated to HIV infection). Patients with complaints of visual loss require a complete eye examination, usually dilation with indirect funduscopy. In patients with fever, three sets of blood cultures, chest radiograph, urinalysis, and urine culture should be obtained.

ED MANAGEMENT

All patients with IDU-related infections should be given tetanus prophylaxis as needed. Localized cutaneous abscesses without vascular involvement may be managed with routine incision and drainage. If there is a possibility of vascular involvement, ultrasound should be obtained first or, if that is unavailable, needle aspiration prior to drainage. Patients with localized infections involving the neck, groin, or vascular structures and those with suspected deep soft-tissue infections such as myositis or pyomyositis should be evaluated by a surgeon. Although antibiotics and hospitalization are not routinely required for cutaneous abscesses that have been drained, patients with HIV infection, neutropenia, vascular involvement, deep space infections, or possible sepsis should be admitted and given parenteral antibiotics. Extensive extremity infections, especially those found in the deltoid area, should be explored in the operating room, as inadequate drainage may prolong hospitalization.

Small uncomplicated abscesses without significant overlying cellulitis require only incision and drainage, as the addition of antibiotics to this treatment has not been shown to improve cure rate or outcome (4). Antibiotic treatment is advised in patients with abscesses that are complicated, have significant overlying edema, or are associated with systemic effects. Antibiotic choice should be guided by local antibiotic resistance and susceptibility patterns. Initial antibiotic therapy for soft-tissue infections can include a penicillinase-resistant synthetic penicillin such as nafcillin (1 g IV q4h), or dicloxacillin (500 mg PO q6h) or a first-generation cephalosporin such as cefazolin (1 g IV q6h) or cephalexin (500 mg PO q6h). The increasing prevalence of MRSA should be considered when choosing empiric antibiotic therapy. For inpatient therapy, vancomycin (1–2 g IV q12h) can be used. For oral therapy, a dual regimen of trimethoprim-sulfamethoxazole (160/800 mg PO q12h) to treat MRSA, combined with cephalexin (500 mg PO q6h) to treat *Streptococcus* species, can be considered. Alternate regimens include linezolid (600 mg PO q12h), though its high cost may preclude widespread use, or clindamycin (300 mg PO q6h), though in many areas MRSA resistance to clindamycin is greater than 50%. An antipseudomonal regimen including an aminoglycoside (APAG) such as gentamicin (traditional dosing 1–2 mg/kg IV q8–24 h with the frequency depending on renal function, and high dose 5–7 mg/kg IV q24h) combined with an agent such as ceftazidime (2 g IV q8h) or cefepime (1–2 g IV q12h) should also be given if enteric organisms or *Pseudomonas* has been identified as part of the local "IDU" flora. Patients with gas-forming or necrotizing infections require *immediate* operative intervention and combination broad-spectrum antibiotic therapy that may include clindamycin, high-dose penicillin G, or vancomycin to treat MRSA and an APAG, and consideration of such adjunctive therapy as intravenous immunoglobulin and hyperbaric oxygen therapy. Such antibiotics as piperacillin/tazobactam (3/0.375 g IV q4–6h) or imipenem (1 g IV q6–8h) can also be considered. Where available, infectious disease consultation should be considered to aid in antibiotic selection and adjunctive therapy for such complex soft-tissue infections as necrotizing fasciitis or myonecrosis associated with *Clostridium.*

Early administration of antitoxin is important in patients with wound botulism. In a retrospective case series, 57% patients who received antitoxin within 12 hours of presentation required mechanical ventilation for a median duration of 11 days whereas 85% of those who received antitoxin at least 12 hours after presentation required mechanical ventilation for a median of 54 days (9).

When associated with infection or vascular injury, needle fragments require urgent removal. Patients who have retained needle foreign bodies but do not have these complications may be given appropriate discharge instructions and referral to a surgeon for elective removal. In general, emergency physicians should not attempt to remove fractured needle fragments. Even if they are palpable, finding them may be difficult, important neurovascular structures nearby may be injured, and migration may occur despite the use of a proximal tourniquet.

Patients with signs and symptoms of intra-arterial injection require aggressive management because of the potential for limb ischemia. Treatment should include antibiotics and anticoagulation with heparin. Consultation with a general or vascular surgeon is essential. Measurement of extremity compartment pressures should also be considered. A variety of off-label treatments have been described in case reports, including IV dextran 40 (20 mL/h) and dexamethasone (4 mg q6h) or the intra-arterial injection of a vasodilator such as papaverine (40–60 mg), phentolamine (2 mg), iloprost, a prostacyclin analogue, and intra-arterial thrombolysis (13). Given the potential morbidity, appropriate infectious disease consultation should guide any treatment plan.

Patients with pseudoaneurysms require blood cultures, preoperative laboratory testing including blood typing, and consultation with a general or vascular surgeon for excision and possible distal revascularization. Hospitalization is usually indicated. Hemorrhage control with direct pressure may be required. Local drainage should not be attempted in the emergency department, as life-threatening hemorrhage may result.

Although many physicians continue to admit all IDU patients with fever as ruling out endocarditis and bacteremia remains problematic, it has been suggested that oral antibiotics might be an acceptable alternative to intravenous therapy when intravenous access is very difficult or high risk (6). However, ciprofloxacin and rifampin have not been studied in patients in whom MRSA infection is prevalent. Pulmonary dysfunction from other causes is treated by supportive measures.

Vertebral osteomyelitis and septic arthritis should be treated with vancomycin and an APAG. Consultation with an orthopedic surgeon should be obtained. Spinal epidural abscess should be managed with urgent surgical drainage and empiric antibiotic therapy with both vancomycin and a third- or fourth-generation cephalosporin such as cefepime or ceftazidime until culture results become available (2).

Patients with cotton fever require only supportive care. This illness usually resolves within 12 to 24 hours. However, given the possibility that a serious medical condition is the etiology of fever, inpatient observation is recommended until the patient is well and the results of blood cultures are known.

CRITICAL INTERVENTIONS

- Consult an appropriate specialist for IDU patients with complicated infections, deep soft-tissue infections, symptomatic retained needle fragments, limb ischemia, or masses in the neck or groin, or with vertebral osteomyelitis, septic arthritis, or visual complaints.
- Consider admitting all IDU patients for intravenous antibiotics until endocarditis and bacteremia can be excluded.
- Consider IDU in patients with multiple unusual infections.

DISPOSITION

Patients with cutaneous abscesses who are otherwise asymptomatic and healthy may be discharged with appropriate instructions and referral for follow-up in 24 to 48 hours. Patients with retained needle foreign bodies can be referred for elective surgery on an outpatient basis unless there are signs of infection. The ability of a patient to comply with outpatient therapy and follow-up should be considered. Most patients with other infectious complications require admission. Concomitant HIV infection should lower the threshold for admission.

Patients should be educated about practices that have been shown to reduce the morbidity and mortality from injection drug use. They should be referred for substance abuse treatment and, if available, to needle-exchange; hepatitis, influenza, and pneumococcal vaccination programs; and for HIV, hepatitis, and sexually transmitted disease screening. Innovative efforts have combined screening for substance use, motivational interviewing, and linkage to drug abuse treatment. Patients can be referred to acupuncture, detoxification, needle exchange programs, outpatient buprenorphine providers, and other resources. Patients who continue to use injection drugs benefit from education about prevention practices, such as antiseptic skin preparation prior to injection, the use of bleach for cleaning needles and syringes, and the use of condoms. Programs that combine medical care with public health services have reduced emergency department visits by 40%, surgical admissions by 43%, and operating room procedures by 71% (5).

COMMON PITFALLS

- Failure to ask about IDU in all patients, including adolescents and older adults
- Failure to consider the possibility of undiagnosed HIV infection
- Labeling patients with IDU as "drug-seekers" or allowing a judgmental attitude to interfere with a careful medical evaluation
- Failure to appreciate that IDU patients with back pain as a result of vertebral infection may render a history of minor trauma and have a normal neurologic examination
- Attributing fever in an IDU to a trivial illness or to cotton fever
- Attempting to drain a soft-tissue mass in proximity to a major blood vessel
- Failure to consider the possibility of arterial injection, compartment syndrome, deep-space infection, or nerve injury in patients with limb complaints
- Failure to appreciate that extensive abscesses cannot be adequately drained in the emergency department

REFERENCES

1. Brancos MA, Peris P, Miro JM, et al. Septic arthritis in heroin addicts. *Semin Arthritis Rheum* 1991;21:81–87.
2. Darouiche RO. Spinal epidural abscess. *N Engl J Med* 2006;355:2012–2020 [Lifelong Learning Self-Assessment article, 2008].
3. Frazee BW, Lynn J, Charlebois ED, et al. High prevalence of methicillin-resistant *Staphylococcus aureus* in emergency department skin and soft tissue infections. *Ann Emerg Med* 2005;45(3):311–320 [Lifelong Learning Self-Assessment article, 2007].
4. Hankin A, Everett WW. Are antibiotics necessary after incision and drainage of a cutaneous abscess? *Ann Emerg Med* 2007;50(1):49–51.
5. Harris HW, Young DM. Care of injection drug users with soft tissue infections in San Francisco California. *Arch Surg* 2002;137(11):1217–1222.
6. Heldman AW, Hartert TV, Ray SC, et al. Oral antibiotic treatment of right-sided staphylococcal endocarditis in injection drug users: prospective randomized comparison with parenteral therapy. *Am J Med* 1996;101(1):68–76.
7. Margaretten ME, Kohlwes J, Moore D, Bent S. Does this adult patient have septic arthritis?. *JAMA* 2007;297(13):1478–1488.
8. Pare JP, Cote G, Fraser RS. Long-term follow-up of drug abusers with intravenous talcosis. *Am Rev Respir Dis* 1989;139(1):133–241.
9. Sandrock CE, Murin S. Clinical predictors of respiratory failure and long-term outcome in black tar heroin-associated wound botulism. *Chest* 2001;120(2):562–566.
10. Swartz MN. Cellulitis. *N Engl J Med* 2004;350:904–912 [Lifelong Learning Self-Assessment article, 2006].
11. Takahashi TA, Merrill JO, Boyko EJ, Bradley KA. Type and location of injection drug use-related soft tissue infections predict hospitalization. *J Urban Health* 2003;80(1):127–136.
12. Weisse AB, Heller DR, Schimenti RJ, et al. The febrile parenteral drug user: a prospective study in 121 patients. *Am J Med* 1993;94(3):274–280.
13. Woodburn KR, Murie JA. Vascular complications of injecting drug misuse. *Br J Surg* 1996;83:1329–1334.

Anticonvulsants and Sedative-Hypnotics

CHAPTER 12

Barbiturates

- Encourage paramedic transport for moderate to severe poisonings.
- Intubate as necessary for respiratory depression or loss of gag reflex.
- Provide intravenous access and supplemental oxygen. (An intravenous fluid bolus is necessary for hypotension.)

CLINICAL PRESENTATION

Significant ingestion of barbiturates is life threatening and typically presents as a depressed level of consciousness ranging from lethargy to deep coma. Patients may also have respiratory depression, which is responsible for most deaths that occur. With the short- and intermediate-acting barbiturates, symptoms usually begin within 1 hour of ingestion, and peak effects are seen within 4 to 6 hours. Patients with chronic lung disease are more susceptible to respiratory depression, even at therapeutic doses. Other clinical findings in overdose include hypothermia, sluggish papillary light reflex, nystagmus, and diminished bowel sounds. Bullous skin lesions, occasionally referred to as "coma blisters," may appear on shoulders, hands, buttocks, and knees. About 40% of patients who present with severe toxicity develop aspiration pneumonia (7). Cardiovascular collapse may be manifested by bradycardia or tachycardia, hypotension, and shock. Drug-induced dilatation of capacitance vessels (venous circulation) with consequent pooling of blood and reduction in effective vascular volume can lead to shock. In patients who have been comatose for a prolonged period, hypothermia and venous thromboembolism occur. Other complications include rhabdomyolysis and acute tubular necrosis secondary to shock and a mixed respiratory and metabolic acidosis. Ethanol and barbiturates have synergistic effects, and there is increased toxicity even when lesser amounts are ingested. Chronic use of barbiturates leads to tolerance and physical dependence as well as withdrawal symptoms when the drug is discontinued. Tolerance can develop with prolonged use and abuse, leading to a progressive increase in doses needed to achieve the desired effect. The withdrawal state is similar to ethanol withdrawal.

Laboratory abnormalities include hypoglycemia, electrolyte disturbances, and alterations in acid–base and fluid balance. The creatine phosphokinase (CPK) may be elevated if the patient has been comatose and immobile for a prolonged period. A chest radiograph may show aspiration pneumonia or pulmonary edema. The electrocardiogram (ECG) is usually normal. The electroencephalogram shows diffuse slowing during barbiturate-induced coma.

The amount of drug required to produce toxic symptoms can vary significantly depending on patient tolerance (8). The therapeutic doses for common barbiturates are given in Table 12.1. For nonaddicted patients, the toxic dose for short-acting barbiturates is about 3 to 6 g (5–8 mg/kg in pediatrics) and for phenobarbital is about 6 to 9 g (8 mg/kg in pediatrics).

Barbiturate addicts may tolerate higher doses. Geriatric patients may be much more sensitive to drug effects and can present with significant findings at lower doses. This may in part be attributed to decreased enzyme activity in the elderly (6).

Barbiturate blood levels are unreliable in predicting duration or severity of an overdose. Plasma barbiturate levels may not accurately reflect brain concentrations, as tissue solubility changes with fluctuations in pH. Chronic abusers tend to develop tolerance to the drug, thus exhibiting few symptoms at levels that would cause severe intoxication in previously unexposed patients (4). Butalbital may cross-react with some enzyme-multiplied immunoassay technique assays for phenobarbital quantification, particularly after large ingestions.

DIFFERENTIAL DIAGNOSIS

Other sedative-hypnotic agents, narcotics, or alcohol intoxication should be included in the differential. Similar presentations may be encountered with gamma-hydroxybutyrate, clonidine, skeletal muscle relaxants, and imidazoline decongestants (e.g., oxymetazoline). An overdose of psychiatric medications such as cyclic antidepressants, trazodone, phenothiazines, and antipsychotics must also be considered. Carbon monoxide poisoning, head trauma, CNS infections, sepsis, hypoglycemia, electrolyte abnormalities, and hypothermia may present similarly to barbiturate overdose and must be excluded.

ED EVALUATION

After initial stabilization, physical examination, basic metabolic panel (electrolytes, blood urea nitrogen, creatinine, bedside glucose), complete blood count, ECG, and urinalysis should be ordered. Blood alcohol and phenobarbital concentrations should be obtained. With pentobarbital and secobarbital overdoses, major toxicity is closely related to the plasma barbiturate concentration and the amount ingested. Coingestion of other CNS depressants has no obvious effect on outcome (5). Urine drug screen and acetaminophen level may be helpful when there is the possibility of co-ingestions.

The initial history is not always obtainable or reliable but, when possible, one should attempt to identify the drug ingested, the approximate amount ingested, the time of ingestion, and the reason for the ingestion (i.e., accidental or intentional).

The physical examination should focus on the vital signs, including rectal temperature and oxygen saturation, and the degree of CNS depression. Absence of bowel sounds suggests ileus; suprapubic percussion may reveal a distended urinary bladder.

TABLE 12.1 Barbiturate Kinetic Data

Drug	Usual Adult Dose (mg)	Onset (h)	Peak (h)	Duration (h)	Half-life (h)	Percentage Protein Binding	Volume of Distribution (L/kg)
Ultra-short-acting							
Thiopental	50–75	<0.1	<0.1	<0.5	3–11	72–86	1.4–6.7
Methohexital	50–120	<0.2	<0.2	<0.5	1–4	83	1–2.6
Short-acting							
Pentobarbital	50–200	0.25	0.5–2	>3–4	15–50	45–70	0.5–1
Secobarbital	100–200	0.25	1–6	>3–4	19–34	45–70	1.5–1.9
Intermediate-acting							
Amobarbital	65–200	<1	2	>4–6	10–40	59	0.9–1.4
Aprobarbital	40–160	<1	12	>4–6	14–34	20	—
Butabarbital	100–200	<1	0.5–1.5	>4–6	66–140	26	—
Butalbital	100–200	—	2	—	61	—	—
Long-acting							
Mephobarbital	50–100	0.5–2	—	>6–12	10–70	40–60	2.6
Phenobarbital	100–320	<0.1	0.5–2	>6–12	80–120	20–50	0.5–0.9
Primidone	300–1,000	—	—	—	3.3–12	20–30	0.4–1.0

Patients with abnormal vital signs or significant CNS depression should have a chest radiograph, ECG, arterial blood gas, liver function tests, and CPK level. Patients in deep coma and those with focal neurologic findings should have a computed tomography scan of the head to rule out cerebral edema or structural causes of coma. A lumbar puncture may be necessary to rule out meningitis.

ED MANAGEMENT

The treatment of barbiturate toxicity is primarily supportive. Patients with depressed respirations and altered mental status require airway management and intubation to support breathing and protect the airway. Blood pressure should be supported initially with intravenous crystalloid, administering 500- to 1,000-mL boluses, and with close monitoring of response. The core temperature should be checked and rewarming instituted if needed. Management decisions should be based on the patient's clinical condition rather than on blood drug levels.

For serious phenobarbital overdose, multiple-dose activated charcoal (MDAC) leads to more rapid recovery and a significant reduction in elimination half-life (1,3). The usual dose is 1 g/kg initially in sorbitol, followed in 2 to 4 hours by 0.5 g/kg in aqueous solution without sorbitol and alternating for 24 hours.

Barbiturates are weak acids with pK_as ranging from 7.2 to 8.5. Increasing the urine pH increases the fraction of ionized drug in the urine and thus decreases the amount of unionized drug available for passive tubular reabsorption. Urine alkalinization can increase the renal clearance of phenobarbital up to 10-fold and can shorten the half-life by one-half to two-thirds (2,9). There are no data to support the use of urine alkalinization for overdose with short- and intermediate-acting barbiturates (10). Urine alkalinization is contraindicated in patients with renal insufficiency and cerebral or pulmonary edema.

Hemodialysis may be used in life-threatening barbiturate overdose (9). Early notification of the nephrology service can expedite initiation of treatment. Both charcoal hemoperfusion and high-flux hemodialysis enhance the elimination of all barbiturates, and high-efficiency hemodialysis with a high blood flow rate may be superior to hemoperfusion (11). As these procedures are invasive and associated with some risk, their use should be reserved for patients with pulmonary edema, cerebral edema, or shock unresponsive to supportive measures.

CRITICAL INTERVENTIONS

- Provide appropriate airway management with supplemental oxygen.
- Treat hypotension with intravenous fluids and vasopressors if necessary.
- Administer MDAC for phenobarbital poisoning.
- Consider early hemoperfusion or hemodialysis for serious phenobarbital ingestions.

DISPOSITION

Nephrology consultation should be obtained when hemodialysis or hemoperfusion is being considered. Awake patients who have ingested short-acting barbiturates and whose symptoms are mild and are not progressing may be observed for 4 to 6 hours and then evaluated for psychiatric admission or discharged. For patients who have ingested long-acting barbiturates, the observation period should be based on both barbiturate levels *and* clinical symptoms. If quantitative serum levels are available (as with phenobarbital), serial levels should be obtained and the patient observed until levels peak and are decreasing. Patients with abnormal vital signs or significant CNS depression should be admitted to an intensive care unit. Patients who require intensive care or extracorporeal elimination measures may need to be transferred if such facilities are unavailable. Advanced life-support measures and gastrointestinal decontamination should be performed prior to transfer.

Psychiatric consultation is indicated for all suspected suicide attempts as soon as the patient is alert enough to be interviewed.

COMMON PITFALLS

- Failure to check for hypoglycemia as a cause of altered mental status
- Failure to protect the airway in a somnolent patient
- Failure to repeat MDAC and failure to check bowel sounds
- Failure to consider barbiturate withdrawal in patient with seizures

ICD 9 CODE

967.0 Poisoning by barbiturates

REFERENCES

1. Boldy DA, Vale JA, Prescott LF. Treatment of phenobarbitone poisoning with repeated oral administration of activated charcoal. *Q J Med* 1986;61(235):997–1002.
2. Ebid A-HIM, Abdel-Rahman HM. Pharmacokinetics of phenobarbital during certain enhanced elimination modalities to evaluate their clinical efficacy in management of drug overdose. *Ther Drug Monit* 2001;23:209–216.
3. Frenia ML, Schauben JL, Wears RL, et al. Multiple-dose activated charcoal compared to urinary alkalinization for the enhancement of phenobarbital elimination. *J Toxicol Clin Toxicol* 1996;34(2):169–175.
4. Goldberg MJ, Berlinger WG. Treatment of phenobarbital overdose with activated charcoal. *JAMA* 1982;247(17):2400–2401.
5. Goldfrank L, Osborn H. The barbiturate overdose. *Hosp Physician* 1977;9:30–34.
6. Greenblatt DJ, Allen MD, Harmatz JS, Noel BJ, Shader RI. Overdosage with pentobarbital and secobarbital: assessment of factors related to outcome. *J Clin Pharmacol* 1979;19(11–12):758–768.
7. Hardman JG, Limbird LE, eds. *Goodman and Gilman's: The Pharmacological Basis of Therapeutics,* 10th ed. New York: McGraw-Hill, 2001.
8. McCarron M, Schulze B, Walberg C, et al. Short-acting barbiturate overdosage. *JAMA* 1982; 248(1):55–61.
9. Palmer BF. Effectiveness of hemodialysis in the extracorporeal therapy of phenobarbital overdose. *Am J Kidney Dis* 2000;36(3):640–643.
10. Proudfoot AT, Krenzelok EP, Vale JA. Position paper on urine alkalinization. *J Toxicol Clin Toxicol* 2004;42 (1):1–26.
11. Quan DJ, Winter ME. Extracorporeal removal of phenobarbital by high-flux hemodialysis. *J Appl Ther Res* 1998;2(1):75–79.

CHAPTER 13

Benzodiazepines

PRE-HOSPITAL CONSIDERATIONS

- Attend to airway and breathing.
- Use a cardiac monitor.
- Provide intravenous access.
- Obtain a rapid glucose determination
- Transport pills and pill bottles in cases of suspected overdose.

CLINICAL PRESENTATION

Manifestations of benzodiazepine (BZD) poisoning include ataxia, lateral nystagmus, hypotonia, drowsiness, slurred speech, and coma. Even when BZDs are given in large doses, a deep coma causing cardiorespiratory depression and loss of deep tendon reflexes is rare. The ultra-short-acting agents are important exceptions, however, and deaths have also been associated with temazepam overdose.

Paradoxical excitement, including hallucinations, hostility, and seizures, have been reported with BZD overdose. Triazolam can produce delirium and psychosis. The elderly and very young children are more susceptible to the central nervous system (CNS) depressant action of BZDs. The toxic dose of flunitrazepam for a child is 0.1 mg/kg. This agent is approximately 10 times as potent as diazepam. Most patients with acute BZD poisoning, however, recover without sequelae within 24 hours. Patients with pre-existing medical conditions such as hepatic disease may be more susceptible to toxicity.

A spectrum of affective disorders (psychosis, agitation, confusion, hallucinations, and delirium) and motor dysfunction (tremors, restlessness, myoclonic jerks, and seizures) may develop on withdrawal from diazepam when taken in daily doses of 60 to 300 mg (see Chapter 58, "Drug Withdrawal"). Seizures are rare and most commonly develop 7 to 8 days after withdrawal (range, 2–12 days). Withdrawal symptoms develop in an average of 3 to 4 days after discontinuation (range, 1–11 days), peak in 5 to 6 days, and resolve by 4 weeks, but minor symptoms may persist for months. Earlier onset and peak and shorter duration of withdrawal may be seen with shorter-acting agents.

DIFFERENTIAL DIAGNOSIS

The presence of deep coma, apnea or significant respiratory depression, hypotension, multiple organ involvement, or a prolonged time for recovery should prompt a search for co-ingestants (e.g., sedatives, narcotics, sympatholytics, cholinergics, or alcohols) or another cause (e.g., CNS lesions, trauma, infection, or metabolic disturbances).

ED EVALUATION

The history should include the time and intent of all agents ingested and the amount and duration of chronic daily BZD documented. The physical examination should focus on vital signs and neurologic and cardiorespiratory function and the ability to protect the airway.

Except for measurement of oxygen saturation, routine laboratory tests are not necessary in the verbally responsive patient. Hematologic and metabolic profiles, urinalysis, and arterial blood gas analysis are recommended for those who are unresponsive to voice. Qualitative or semiqualitative BZD analysis of the blood and urine by immunoassay or thin-layer chromatography may confirm the presence of the drug but does not further guide clinical management. It should be noted, however, that immunoassay screening techniques will detect only BZDs that are metabolized to desmethyldiazepam or oxazepam and that most BZDs are not detected in thin-layer chromatography of the urine as a result of low drug concentrations.

ED MANAGEMENT

Advanced life support measures should be instituted as necessary. Supportive therapy is usually all that is necessary when a BZD is the sole agent involved. Gastrointestinal decontamination should be considered for patients within 1 hour of ingestion. Forced diuresis and hemodialysis are ineffective in enhancing BZD elimination because of high protein binding and volume of distribution. In uncomplicated cases, full recovery can be expected within 12 to 24 hours.

Flumazenil (Romazicon) is available in 5-mL and 10-mL vials containing 0.1 mg/mL. It is a specific competitive BZD receptor antagonist that reverses BZD-induced CNS depression. It also appears to be effective in reversing the sedative effects of zolpidem and endogenous BZD receptor agonists associated with hepatic encephalopathy. It does not antagonize other portions of the gamma-aminobutyric acid receptor (e.g., barbiturate, ethanol, and general anesthetic binding sites) and does not affect the bioavailability, plasma concentration, or elimination half-life of BZDs. Most important, it does not reverse BZD-induced hypoventilation. Airway protection and mechanical ventilation are definitive treatment for respiratory distress or failure.

In intravenous doses of 0.1 to 0.2 mg, flumazenil is partially antagonistic. In doses of 0.4 to 1.0 mg, onset of action and reversal of the CNS effects are evident within 1 to 2 minutes. An 80% response occurs within 3 minutes, and the peak effect is noted within 6 to 10 minutes. Duration and degree of reversal is related to the dose and the plasma concentration of BZD. Because flumazenil has a shorter duration of action than most BZDs, the effects from the initial exposure may recur. A 1-mg bolus usually lasts about 60 minutes but can last as long as 6 hours.

Indications for flumazenil include reversal of the sedative effect of BZDs when they have been used therapeutically (e.g., for conscious sedation) and for the management of accidental or intentional BZD overdose. In overdoses, flumazenil is best reserved for patients with pure, acute BZD overdose who are verbally unresponsive and have no history of seizures or long-term BZD use, as reversal may precipitate acute withdrawal. The use of flumazenil as a diagnostic and therapeutic tool in patients in coma of uncertain etiology is not recommended.

The suggested treatment protocol for using flumazenil in patients with known or suspected BZD overdose is shown in Figure 13.1. It may be repeated in boluses of 0.1 mg or administered as an infusion of 0.1 to 0.5 mg/h if necessary.

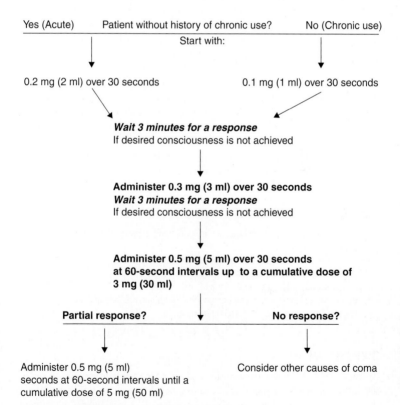

FIGURE 13.1   Flumazenil dosing for acute benzodiazepine exposure.

Patients who respond to flumazenil should be monitored for resedation. Furthermore, because flumazenil does not reverse hypoventilation, patients who awaken must often be repeatedly reminded to breathe (i.e., "take a deep breath"), and the adequacy of ventilation must be frequently reassessed. Emergence reactions after flumazenil administration (e.g., anxiety, agitation, confusion) are common, particularly when flumazenil is given in higher doses or more rapidly than recommended.

Flumazenil has no significant intrinsic pharmacologic activity. It may cause withdrawal and seizures in BZD-dependent patients, and it should be used in such patients with extreme caution. Lower than recommended doses and slower administration should be used if the benefits are felt to outweigh the risks. Seizures have also been reported after flumazenil in patients intoxicated with cyclic antidepressants, cocaine, or isoniazid and in those with CNS trauma. Because BZDs have a therapeutic role as anticonvulsants, flumazenil should not be given to such patients. Serious cyclic antidepressant poisoning is an absolute contraindication to using flumazenil and QRS interval prolongation with an unknown or mixed overdose should be considered a contraindication to flumazenil administration. A flumazenil-related dystonic reaction has also been reported. Naloxone, physostigmine, and stimulants such as aminophylline or theophylline are not indicated in the treatment of BZD poisoning.

Stopping the use of BZDs in any patient who has been maintained on these drugs longer than 6 weeks should be accomplished gradually over a minimum of 3 weeks and up to 2 to 3 months, depending on previous dosage and duration of treatment. Benzodiazepine withdrawal is managed by institution of oral diazepam (10–60 mg) for several days, followed by tapering the dose by 10% daily, usually over several weeks. Physician visits every 5 to 7 days are necessary to assess both physical symptoms and coping mechanisms.

CRITICAL INTERVENTIONS

- Protect the airway and provide ventilatory support in patients with significant CNS depression.
- Titrate the dose of flumazenil to the desired effect, beginning with low doses and waiting at least 3 minutes for a response before administering incremental doses, particularly in patients with a history of BZD use.
- Realize that most cases of poisoning with BZDs alone are mild and usually require only emergency department observation.

DISPOSITION

Patients with mild clinical toxicity (lethargic or asleep but who respond to verbal stimuli) can often be observed in the emergency department until they recover. Psychiatric evaluation should be performed before discharge unless the exposure is accidental.

Patients who respond only to painful stimulation, regardless of whether flumazenil is given, probably require 12 or more hours of monitoring and treatment. If emergency department observation is not possible, these patients should be admitted to an intensive care unit.

Outpatient referral and follow-up are indicated for patients who have evidence of chronic abuse, dependence, or psychological problems such as depression and do not require inpatient therapy.

Transfer is rare and indicated only if the initial facility lacks the equipment or personnel for caring for intubated patients.

COMMON PITFALLS

- Failure to consider co-ingestants or other causes of CNS dysfunction in patients with severe CNS depression
- Failure to appreciate that immunoassay screening techniques do not detect all BZDs
- Failure to appreciate that flumazenil can precipitate seizures in patients with chronic BZD use, history of seizures, or the co-ingestion of drugs known to cause seizures
- Administering flumazenil to overdose patients with cardiac conduction delays on electrocardiography
- Failure to appreciate that recurrent toxicity can develop after flumazenil administration and that continued observation is necessary

ICD 9

969.4 Poisoning by benzodiazepine-based tranquilizers

CHAPTER 14

Gamma Hydroxybutyrate

PRE-HOSPITAL CONSIDERATIONS

- Transport all pills and pill bottles and drug paraphernalia involved in overdose for identification in the emergency department (ED).
- Keep in mind that gamma hydroxybutyrate (GHB) precursors (gamma butyrolactone, 1,4 butanediol, gamma hydroxyvalerate, and gamma valerolactone) have the same effects as GHB.

CLINICAL PRESENTATION

Although there is significant variability of GHB effects, the characteristic presentation of acute GHB toxicity is dose-related central nervous system (CNS) depression, manifested as somnolence, lethargy, hypothermia, bradycardia, respiratory depression, coma, and death (2,4,9). The onset of coma may be rapid and abrupt, with Glasgow Coma Scale (GCS) scores of 3 to 8, but symptoms typically resolve within several hours. Hypotension and bradycardia have been noted to correlate with low GCS scores and co-ingestion of ethanol or other depressants (4). A biphasic stimulant-sedative effect of GHB has been documented with GHB administration (1), and stimulant effects such as psychomotor agitation are commonly seen in acute toxicity cases, even in the absence of stimulant co-intoxicants (4,9). Agitation may occur before coma, in rapid alternation with somnolence or coma (cycles of 2–3 minutes each), in response to interventions such as intubation, or as emergence delirium. It may also take the form of self-injurious behaviors (i.e., banging face or head on wall, floor). Gastrointestinal effects include urinary and fecal incontinence and nausea and vomiting, the incidence of which may be increased with alcohol co-ingestion (4). Myoclonus and/or seizure-like effects may occur; far less commonly, true seizures have been reported (5). Ophthalmologic effects include blurred or distorted vision, loss of peripheral vision, disconjugate gaze, and nystagmus (1,5). Although controlled study has shown pupillary dilation with GHB administration (1), pupillary reactions in GHB toxicity cases are variable, probably owing to effects of co-intoxicants. Rare cases of cardiac arrhythmias and atrial fibrillation have been reported in acute GHB toxicity (5) and after administration of physostigmine for purported antidotal effects (11). Additional effects include ataxia, sudden loss of muscle control, dizziness, confusion, headache, and amnesia, which is of special significance in cases of GHB-facilitated sexual assault (2,5,8).

This onset of GHB toxicity is rapid, typically within 15 to 20 minutes after ingestion, and often abrupt, owing to the steep dose-effect of GHB; 20 to 30 mg/kg produces euphoria, whereas doses >60 mg/kg may result in coma (2,7). Recreational doses for euphoria are estimated at approximately 2 to 3 g but vary widely, with dependent users dosing more frequently and with significantly larger amounts (3). Clinical effects typically peak approximately 30 to 60 minutes postingestion (5). Duration of effects is dose-dependent, typically from 2 to 4 hours in nonintubated patients (4). Intubation times may be longer, particularly in cases with co-intoxicants. As with abrupt onset of effects, sudden awakening is characteristic of recovery from GHB effects (4).

GHB ingestion has been associated with fatalities, both with and without co-intoxicants. In a series of 224 GHB-associated fatalities, 211 resulted from cardiopulmonary arrest, and 13 resulted from fatal trauma (motor-vehicle collisions, drownings, and smoke inhalation); 34% of the deaths occurred in the absence of co-intoxicants. Aspiration and asphyxia are less common causes of death. Forensic analysis of GHB death is complicated by endogenous GHB, levels of which rise over time by as much as 50 mg/L after death from any cause. Thus, death with levels <50 mg/L must be confirmed by history, and GHB deaths may occur, with no co-intoxicants, at very low measured levels. The lowest reported level associated with confirmed death, without co-intoxicants, was 18 mg/L; thus, levels associated with death can fall within the postmortem endogenous range.

The risks of GHB use and toxicity are heightened by its unpredictability, owing to its steep dose response, abrupt onset, inter-individual variability of effects, effects of food on absorption, and availability in a wide array of forms and concentrations, often unknown to the user. Adverse effects of GHB and its analogs may be compounded by toxic contaminants and additives. Accidental ingestions have been reported among users mistaking it for water. Risk is further compounded by a high rate of co-intoxicant use. Acute GHB toxicity case series document from 22% to 73% of patients presenting with ethanol co-intoxication and 28% to 86% presenting with illicit drug co-intoxication (4,11). Co-ingestion with alcohol or other CNS depressants may potentiate respiratory depressants of GHB.

The risks of GHB use are increased by its promotion as healthful, "natural," and "nontoxic" and by widespread misinformation on Internet Web sites and supplement labels that advised users to "sleep it off" in case of GHB overdose in the absence of depressant co-intoxicants (8). Of 224 GHB-associated fatalities, all of the decedents sustained cardiopulmonary arrest prior to arrival at an ED; in many cases, witnesses failed to notify emergency medical services, often despite known GHB ingestion and witnessed adverse effects including loss of consciousness. As there have been no deaths among GHB toxic patients transported prior to arrest, many of those deaths were probably preventable had medical assistance been promptly sought (10).

GHB is used to facilitate sexual assault because of the rapid onset, disinhibitory and amnestic effects, failure of routine toxicology tests to detect GHB, and rapid clearance from blood (4–6 h) and urine (6–12 h). Victims typically present late, beyond the window of detection; thus, a negative test for GHB does not mean that GHB was not used. Amnesia may or may not be associated with loss of consciousness, and victims may or may not remember the actual assault or assailant. GHB use should be suspected in patients presenting with unexplained lapses in memory of events, sudden onset of intoxication disproportionate to ethanol consumption or recorded ethanol level, missing or disheveled clothing, uncharacteristic behaviors, and symptoms consistent with GHB toxicity (sedation, agitation, coma) (8).

Chronic GHB use has resulted in the development of dependence and withdrawal, which may be lethal. Dependent GHB users typically dose multiple times daily, with reported ingestions of up to 144 g/day (3). The onset of withdrawal symptoms is rapid, generally within 1 to 6 hours of the last dose. GHB withdrawal presents with tremor, anxiety, agitation, diaphoresis and insomnia. Symptoms may progress rapidly (within 24 hours) to hallucinations, delusions, and delirium and may be confused with other withdrawal syndromes, head injury, CNS infection, anticholinergic or sympathomimetic poisoning, seizures, pheochromocytoma, serotonin syndrome, neuroleptic malignant syndrome, thyroid storm, and functional psychosis.

In contrast with the severe autonomic disturbance documented for ethanol and sedative-hypnotic withdrawal, tachycardia and hypertension may be transient and mild in severe GHB withdrawal, despite profound delirium (3,6). Severe and refractory agitation may increase the risk of hyperthermia, rhabdomyolysis, and disseminated intravascular coagulation; elevated CPK levels have been reported in cases of severe GHB withdrawal. Death or intensive care unit (ICU) stays of up to 15 days have been reported among patients hospitalized for treatment of GHB withdrawal (3). Ongoing insomnia, depression, anxiety, and cognitive deficits may persist for weeks to months after detoxification (6). Owing to frequent, chronic dosing, dependent GHB users are also at increased risk of overdose and trauma resulting from motor vehicle collisions and falls. Co-dependency of GHB and other drugs (e.g., methamphetamine, ethanol) is common.

DIFFERENTIAL DIAGNOSIS

Important indicators of GHB intoxication are abrupt onset and cleaning of effects and characteristic presentations with coma with psychomotor agitation. Physicians should question witnesses and paramedics on the scene and observe carefully for details of onset and course of altered mental status, specifically: (a) rapid and abrupt onset of altered mental status and coma, particularly when known by witnesses to be disproportionate to the amount of alcohol or drugs consumed; (b) periods of psychomotor agitation occurring prior to onset of coma, agitation in rapid alternation with somnolence or coma (2- to 3-minute cycles), agitation in response to interventions such as intubation, emergence delirium after coma, and self-injurious behaviors; and (c) rapid and abrupt clearing of effects. Physicians should also question paramedics as to circumstances prior to arrival: Dance clubs, raves, parties, and bars are common venues for use of GHB and other "club drugs," alone or in combination.

The differential diagnosis can be divided into two categories: (a) obtundation, stupor, and coma and (b) psychomotor agitation.

Etiologies of obtundation, stupor, and coma include intoxication with ethanol and licit or illicit drugs including opiates, barbiturates, beta blockers, carbamazepine, centrally acting antihypertensives such as clonidine, cholinergics, imidazolines, muscle relaxants, and sedative-hypnotics such as benzodiazepines. Carbon monoxide poisoning and CNS infections (meningitis, encephalitis) must be considered along with head trauma, intracranial hemorrhage, and increased intracranial pressure due to stroke or other causes. Metabolic and electrolyte disturbances such as hyperglycemia, hypo- and hypernatremia, renal or liver failure, and postictal state must also be considered. Profound metabolic disturbances such as acidosis, hypoxia, and shock may also result in altered mental status.

Etiologies of psychomotor agitation may include ethanol, sympathomimetic drugs of abuse (PCP, amphetamines, methamphetamines), cocaine, or hallucinogens. Psychiatric disorders and withdrawal from ethanol or other sedative-hypnotic drugs must be considered.

ED EVALUATION

The emergency department (ED) history should focus on the nature, timing, and amount of any drug(s) or ethanol consumed; the timing and abruptness of symptom onset; symptom course; past medical and psychiatric history; and regular medications. Physical examination should include assessment of vital signs, cardiopulmonary function, and neurologic status. Assessment and frequent monitoring of respiratory status (airway patency and protection, adequacy of ventilation) is of primary concern, particularly in coma. Pulse oximetry is recommended. Arterial blood gases may detect hypoventilation.

GHB is not detected on routine toxicologic screens. Confirmation requires targeted analysis with gas chromatography/mass spectrometry, which may take a number of days and thus does not help ED management. GHB is no longer detectable in the blood (and urine) at 4 to 6 hours (6–12 hours) after ingestion; its only metabolites are CO_2 and H_2O. Blood ethanol and drug screens and blood urea nitrogen (BUN), creatinine, electrolytes, fingerstick glucose, and urinalysis are usually unnecessary but may rule out or confirm other drugs. Tests indicated in cases of GHB withdrawal may also include electrolytes, BUN, creatinine, glucose, complete blood count with differential, coagulation studies, transaminases and liver function tests, creatine phosphokinase (CPK), urine drug screen, and drug levels (i.e., anticonvulsants, antidepressants), as indicated.

ED MANAGEMENT

Management of acute GHB intoxication is supportive. Airway protection, adequate oxygenation, and prevention of aspiration are critical. Frequent monitoring is necessary, and intubation and mechanical ventilation may be indicated. Sedation may be necessary for agitation. Because many patients recover rapidly and spontaneously, a conservative approach to intubation may be appropriate. However, the low frequency of reported intubation complications must be weighed against the potentially lethal risk of respiratory depression. Rapid-sequence intubation using succinylcholine is recommended; otherwise, intubation attempts of an apparently comatose patient may trigger agitation. Bradycardia is typically asymptomatic, and the few reported cases of atrial fibrillation have resolved spontaneously. The use of atropine may be necessary.

Physical and/or chemical restraints may be indicated for control of agitation. Benzodiazepines such as lorazepam (1–3 mg IV or IM) or butyrophenones such as droperidol (2.5–5.0 mg IV or IM) or haloperidol (5–10 mg IM) may be administered.

Though myoclonic movements have been well documented, seizures are rare. Although causality is not apparent, in the absence of definitive data it is likely that benzodiazepines such as lorazepam 2 to 4 mg IV or midazolam 2 to 4 mg IV could be employed for seizure control. CPK levels, cardiac enzymes, and urine myoglobin may be indicated to monitor for rhabdomyolysis.

Gastric lavage and activated charcoal are not indicated, owing to GHB's rapid absorption. There are no proven antidotes or reversal agents for acute GHB intoxication. Naloxone should be considered only in cases of suspected co-ingestion of opioids. Flumazenil has been shown to be ineffective in reversing coma (5). Although physostigmine has been suggested as a treatment, it is not recommended because of lack of efficacy, potential adverse effects and good outcomes with supportive care (5,11).

For forensic evidence in cases of suspected GHB-facilitated sexual assault, 100 ml of first-catch urine should be collected and refrigerated. If a blood specimen is necessary, 10 to 30 ml should be obtained in a gray-top tube (with sodium fluoride and potassium oxalate) and refrigerated. Established chain of evidence procedures should be followed.

GHB withdrawal requires aggressive supportive care and is very similar to management of severe delirium tremens. Agitation and delirium must be controlled and efforts made to prevent hyperthermia, rhabdomyolysis, renal failure, injury, and other complications. Long-acting sedatives such as diazepam (10 mg IV per dose, and titrated to restfulness) are recommended. Propofol may be used for intubated patients, starting with an IV infusion of 5 μg/kg/min (0.3 mg/kg/h) for 5 to 10 minutes until sedation is achieved, and maintaining infusion rates of 5 to 50 μg/kg/min. Barbiturates such as pentobarbital (100- to 200-mg IV increments) or phenobarbital (250-mg IV increments), titrated for symptom control, may also be utilized (6). Close monitoring and continuous pulse oximetry are critical after administration of all the sedative agents described earlier, and intubation and mechanical ventilation are frequently necessary.

CRITICAL INTERVENTIONS

- For acute GHB toxicity:
  - Use intubation and mechanical ventilation for airway protection.
  - Treat agitation with benzodiazepines and/or butyrophenones such as droperidol or haloperidol.
  - Monitor for rapid development of GHB withdrawal.
  - Question for history of known or suspected GHB use.
- For GHB withdrawal:
  - Provide adequate sedation.

DISPOSITION

The majority of cases of acute GHB toxicity resolve spontaneously without complications within 2 to 6 hours. After close observation, patients may often be discharged from the ED when they are clinically stable and mental status has fully normalized. In cases of coma requiring intubation and mechanical ventilation, admission to the ICU may be necessary; however, as with patients managed in the ED, recovery in the ICU may be rapid and abrupt, and patients may self-extubate. Complications such as aspiration or associated trauma may also necessitate ICU admission. Signs of GHB withdrawal may develop rapidly after the patient wakes up. This may begin in the ED or in the ICU in patients who have presented with acute toxicity. It is essential to counsel patients regarding the potentially lethal risks of GHB. For habitual users, referral for substance abuse counseling and treatment is critical.

COMMON PITFALLS

- Assuming that a negative toxicology screen rules out GHB; GHB is not included on standard hospital toxicology screens.
- Confusing the diagnosis of GHB intoxication with other drugs: agitation resulting from GHB toxicity, in particular may be mistakenly attributed to stimulants such as methamphetamine, cocaine, PCP, and so on
- Missing GHB-facilitated sexual assault in patients presenting with altered mental status or unexplained memory loss
- Failure to note early signs of GHB withdrawal after awakening from acute toxicity

ICD 9

968.4 Poisoning by other and unspecified general anesthetics

REFERENCES

1. Abanades S, Farre M, Barral D, et al. Relative abuse liability of gamma-hydroxybutyric acid, flunitrazepam, and ethanol in club drug users. *J Clin Psychopharmacol* 2007;27:625–638.
2. Dyer JE. Gamma-hydroxybutyrate: a health-food product producing coma and seizure-like activity. *Am J Emerg Med* 1991;9:321–324.

3. Dyer JE, Roth B, Hyma BA. Gamma-hydroxybutyrate withdrawal syndrome. *Ann Emerg Med* 2001;37:147–153.

4. Liechti ME, Kupferschmidt H. Gamma-hydroxybutyrate (GHB) and gamma-butyrolactone (GBL): analysis of overdose cases reported to the Swiss Toxicological Information Centre. *Swiss Med Wkly* 2004;134:534–537.

5. Mason PE, Kerns WP. Gamma hydroxybutyric acid (GHB) intoxication. *Acad Emerg Med* 2002;9:730–739.

6. Miotto K, Roth B. *GHB withdrawal syndrome.* Austin, TX: Texas Commission on Alcohol and Drug Abuse, 2001:3–10.

7. Snead OC 3rd, Gibson KM. Gamma-hydroxybutyric acid. *N Engl J Med* 2005;352:2721–2732.

8. Zvosec DL, Smith SW, McCutcheon JR, et al. Adverse events, including death, associated with the use of 1,4-butanediol. *N Engl J Med* 2001;344:87–94.

9. Zvosec DL, Smith SW. Agitation is common in gamma-hydroxybutyrate toxicity. *Am J Emerg Med* 2005;23:316–320.

10. Zvosec DL, Smith SW, Porrata T, et al. Preventable deaths from gamma hydroxybutyrate ingestion. *Ann Emerg Med* 2006;48:S75.

11. Zvosec DL, Smith SW, Litonjua R, Westfal RE. Physostigmine for gamma-hydroxybutyrate coma: inefficacy, adverse events, and review. *Clin Toxicol* 2007;45:261–265.

CHAPTER 15

Muscle Relaxants and Other Sedative–Hypnotic Agents

PRE-HOSPITAL CONSIDERATIONS

- Transport all pills and pill bottles in overdose for identification in the emergency department.

CLINICAL PRESENTATION

The onset of toxicity is expected to occur within 1 to 2 hours for most sedative–hypnotic agents and skeletal muscle relaxants. Delays are possible, especially with agents that have anticholinergic properties such as orphenadrine and cyclobenzaprine. Central nervous system (CNS) depression is the most common toxic effect. The extent of the CNS depression depends on the potency of the agent, the dose ingested, and the presence of alcohol or other CNS depressants.

Baclofen overdose is associated with profound CNS depression. Autonomic disturbances (e.g., bradycardia or tachycardia, hypotension, or hypertension) occur less frequently. Pupillary response is inconsistent, and both mydriasis and miosis have been reported. Seizures and cardiac dysrhythmias have been reported. Serum concentrations do not correlate with toxicity. Elimination of baclofen is slow after an overdose. In a series of adolescents with acute baclofen toxicity, mechanical ventilation was required for up to 60 hours after ingestion (7).

Seizures have been described 36 hours after the ingestion of 420 mg of buspirone (2). Serotonin syndrome (see Chapter 48, "Serotonin Reuptake Inhibitors and the Serotonin Syndrome") may occur in patients concurrently taking buspirone and selective serotonin reuptake inhibitor, trazodone, or St. John's Wort.

Carisoprodol primarily produces CNS depression in overdose. Tremor, myoclonus, muscle rigidity, tachycardia, and hypertension have also been reported (1). Physical dependence can occur after chronic use, and withdrawal can occur after abrupt discontinuation.

Manifestations of chloral hydrate overdose resemble those of barbiturates, with coma, miosis, and hypotension. Chloral hydrate is also a gastrointestinal irritant and commonly causes nausea and vomiting. Hemorrhagic gastritis and gastric necrosis occur rarely. As a halogenated hydrocarbon, it can also cause hepatic injury, renal failure, and cardiotoxicity. It reduces myocardial contractility, shortens the refractory period, sensitizes the myocardium to circulating catecholamines, and can precipitate cardiac dysrhythmias (see Chapter 36, "Hydrocarbons").

Cyclobenzaprine produces profound CNS depression and has significant anticholinergic effects. Confusion, agitation, and hallucinations can occur in overdose. Hallucinations can occur after therapeutic doses, especially in older adults. Although it is structurally similar to amitriptyline, serious cardiovascular effects have not been noted. In a retrospective review of cyclobenzaprine exposures reported to five regional poison centers, the most common toxic effects in patients older than 10 years of age were lethargy and tachycardia (9).

Prolonged coma is the predominant effect of severe ethchlorvynol and glutethimide overdose. Glutethimide also has anticholinergic properties that contribute to toxicity. Meprobamate overdose is associated with hypotension most likely owing to depressed myocardial function and has a tendency to clump in the stomach, forming a pharmacobezoar (4). Methaqualone commonly causes muscle hyperactivity, including hyperreflexia, twitching, and clonus, in addition to CNS depression. Hypotension and respiratory depression occur infrequently.

Orphenadrine overdose commonly results in both peripheral and central anticholinergic effects. Generalized seizure activity is reported commonly. Ventricular tachycardia and prolongation of the QRS interval have been reported and are likely the result of sodium channel blockade.

Ramelteon was approved for use in 2005, and there is limited information about overdose. Possible serotonin syndrome was associated with ingestion of thirty 8-mg ramelteon tablets in a woman on escitalopram (8).

Tizanidine overdose commonly results in lethargy and bradycardia, similar to clonidine. Hypotension, agitation, confusion miosis and coma have also been observed. A 2-year-old child became lethargic and bradycardic (heart rate, 40 bpm) after ingesting 16 mg. The duration of symptoms is usually <24 hours (10).

Eszopiclone, zolpidem, and zaleplon appear to be well tolerated in overdose. A review of eszopiclone (N = 60), zolpidem (N = 2,918) and zaleplon (N = 201) ingestions found drowsiness as the most common clinical effect (5,6). Tachycardia and slurred speech were noted in 5% to 10% with zolpidem and zaleplon. Agitation and irritability occurred in 5% of eszopiclone exposures. The patients who took zolpidem and zaleplon had mild CNS effects, including dizziness, slurred speech, and lethargy. Few patients complain of nausea, vomiting, and abdominal discomfort. Deep sedation is rare. Toxic effects from chlorzoxazone, metaxalone, and methocarbamol are primarily CNS depression.

DIFFERENTIAL DIAGNOSIS

Poisoning by alcohols, anticonvulsants, barbiturates, benzodiazepines, β blockers, calcium channel blockers, centrally acting antihypertensives, cyclic antidepressants, opioids, and skeletal muscle relaxants can cause similar signs and symptoms. Hypotension out of proportion to the degree of CNS depression suggests meprobamate, a cardiovascular agent, or a cyclic antidepressant. Cyclic coma suggests glutethimide ingestion or formation of a gastric pharmacobezoar. CNS infection and trauma, hypoglycemia, hypernatremia, hypercalcemia, and hypermagnesemia should also be considered. Ingestion of plants, mushrooms, and many different nonprescription and prescription medications can all cause anticholinergic symptoms.

ED EVALUATION

The history should include the time and amount of drug(s) ingested, the time and the nature of symptoms, and medical history, including the pattern and extent of muscle relaxant or sedative–hypnotic drug use. The physical examination focuses on vital signs and the neurologic and cardiopulmonary status.

Symptomatic patients should have baseline laboratory testing as indicated by clinical severity, including oxygen saturation or arterial blood gas analysis. Complete blood count, serum electrolytes, blood urea nitrogen, creatinine, and glucose concentrations, urinalysis, an electrocardiogram, a chest radiograph, and liver function tests may be helpful. Patients with deep coma should be evaluated for rhabdomyolysis by serum creatine phosphokinase and urine myoglobin tests. Comprehensive urine toxicology screening tests may confirm the presence of some muscle relaxants and sedative–hypnotic agents. Drugs-of-abuse immunoassays will not detect these agents. Cyclobenzaprine can cross-react with some toxicology assays to give a positive tricyclic antidepressant result. Quantitative serum drug levels are neither readily available nor clinically useful.

ED MANAGEMENT

Therapy involves stabilization and support of vital signs and early decontamination with activated charcoal. Patients normally respond well to good supportive measures. If a patient starts to deteriorate after apparent recovery or is deteriorating despite good supportive care, a pharmacobezoar should be suspected. Endoscopy may be necessary to remove the bezoar (4). If hypotension fails to respond to fluids or if the patient is already fluid-overloaded, a trial of dopamine and epinephrine is indicated. Unless there is hypoxic injury, full recovery can be expected once these drugs have been eliminated. Partial or full cardiopulmonary bypass and intra-aortic balloon pump therapy should be considered for hemodynamically unstable patients.

Patients with methaqualone poisoning may require pharmacologic paralysis for control of neuromuscular hyperactivity. Flumazenil, the benzodiazepine antagonist, has reversed CNS depression from zolpidem, zaleplon, and zopiclone (3). Routine use of flumazenil in the management of overdoses due to these agents requires caution, as detailed in the discussion of its role in treatment of benzodiazepine toxicity (see Chapter 13, "Benzodiazepines"). Sodium bicarbonate should be the first line of treatment for dysrhythmias or conduction disturbances associated with orphenadrine. Physostigmine may be useful to control severe anticholinergic effects associated with orphenadrine. There is no specific antidote for baclofen toxicity.

The anticholinergic properties of cyclobenzaprine, glutethimide, and orphenadrine may slow absorption and lead to delayed gastric emptying, so activated charcoal may be useful hours after ingestion. Fluids should be given with caution in treating the hypotensive effects of meprobamate, because its myocardial depressant properties increase the risk of pulmonary edema. The use of extracorporeal elimination may be useful in the treatment of life-threatening meprobamate overdoses unresponsive to supportive measures.

Ventricular dysrhythmias from chloral hydrate are often refractory to treatment. Lidocaine, magnesium (especially for torsades de pointes), β blockers, and overdrive pacing have been used with success. Excess stimulation or manipulation of the patient, as well as catecholamine pressor agents, should be avoided to decrease the risk of precipitating refractory dysrhythmias. Hemodialysis may be considered in chloral hydrate toxicity with profound hypotension and unstable dysrhythmias.

CRITICAL INTERVENTIONS

- Establish intravenous access, institute cardiac monitoring, and assess and maintain airway patency and respirations with endotracheal intubation and mechanical ventilation as necessary.
- Administer dopamine and epinephrine for hypotension refractory to intravenous crystalloid.
- Administer intravenous sodium bicarbonate for dysrhythmias or conduction disturbances as a result of orphenadrine.
- Consider the use of flumazenil in selected cases as a reversal agent for zolpidem, zaleplon, and chlorzoxazone.
- Consider cardiopulmonary bypass, intra-aortic balloon pump, and hemodialysis in severe poisoning refractory to standard therapy.

DISPOSITION

Patients with mild symptoms may be observed in the emergency department until asymptomatic. Patients with moderate or severe symptoms require intensive care admission for close monitoring, and supportive care is necessary. Patients with unstable vital signs should be transferred to a facility that is capable of intensive care for poisoning victims. Advanced life-support equipment and staff should accompany the patient during transfer.

COMMON PITFALLS

- Failure to consider gastric drug bezoar and continuing drug absorption in patients with progressive, prolonged, or cyclic coma (particularly due to glutethimide and meprobamate)

- Failure to appreciate that meprobamate can cause hypotension in the absence of severe CNS depression
- Failure to appreciate that buspirone, methaqualone, carisoprodol, and agents with anticholinergic properties such as cyclobenzaprine, glutethimide, and orphenadrine can cause neuromuscular hyperactivity or seizures in addition to CNS depression
- Failure to monitor for pulmonary edema, especially in patients who require fluid resuscitation
- Failure to anticipate and treat withdrawal syndromes in patients who are chronically taking muscle relaxants and sedative–hypnotics
- Failure to appreciate that chloral hydrate–induced ventricular dysrhythmias are exacerbated by endogenous and exogenous catecholamines and may respond to β-blocker therapy

ICD 9

967.9 Poisoning by unspecified sedative or hypnotic

REFERENCES

1. Bramness JG, Mørland J, Sørlid HK, Rudberg N, Jacobsen D. Carisoprodol intoxications and serotonergic features. *Clin Toxicol* 2005;43:39–45.
2. Catalano G, Catalano MC, Hanley PF. Seizures associated with buspirone overdose: case report and literature review. *Clin Neuropharmacol* 1998;21:347–350.
3. Cienki JJ, Burkhart KK. Zopiclone overdose responsive to flumazenil. *Clin Toxicol* 2005;43:385–386.
4. Davis RN, Rettmann JA, Christensen B. Relapsing altered mental status secondary to a meprobamate bezoar. *J Trauma* 2006;61:990–991.
5. Forrester MB. Comparison of zolpidem and zaleplon exposures in Texas,1998–2004. *J Toxicol Environ Health* 2006;69:1883–1892.
6. Forrester MB. Esopiclone ingestions reported to Texas poison control centers,2005–2006. *Hum Exp Toxicol* 2007;26:795–800.
7. Perry HE, Wright RO, Shannon MW, Woolf AD. Baclofen overdose: drug experimentation in a group of adolescents. *Pediatrics* 1998;101:1045–1048.
8. Simpson SE, Greenberg MI. Serotonin syndrome associated with ramelteon overdose. *Clin Toxicol* 2007;45:630–631.
9. Spiller HA, Winter ML, Mann KV, et al. Five-year multicenter retrospective review of cyclobenzaprine toxicity. *J Emerg Med* 1995;13:781–785.
10. Spiller HA, Bosse GM, Adamson LA. Retrospective review of tizanidine (Zanaflex) overdose. *J Toxicol Clin Toxicol* 2004;42:593–596.

CHAPTER 16

Phenytoin

- Differentiate phenytoin-induced altered mental status from other potentially serious causes (head trauma is common in the seizure population).
- Collect and transport pills and pill bottles to aid in identification and quantification of ingestion.

CLINICAL PRESENTATION

The predominant signs and symptoms of acute or chronic oral phenytoin overdose are related to central nervous system (CNS) dysfunction. Effects such as nystagmus, nausea, vomiting, tremor, ataxia, diplopia, and dysarthria often reflect cerebellar and vestibular impairment; toxicity usually correlates with increasing plasma concentrations. However, individual variations in drug response, baseline neurologic status, and protein binding all influence the threshold for toxicity. Although some patients may tolerate and therapeutically require phenytoin levels >20 μg/mL, patients with underlying brain disease may become toxic at only slightly elevated drug levels. Although nystagmus is common as concentrations rise >20 μg/mL, the absence of this finding does not rule out toxicity. Horizontal, vertical, bidirectional, or alternating nystagmus can be noted with significant poisoning but may disappear as CNS depression and depth of coma increase (3). At levels >30 μg/mL, ataxia, slurred speech, and tremor are common. As levels rise to >40 μg/mL, confusion, lethargy, and stupor may occur. Although progressive CNS depression is typical, fluctuating agitation and lethargy have also been described. With levels >50 μg/mL, marked CNS depression and coma predominate; profound CNS depression is associated with hyporeflexia and depression of cranial nerve reflexes. A number of infrequently encountered CNS findings have also been described, including choreo-athetosis, ballismus, opisthotonus, and dystonias (4). Focal neurological deficits may be precipitated in patients with prior hypoxic or ischemic brain injury. Although rarely described, "paradoxical" seizures have been noted with phenytoin levels >30 to 50 μg/mL, typically in the setting of a pre-existing seizure disorder. In the setting of acute overdose, seizures should prompt a search for co-ingestants or physiologic derangements. Additionally, although cerebellar atrophy has been reported following acute overdose, it remains unclear whether this results from phenytoin itself, the underlying chronic seizure disorder, or unknown other causes (2).

Cardiovascular toxicity is not a clinical concern following oral overdose, but it is the major toxicity seen with rapid administration of intravenous (IV) phenytoin. Hypotension, apnea, bradycardia, asystole, and ventricular dysrhythmias may complicate the use of phenytoin infusion at rates in excess of 50 mg/min (rates as low as 25 mg/min have been recommended for patients >50 years of age). Associated electrocardiographic (ECG) changes may include ST segment and T wave changes, as well as atrioventricular blocks. Although the propylene glycol diluent in phenytoin injection solution is believed to be the primary mediator of cardiovascular toxicity, there may be other mechanisms. Bradyasystolic arrest has occurred in infants following several-fold overdoses of IV fosphenytoin, which does not contain propylene glycol. The cardiotoxicity associated with IV phenytoin is usually transient and is expected to dissipate when the infusion is stopped.

Extravasation of phenytoin can cause skin and soft tissue necrosis, compartment syndrome, and gangrene, which may lead to limb loss. Death has also been reported caused by complications of inadvertent intra-arterial administration of phenytoin in an elderly patient. "Purple glove syndrome," which consists of progressive limb edema, bluish discoloration, pain, and blistering, may follow IV administration of phenytoin on a delayed basis, even in the absence of evidence of extravasation. This syndrome has not been reported with fosphenytoin use. Previously described risk factors for "purple glove syndrome" include advanced age, use of large repeated doses, small gauge IV catheter use, and use of the same infusion site for multiple doses (1).

An idiosyncratic anticonvulsant hypersensitivity syndrome may be noted in patients taking phenytoin, typically developing weeks to months after the initiation of therapy. This syndrome often produces multisystem involvement and may present with fever, rash, hepatitis, eosinophilia, blood dyscrasias, pneumonitis, myositis, vasculitis, and/or nephritis. Anticonvulsant hypersensitivity syndrome is thought to occur from the generation of toxic arene metabolites of aromatic anticonvulsants (carbamazepine, phenobarbital, and phenytoin) and is potentially life threatening. Additional adverse effects of phenytoin include Stevens-Johnson syndrome, toxic epidermal necrolysis, and drug-induced lupus (6).

Death is rare after acute oral overdoses of phenytoin. Most fatalities involve coingestants or respiratory failure and its associated complications, and many of the deaths reported in the medical literature predate modern intensive care and supportive care (5). Reported fatal cases are usually associated with phenytoin levels in excess of 120 μg/mL (2).

DIFFERENTIAL DIAGNOSIS

The differential diagnosis of phenytoin intoxication includes other processes that can produce the typical constellation of nystagmus, ataxia, dysarthria, and mental status changes. Other anticonvulsants can produce similar signs and symptoms and are often utilized by patients with epilepsy, so poisoning with these agents should be considered. Similarly, an overdose of sedative-hypnotic agents, ethanol, muscle relaxants, or psychiatric medications can produce a comparable clinical presentation. Intoxication with lithium, cyclic antidepressants, or the selective serotonin-reuptake inhibitors is another possibility. Although ECG changes are very rare following oral phenytoin overdose, ECG screening may provide additional information when the ingestion of psychotropic medications is being entertained. CNS pathology, particularly cerebellar infarction, hemorrhage, or neoplasm, should also be considered. Other diagnostic considerations include hypoglycemia, Wernicke encephalopathy, extrapyramidal disorders, seizure disorders, and postictal states.

ED EVALUATION

The time and quantity of ingestion should be the primary historical focus, but a history of seizure disorder and of other medication use should also be sought. The examination should focus on the neurological system. The clinician should note the presence or absence of altered mentation, nystagmus, slurred speech, and ataxia.

Serum glucose and an ECG should be obtained in patients with an altered mental status or in whom there may have been a coingestion of other substances. Routine laboratory studies can be obtained. If the patient has a known seizure disorder but is taking unknown medications, phenytoin, phenobarbital, carbamazepine, and valproic acid are commonly prescribed medications for which blood levels can be measured. If medications are known, levels of the specific agent should be ordered. When levels are positive and the patient is either unreliable or may have attempted suicide, two levels can establish a peak and declining trend. These levels should be clinically correlated with the patient's condition.

ED MANAGEMENT

Patients who develop hypotension or bradycardia during IV infusion should have the drip immediately discontinued. The drip rate and concentration should be checked. When vital signs are normalized, a slower infusion rate can then be continued with cardiac monitoring.

For oral overdose, the patient's airway, breathing, and circulation (ABCs) should be monitored and stabilized appropriately. Oral phenytoin overdose is rarely fatal with good supportive care, and cardiovascular toxicity is unlikely. An initial ECG should be obtained to establish normal intervals, and cardiac monitoring should be initiated if there are any abnormalities. If there is significant neurological impairment, the patient should be protected from falls and should have frequent neurological checks done.

A single dose of activated charcoal is a good method for gastric decontamination because oral absorption may be delayed. The use of multiple doses of charcoal, although of theoretical value, has not been proven to be consistently effective. If the patient has an underlying seizure disorder, care should be taken not to let the phenytoin level decrease to less than the therapeutic range. Phenytoin should be administered before this absence occurs.

Hemodialysis and charcoal hemoperfusion are not useful in phenytoin overdose.

CRITICAL INTERVENTIONS

- Obtain serial phenytoin levels to establish a peak and declining trend.
- When loading phenytoin IV, use continuous cardiac monitoring and avoid extravasation.
- Stop infusions if there is evidence of bradycardia or hypotension.

DISPOSITION

Patients with no or minimal toxicity after a suicidal ingestion and a therapeutic peak phenytoin concentration can be cleared for psychiatric evaluation. Patients with elevated peak phenytoin levels and moderate to severe symptoms require hospitalization prior to being cleared for psychiatric hospitalization. Patients admitted after oral phenytoin overdose can be admitted to nonmonitored settings but should go to a setting where fall precautions can be instituted and frequent neurological checks can be performed. The rare severely intoxicated patient will require an intensive care setting (2).

Nonsuicidal patients with mild symptoms and a reliable family support system can be discharged home with instructions to prevent falls. The family should also be counseled on holding doses for the next day or two as appropriate. More seriously intoxicated patients should be admitted to the hospital as above for supportive treatment.

COMMON PITFALLS

- Exceeding phenytoin IV infusion rates of 25 to 50 mg/min, causing hypotension and/or bradycardia
- Causing phenytoin toxicity by not checking a drug level prior to giving a loading dose
- Admitting all oral phenytoin overdoses to a telemetry setting. Cardiac toxicity is extremely rare, and this is generally not necessary.
- Failing to diagnose phenytoin toxicity and proceeding with evaluation for other acute neurological conditions
- Failing to recognize the anticonvulsant hypersensitivity syndrome
- Failing to recognize the purple glove syndrome

ICD 9

966.1 Poisoning by hydantoin derivatives

REFERENCES

1. Chokshi R, Openshaw J, Mehta NN, et al. Purple glove syndrome following intravenous phenytoin administration. *Vasc Med* 2007;12:29–31.
2. Curtis DL, Piibe R, Ellenhorn MJ, et al. Phenytoin toxicity: a review of 94 cases. *Vet Hum Toxicol* 1989;31:164–165.
3. LoVecchio F. Phenytoin. In: Brent J, Wallace KL, Burkhart KK, et al., eds. *Critical Care Toxicology,* 1st ed. Philadelphia, PA: Elsevier, Mosby, 2005:553–558.
4. McNamara JO. Pharmacotherapy of the epilepsies (Chapter 19). In: Brunton LL, Lazo JS, Parker KL, eds. *Goodman & Gillman's The Pharmacological Basis of Therapeutics,* 11th ed. http:www.accesspharmacy.com/content.aspx?aID=939716.
5. Mellick LB, Morgan JA, Mellick GA. Presentations of acute phenytoin overdose. *Am J Emerg Med* 1989;7(1):61–67.
6. Morkunas AR, Miller MB. Anticonvulsant hypersensitivity syndrome. *Crit Care Clin* 1997;13: 727–739.

CHAPTER 17

Valproic Acid

PRE-HOSPITAL CONSIDERATIONS
- Differentiate valproic acid-induced altered mental status from other potentially serious causes (head trauma is common in the seizure population).
- Collect and transport pills and pill bottles to aid in identification and quantification of ingestion.

CLINICAL PRESENTATION

Central nervous system depression (CNS) is the predominant finding in valproic acid toxicity. With severe intoxication, coma is common, and seizures may rarely occurs. Cerebral edema has been reported in both acute and chronic intoxications (6). Hemodynamic instability and shock are seen with massive overdose. Nausea and vomiting may occur; more significant gastrointestinal findings are pancreatitis and hepatotoxicity. Pancreatitis is seen in both acute ingestion and chronic therapy, whereas hepatotoxicity is rare in acute ingestions. Metabolic effects are seen with more severe toxicity and may include hypernatremia, anion gap metabolic acidosis, and lactic acidosis.

Serum levels >100 μg/mL are considered toxic. Although higher levels do not correlate exactly with clinical findings, some generalizations can be made. Levels <450 μg/mL are associated with less serious toxicity, and those >850 μg/mL with critical illness (5). This leaves a wide range with variable prognosis, though it is clear that patients with levels between 450 μg/mL and 850 μg/mL may also be critically ill. Interpretation of these values is complicated by delayed peaks in serum levels, which mandates serial testing regardless of the presence or absence of symptoms.

ED EVALUATION

Because valproic acid overdose primarily manifests as CNS depression, the airway must be carefully assessed. After completion of the primary survey and appropriate interventions, a detailed history should include whether the ingestion was accidental or intentional, the potential for co-ingestants, other medications the patient has had access to, time of ingestion, and apparent acute versus chronic ingestion. Physical examination should focus on mental status. When there is an altered mental status, a direct history may be difficult to obtain, so paramedics, friends, family, and old medical records are often most helpful for this purpose.

In patients with significant toxicity, the laboratory evaluation should include a complete blood count, chemistry panel with anion gap calculation, liver function tests, lactate, valproic acid, and ammonia levels. An acetaminophen level should be measured in intentional ingestions. Electrocardiograms are useful for patients with abnormal vital signs and those with potential for a cardiotoxic co-ingestant.

DIFFERENTIAL DIAGNOSIS

The list of agents that can cause altered mental status is extensive. Valproic acid intoxication can mimic most other CNS depressant drugs. Postictal states, metabolic derangements, CNS lesions, trauma, hypoglycemia and hypoxia may present similarly. The key to arriving at the correct diagnosis is a good history, exclusion of alternate etiologies, and a serum valproic acid level.

ED MANAGEMENT

Aggressive supportive care and strict attention to airway and breathing is critical, with intubation and ventilation for any evidence of airway compromise or respiratory depression. Prior to definitive airway management, naloxone and either bedside glucose testing or empiric dextrose administration is appropriate in the undifferentiated comatose patient. Naloxone has been reported to improve valproic acid-induced CNS depression, but a beneficial effect is not routinely expected (6).

Early decontamination may prevent absorption and subsequent toxicity. However, an intact airway and mental status are required for this. Activated charcoal is the preferred mode of decontamination as it readily adsorbs valproic acid. A dose of 1 g/kg may provide a reasonable initial dose; however, repeat dosing may be indicated if continued absorption is occurring. Gastric lavage may be considered in patients presenting within 1 hour of a life-threatening overdose, although this intervention has not definitively been shown to improve outcome and may cause harm.

Enhanced elimination may result in lowering of drug levels, especially in cases where the valproic acid concentration is excessive (>850 μg/mL) and saturation of protein binding has resulted in free drug available for elimination. However, it has never been proven to have greater benefit than aggressive supportive care alone. High-flux hemodialysis is as effective as charcoal hemoperfusion and is the preferred modality if dialysis is indicated (1). Hemodialysis may be considered when there is renal insufficiency, persistent hemodynamic instability, or significant metabolic acidosis unresponsive to volume repletion. Multiple-dose activated charcoal can also enhance elimination of valproic acid when levels are excessive, protein binding is saturated, and enough free drug is available (2). L-carnitine may hasten resolution of coma in patients with valproic acid intoxication associated with hyperammonemia (4). It is prescribed for pediatric patients chronically taking valproic acid to avoid hepatotoxicity. Carnitine depletion that occurs after acute massive overdose leads to urea accumulation and hyperammonemia, which contributes to altered mental status. L-carnitine supplementation after overdose is intended to correct this imbalance. It has a benign side effect profile and is a reasonable intervention despite the lack of clear evidence of its efficacy. Dosing recommendations vary, but 100 mg/kg intravenously (up to 6 g) over 30 minutes, followed by 15 mg/kg every 4 hours, is appropriate. The end point is clinical improvement or 3 days of therapy.

CRITICAL INTERVENTIONS

- Use aggressive airway management for severely poisoned patients.
- For patients with elevated levels or symptoms, order electrolyte panel, liver function panel, ammonia level, and pancreatic enzymes.
- Monitor the anion gap and lactate in critically ill patients.
- Obtain serial valproic acid levels in all patients with acute overdose.
- Consider administration of L-carnitine.

DISPOSITION

All patients with evidence of mental status decline or respiratory insufficiency warrant an intensive care unit admission with continuous cardiac monitoring and airway assessment. In suicidal patients, clearance for psychiatric admission cannot occur until a downward trend in valproic acid concentration is confirmed. Both therapeutic and subtherapeutic concentrations have been reported to steadily rise, with concurrent signs of significant poisoning after acute overdose (3). Patients should not be discharged until serum levels are falling based on serial levels, are in the therapuetic range, and the patient is asymptomatic.

COMMON PITFALLS

- Failure to detect a delayed rise of valproic acid levels. Serial levels are required.
- Failure to consider delayed onset of toxicity
- Premature medical clearance
- Failure to work up patients completely for alternate etiologies of abnormal mental status

ICD 9

966.3 Poisoning by other and unspecifed anticonvulsants

REFERENCES

1. Al Aly Z, Yalamanchili P, et al. Extracorporeal management of valproic acid toxicity: a case report and review of the literature. *Semin Dial* 2005;18(1):62–66.
2. Farrar HC, Herold DA, et al. Acute valproic acid intoxication: enhanced drug clearance with oral-activated charcoal. *Crit Care Med* 1993;21(2):299–301.

3. Ingels M, Beauchamp J, et al. Delayed valproic acid toxicity: a retrospective case series. *Ann Emerg Med* 2002;39(6):616–621.

4. Lheureux PE, Penaloza A, et al. Science review: carnitine in the treatment of valproic acid-induced toxicity—what is the evidence? *Crit Care* 2005;9(5):431–440.

5. Spiller HA, Krenzelok EP, et al. Multicenter case series of valproic acid ingestion: serum concentrations and toxicity. *J Toxicol Clin Toxicol* 2000;38(7):755–760.

6. Sztajnkrycer MD. Valproic acid toxicity: overview and management. *J Toxicol Clin Toxicol* 2002;40(6):789–801.

CHAPTER 18

Carbamazepine

PRE-HOSPITAL CONSIDERATIONS

- Do *not* administer ipecac.
- Intubate if significant respiratory depression or airway compromise is evident.
- Secure intravenous access.
- Obtain complete information about all products potentially ingested.

CLINICAL PRESENTATION

The clinical manifestations of carbamazepine (CBZ) toxicity involve four main areas: central nervous system (CNS), ocular, cardiac, and motor (7). Although a sequential progression is classically described, individual patients may present at any stage and may, at times, progress rapidly to profound coma and cardiac instability (6). Initial CNS symptoms include restlessness, confusion, excitation, and aggression. Dizziness, ataxia, nystagmus, diplopia, nausea, and vomiting are often present. As toxicity progresses, drowsiness, coma, and respiratory depression may occur, often after some hours (3,8). Hypotension, global hypokinesia, and cardiac rhythm disturbances may be seen in severe poisoning (2,5,6). Loss of P waves, premature ventricular beats, QRS prolongation, and complete atrioventricular block have been described (5), as have bradycardia, Adams-Stokes syncope, and ventricular standstill (2). Prolongation of the age-adjusted QRS interval is common in children (5). Severely poisoned patients may have fixed and dilated pupils and disconjugate gaze (2).

Abnormal motor findings include tremor, choreoathetoid movements, and hemiballismus. Reflexes may initially be hyperactive with clonus. Seizures can occur, usually in patients with an underlying seizure disorder (9). The electroencephalogram may show occipital δ activity (usually suggestive of a brainstem disorder) (5). In the deeply comatose patient, adynamic ileus, hypothermia, and pulmonary edema may be present (3). Complications include aspiration, resistant status epilepticus, and the sequelae of hypoxia and seizures (2,8). Hyponatremia may result from an antidiuretic effect in either acute or chronic overdoses (7). Acute intoxication may result in hypokalemia.

Confusion, lethargy, and ataxia are usually associated with peak plasma CBZ concentrations of about 20 μg/mL. Coma, hypotension, dysrhythmias, seizures, and death typically occur in patients with peak plasma concentrations above

40 μg/mL (4,5,8,9). It is important to note that these concentrations represent peak concentrations, which may occur hours or days after ingestion. Initial drug levels correlate only weakly with clinical course and are imperfect prognosticators of outcome (3,7,10). Because of the long half-life after overdose and continued absorption over many hours, the clinical course is typically prolonged (2,3,5). Severely poisoned patients may require more than a week to make a full recovery. Cyclic coma has been described, in which partial recovery is followed by a relapse into a coma, presumably as gastrointestinal absorption resumes after ileus resolves (4,9).

DIFFERENTIAL DIAGNOSIS

Mild poisoning may resemble hypoglycemia, neurologic disease, serotonin syndrome, or intoxication by ethanol. In severe poisoning, the clinical picture may mimic overdose with cyclic antidepressants, anticholinergic agents, or other anticonvulsants. Other physiologic depressants, coexistent trauma, and co-ingestions should also be considered. A prolonged postictal state in a patient with a history of seizures should raise suspicion for poisoning with CBZ or another anticonvulsant.

ED EVALUATION

A directed history should be obtained from the patient, prehospital care providers, or available friends and family members. Recent dosing changes or newly prescribed medications that may inhibit CBZ metabolism should be identified. The physical examination should include a full set of vital signs; pupil position, size, and reactivity; bowel sounds; and a focused neurologic examination, including level and content of consciousness, responsiveness to stimuli, reflexes, motor tone, and cerebellar function. A 12-lead electrocardiogram (ECG), cardiac monitoring, and serum electrolyte and glucose determinations are indicated in symptomatic patients. Comprehensive toxicology testing and computed tomography scanning of the head may be necessary in cases of diagnostic uncertainty.

Frequent measurements of serum CBZ concentrations are mandatory to detect continued absorption in patients with acute overdose. Serial levels should be obtained until the patient is asymptomatic and levels have clearly peaked and fallen into the therapeutic range of 4 to 12 μg/mL. Rebounds in CBZ levels coinciding with clinical deterioration are well described. Serum CBZ and CBZ-10,11 epoxide (CBZ-E) concentrations can be separately determined by high-performance liquid chromatography. Immunologic assays used in most centers cannot distinguish between CBZ-E and the parent compound, but quantification of CBZ-E is not necessary for clinical care of the patient (3,10).

ED MANAGEMENT

As always, stabilization of the airway has the highest priority. Most deaths from CBZ overdose are secondary to complications such as pulmonary aspiration and respiratory depression. Level of consciousness and vital signs should be monitored. Hypotension should be managed with intravenous fluids and, if necessary, invasive monitoring and pressors such as norepinephrine. Central venous pressure monitoring is recommended in such patients to avoid fluid overload, which can result from CBZ's antidiuretic effect. Wide-complex cardiac dysrhythmias should be treated with hypertonic sodium bicarbonate as described for cyclic antidepressants (see Chapter 44, "Cyclic Antidepressants"). Aggressive resuscitation efforts, including prolonged chest compressions and extracorporeal circulatory support, have been used successfully for severe cardiogenic shock (2,5).

Activated charcoal (AC) is recommended for all symptomatic patients regardless of time to presentation, and for those with significant recent ingestions by history. Multiple-dose activated charcoal (MDAC) therapy enhances the elimination of both CBZ and CBZ-E and should be instituted for patients with significant symptoms or CBZ levels above 20 μg/mL (1). This treatment should be continued until levels have fallen into the therapeutic range or lower for patients not dependent on the anticonvulsant properties of CBZ. Ileus after massive overdose may preclude or complicate MDAC (2,3).

Forced diuresis, peritoneal dialysis, and continuous renal replacement therapies are of limited value in CBZ poisoning (2). CBZ and CBZ-E are both filtered efficiently by either conventional or high-flux hemodialysis, but only a relatively small proportion of the body burden is removed. Although charcoal hemoperfusion also clears CBZ from the blood (2,3), this modality has been abandoned in most centers. Extracorporeal removal should only be considered for patients with significant dysrhythmias, hypotension, or prolonged coma and extremely elevated CBZ levels despite MDAC.

CRITICAL INTERVENTIONS

- Obtain serial serum CBZ concentrations until values clearly peak and then fall into the therapeutic range.
- Check for other drugs that affect CBZ metabolism.
- Administer MDAC in patients with significant symptoms or CBZ concentrations above 20 μg/mL.

DISPOSITION

Patients who are symptomatic or who have a CBZ level >15 μg/mL should be admitted. Those with moderate or severe clinical toxicity, rising drug levels, or an abnormal ECG should be treated in an intensive care unit. Patients with intentional overdose should be evaluated for suicide risk.

COMMON PITFALLS

- Failure to appreciate that CBZ absorption is slow and erratic and that peak levels may not be seen for many hours or days after acute overdose

- Failure to appreciate that although CBZ is an anticonvulsant, overdosage can cause or exacerbate seizures
- Failure to appreciate that CBZ is structurally similar to cyclic antidepressants and can cause similar CNS and cardiovascular toxicity
- Failure to appreciate that AC and MDAC may be useful, even many hours after ingestion
- Failure to appreciate that CBZ has active metabolites and that toxicity may take days to resolve

ICD 9

966.3 Poisoning by other and unspecified anticonvulsants

REFERENCES

1. Brahmi N, Kouraichi N, Thabet H, Amamou M. Influence of activated charcoal on the pharmacokinetics and the clinical features of carbamazepine poisoning. *Am J Emerg Med* 2006;24(4):440–443.
2. Cameron RJ, Hungerford P, Dawson AH. Efficacy of charcoal hemoperfusion in massive carbamazepine poisoning. *J Toxicol Clin Toxicol* 2002;40(4):507–512.
3. Graudins A, Peden G, Dowsett RP. Massive overdose with controlled-release carbamazepine resulting in delayed peak serum concentrations and life-threatening toxicity. *Emerg Med* 2002;14(1): 89–94.
4. Hojer J, Malmlund HO, Berg A. Clinical features in 28 consecutive cases of laboratory confirmed massive poisoning with carbamazepine alone. *J Toxicol Clin Toxicol* 1993;31(3):449–458.
5. Megarbane B, Leprince P, Deye N, et al. Extracorporeal life support in a case of acute carbamazepine poisoning with life-threatening refractory myocardial failure. *Intensive Care Med* 2006;32(9): 1409–1413.
6. Mordel A, Sivilotti MLA, Linden CH. Fatal TCA-like cardiotoxicity following carbamazepine overdose. *J Toxicol Clin Toxicol* 1998;36:472.
7. Schmidt S, Schmitz-Buhl M. Signs and symptoms of carbamazepine overdose. *J Neurol* 1995; 242(3):169–173.
8. Spiller HA, Carlisle RD. Status epilepticus after massive carbamazepine overdose. *J Toxicol Clin Toxicol* 2002;40(1):81–90.
9. Spiller HA, Krenzelok EP, Cookson E. Carbamazepine overdose: a prospective study of serum levels and toxicity. *J Toxicol Clin Toxicol* 1990;28(4):445–458.
10. Winnicka RI, Topaciski B, Szymczak WM, et al. Carbamazepine poisoning: elimination kinetics and quantitative relationship with carbamazepine 10,11-epoxide. *J Toxicol Clin Toxicol* 2002;40(6): 759–765.

CHAPTER 19

Other Anticonvulsants

PRE-HOSPITAL CONSIDERATIONS

- Differentiate anticonvulsant-induced altered mental status from other potentially serious causes (head trauma is common in the seizure population).
- Collect and transport pills and pill bottles to aid in identification and quantification of ingestion.

CLINICAL PRESENTATION

Although the chemistry and pharmacology of each of the new anticonvulsants is unique, central nervous system (CNS) effects usually predominate in overdose. Common symptoms include dizziness, nystagmus, diplopia, somnolence, and lethargy. However, complications that are not limited to predictable effects on the CNS system can also occur.

Felbamate   Common effects of felbamate in overdose include somnolence, ataxia, vomiting, abdominal pain, and tachycardia. Documented fatalities from aplastic anemia and hepatic failure have occurred with therapeutic use. In one case, death from massive hepatic necrosis occurred within 40 days of the initiation of therapy (5). At least 10 deaths related to aplastic anemia have been reported to the manufacturer.

Gabapentin   Isolated gabapentin overdose in otherwise healthy patients generally causes only mild toxicity. In a case series of 20 exposures to gabapentin ranging from 50 mg to 35,000 mg, drowsiness, dizziness, nausea and vomiting, tachycardia, and hypotension were the most common effects reported in symptomatic patients. Clinical effects were noted to occur within 5 hours, and they resolved within 10 hours in most patients (5). In patients with renal impairment, however, the half-life of gabapentin may be greatly prolonged. There are several reports of toxicity including respiratory failure and coma in hemodialysis patients receiving therapeutic doses (5).

Lamotrigine   The most common symptoms of lamotrigine overdose include nystagmus, somnolence, ataxia, and lethargy. However, stupor, transient coma, and seizures; electrolyte imbalances (hypokalemia); and intraventricular conduction abnormalities (QRS widening and PR prolongation) have also occurred (5).

Up to 10% of patients develop a severe rash including Stevens-Johnson syndrome and toxic epidermal necrolysis, which are occasionally fatal (2,4,6). Multiorgan involvement and disseminated intravascular coagulation have also been reported with the addition of lamotrigine to existing anticonvulsant therapies (5).

Levetiracetam Levetiracetam overdose data are limited. A 38-year-old woman became obtunded with respiratory depression requiring intubation after ingesting 30 g. She was extubated the following day and eventually recovered without sequelae (5). Two children who accidentally received high doses of levetiracetam had only mild itching and decreased muscle tone (1). The manufacturer reports that somnolence, agitation, aggression, depressed level of consciousness, respiratory depression, and coma have been observed after overdose.

Oxcarbazepine Aside from somnolence and lethargy, the more serious effects in oxcarbazepine overdose include bradycardia and hypotension. Hyponatremia (reported at a greater frequency than with carbamazepine) may result in seizures (5). Dose-related oculogyric crises have also been reported (5).

Pregabalin During clinical development, the highest reported pregabalin overdose (8 g) resulted in no permanent complications (5). During initial clinical trials, a decreased platelet count, mild PR prolongation, elevation in liver transaminases, and creatinine kinase were reported (5).

Tiagabine There are multiple reports of coma and status epilepticus with tiagabine overdose. Both convulsive and nonconvulsive status epilepticus occur in 5% of ingestions (5).

Topiramate Seizures, coma, and metabolic acidosis are the more serious effects in topiramate overdose but recovery is typical (5).

Vigabatrin Drowsiness and fatigue are common adverse effects during therapeutic use of vigabatrin. Visual disturbances, including visual-field constriction, alterations in color perception, and retinal disorders, have been reported to occur with chronic therapy. Psychotic behavior including delusions, auditory and visual hallucinations, extreme aggression, and paranoia have been reported with therapeutic use in epileptic patients (5). Symptoms resolved with discontinuation of the drug.

Zonisamide Bradycardia, hypotension, respiratory depression, and coma have been reported in zonisamide overdose. There are several reports of psychotic reactions after initiating zonisamide that resolve after discontinuation of the drug. Hyperthermia and oligohidrosis have been reported in the pediatric population (4). Zonisamide's labeling includes a warning for potentially fatal reactions to sulfonamides.

It should be noted that overdoses with the anticonvulsants are complicated by the fact that patients are often taking multiple medications or have co-ingested other substances such as ethanol. The potential for complications increases with the use of more than one agent, including the risks of dose-dependent adverse effects, idiosyncratic reactions, drug-drug interactions, and long-term effects. Metabolic disturbances from cytochrome P450 and from competition by drugs for similar neuroreceptors may contribute to the clinical presentation (3).

DIFFERENTIAL DIAGNOSIS

Numerous agents can cause CNS depression similar to that caused by the newer anticonvulsants. These include the traditional anticonvulsants (carbamazepine, phenobarbital, phenytoin, and valproic acid), tricyclic antidepressants, antihistamines, alcohols, benzodiazepines, β-blockers, barbiturates, muscle relaxants, neuroleptics, opioids, and sedative–hypnotics. Medical causes such as electrolyte abnormalities, infection, or trauma should be considered and differentiated from drug-induced CNS depression.

ED EVALUATION

As quantitative levels of these agents are not readily available to guide emergency department (ED) management, every effort should be made to obtain historical information about the time of ingestion and type and amount of drug(s) taken, any treatment in the field, the onset and nature of symptoms, existing medical or psychiatric problems, and current drug therapy, particularly if the patient is on multiple medications for epilepsy. A rapid glucose concentration and vital signs, including temperature and pulse oximetry, should be obtained. The physical examination should focus on the vital signs, cardiopulmonary status, and neurologic assessment. An electrocardiogram should be obtained, and the patient should be placed on a cardiac monitor. Cardiac conduction intervals should be evaluated in all patients, especially with lamotrigine or zonisamide overdoses. Arterial blood gases, chemistry panel, ammonia, complete blood count, toxicology testing, chest radiograph, computed tomography, and lumbar puncture should be ordered as clinically indicated to search for other causes. Recognition of a toxidrome may be helpful, and co-ingestants should always be considered.

ED MANAGEMENT

Symptom-based supportive therapy is the most important ED management consideration in cases of overdose with the second-generation antiepileptic drugs. Attention to airway, breathing, and circulation should be a primary concern. Respiratory depression and/or coma may require endotracheal intubation for airway protection. Hypotension is usually responsive to intravenous crystalloids but may require pressors, particularly if co-ingestants are contributory. Intravenous sodium bicarbonate boluses should be given for QRS interval prolongation. Seizure precautions should be implemented for symptomatic patients, especially those with altered mental status. Benzodiazepines should be the first-line treatment for seizures, followed by phenobarbital for cases refractory to benzodiazepines.

Decontamination with oral activated charcoal may be considered for the awake patient with a protected airway, if there is a potentially toxic ingestion. Invasive decontamination procedures such as gastric lavage are likely to be of more risk than benefit and should be reserved for life-threatening ingestions when no contraindication exists. There is no role for multiple-dose activated charcoal.

Hemodialysis may enhance the elimination of gabapentin, levetiracetam, and possibly oxcarbazepine and topiramate. Hemodialysis should also be considered for patients with severe acid-base and electrolyte disturbances.

CRITICAL INTERVENTIONS

- Provide airway protection and respiratory support as clinically indicated.
- Administer intravenous fluids for hypotension.
- Administer boluses of intravenous sodium bicarbonate for prolonged QRS interval.
- Administer benzodiazepines as first-line agents for seizures.

DISPOSITION

A poison control center or toxicologist should be consulted for guidance with the management of overdose from the newer antiepileptics. Patients who remain completely asymptomatic after an observation period of 8 hours may be cleared, unless a co-ingestant (e.g., acetaminophen) requires further management. With felbamate, serial evaluation for crystalluria and changes in renal function may require a longer period of observation. Patients with CNS or respiratory depression, hemodynamic instability, or cardiac conduction disturbances should be admitted to an intensive care unit. A psychiatric evaluation should be obtained for all suspected suicidal ingestions. Substance abuse counseling is recommended for cases wherein a substance has been misused or abused (e.g., for recreational purposes). Patients and their families should be educated in cases where an unintentional exposure occurred to prevent another accidental exposure.

COMMON PITFALLS

- Failure to consider that, although rare, significant CNS depression can occur after overdose with newer antiepileptics
- Failure to weigh the risks and benefits involved in using invasive decontamination measures for overdoses

- Failure to consider that topiramate and zonisamide can paradoxically cause seizures
- Failure to consider that cardiac conduction disturbances can occur, especially after lamotrigine and zonisamide overdose
- Failure to note black box warnings for felbamate (aplastic anemia, hepatic failure)
- Failure to consider potentially severe rashes, especially with zonisamide, lamotrigine, and oxcarbazepine
- Failure to consider the risks of medical comorbidities, drug interactions, and adverse effects

ICD 9

966.3 Poisoning by other and unspecified anticonvulsants

REFERENCES

1. Awaad Y. Accidental overdosage of levetiracetam in two children caused no side effects. *Epilepsy Behav* 2007;11(2):247.
2. Czapinski P, Blaszczyk B, Czuczwar SJ. Mechanisms of action of antiepileptic drugs. *Curr Topics Med Chem* 2005;5(1):3–14.
3. Johnson WW. Cytochrome P450 inactivation by pharmaceuticals and phytochemicals: therapeutic relevance. *Drug Metab Rev* 2008;40(1):101–147.
4. LaRoche SM, Helmers SL. The new antiepileptic drugs scientific review. *JAMA* 2004;291(5): 605–614.
5. Thomson Micromedex HealthCare Series. Available at: www.micromedex.com. Last accessed March 12, 2008.
6. Yoon Y, Jagoda A. New antiepileptic drugs and preparations. *Emerg Med Clin North Am* 2000; 18(4);755–765.

Anti-Infective Agents and Biocides

CHAPTER 20

Antimalarial Drugs

CLINICAL PRESENTATION

Cinchonism is characterized by tinnitus, hearing loss, nausea, vomiting, vertigo, ataxia, diaphoresis, headache, flushing, lethargy, and hypotension (1,4). It is the most common early feature of quinine overdose, usually occurring within 4 hours of ingestion but as early as 2 hours and as late as 8 to 12 hours. Cinchonism can be seen with acute or chronic poisoning and is noted in about 75% of patients.

Cardiac toxicity after quinine overdose is typically mild, with sinus tachycardia and minor electrocardiographic (ECG) changes. However, ventricular arrhythmias, including torsades de pointes, significant conduction disturbances, and complete atrioventricular dissociation have been reported (1). Specific ECG abnormalities include prolonged P-R and Q-T intervals, ST- and T-wave changes, U waves, bundle-branch blocks, and QRS interval widening. With massive exposures, convulsions, coma, respiratory depression, adult respiratory distress syndrome, and cardiac arrest may occur.

Visual disturbances can be delayed for 6 to 24 hours after ingestion and may present with progressive blurring of vision or sudden blindness. Dilated pupils that become fixed before vision loss occurs have been reported. Peripheral visual-field defects, color misperceptions, diplopia, and poor dark adaptation can precede the development of total blindness or can be transient (1). The fundus is usually normal at the onset of visual defects, but retinal arteriole constriction, macular edema, and a cherry-red macular spot can develop within hours, evolving into optic atrophy (1). Laboratory findings may include hypoglycemia, hypokalemia, and thrombocytopenia (4). The hypoglycemia may occur as a result of quinine-induced insulin secretion (1). Quinine seldom induces abortion but is associated with fetal abnormalities and maternal deaths.

Chloroquine toxicity differs in presentation with a rapid onset of symptoms, severe cardiovascular (CV) effects, greater respiratory depression, marked hypokalemia, and milder and transient ocular and auditory toxicity (4). CV collapse is common within 2 hours in serious overdoses and is a result of marked myocardial depression and ventricular dysrhythmias (4). Toxicity can be predicted by a prolonged QRS interval and hypokalemia, probably from intracellular shifts (4). Toxic effects are usually short-lived, despite persistently high plasma levels of the drug.

Other quinoline derivatives, such as primaquine, do not have severe CV toxicities but are associated with gastrointestinal (GI) distress, hemolytic anemia, and methemoglobinemia (4).

Mefloquine overdoses have neuropsychiatric manifestations including headache, dizziness, vertigo, seizures, affective disorder, anxiety, and hearing loss, and sleep disturbances have occurred along with prolongation of the QTc interval (5). Nausea, vomiting, diarrhea, abdominal pain, and transient elevations in transaminase levels may be a posthepatic syndrome caused by drug-induced liver damage coupled in some with thyroid inhibition. Because of the prolonged $t_{1/2}$, these adverse events can persist for weeks. Mefloquine (Lariam) dispensed in error to patients who had been prescribed terbinafine (Lamisil) for onychomycosis has been reported to cause prolonged symptoms (5).

Of the dihydrofolate reductase inhibitors, pyrimethamine is the most toxic and may cause ataxia, seizures, coma, blindness, and deafness and folate deficiency with megaloblastic anemia (4). Proguanil, another dihydrofolate reductase inhibitor, is one of the safest antimalarial drugs (4). GI distress with vomiting, diarrhea, and abdominal pain coupled with headaches, nausea, and hematuria has been reported with ingestions of 1 g or more. Therapeutic doses of proguanil have been associated with mouth ulcerations, GI distress, rash, and anemia.

Dapsone, another dihydrofolate reductase inhibitor, may cause acute methemoglobinemia and hemolytic anemia (4). A series of five human immunodeficiency virus patients developed methemoglobinemia while on primaquine and dapsone.

Massive doxycycline overdoses have resulted in precipitation of calcium and hypocalcemic death in animals. In humans, precipitation of calcium can lead to staining of teeth in children younger than 8 years. Doxycycline has been associated with Sweet's syndrome, which is characterized by nonpruritic, painful, reddish nodules on the head, neck, chest, or upper limbs usually with fever, general malaise, and leukocytosis. Phototoxicity and esophageal ulcerations have also been reported with doxycycline.

Atovaquone, a novel hydroxynaphthoquinone, has produced minimal effects with overdoses up to 31.5 g. In one case, methemoglobinemia was reported, but an unknown amount of dapsone was also ingested (3).

DIFFERENTIAL DIAGNOSIS

Quinoline derivative toxicity may resemble other agents that cause visual, auditory, or cardiac effects. Methanol, ergot derivatives, and heavy metals (e.g., lead and mercury) are in the differential diagnosis of visual disturbances from an unknown agent. Unlike the quinolones, methanol is usually associated with a marked anion gap acidosis and osmolal gap. Manifestations of cinchonism are similar to those of salicylate toxicity, but the latter also causes an elevated anion gap, acid-base imbalances, and no visual effects. Quinidine, an isomer of quinine, causes similar cardiac effects but no visual deficits (4). Many drugs such as the cyclic antidepressants can cause similar CV and ECG effects but are not linked to auditory or visual changes. In patients with unexplained thrombocytopenia, drug-induced (e.g. quinine, quinidine) immune mediated causes should always be considered.

ED EVALUATION

In the overdose or toxic patient who presents with visual, auditory, neuropsychiatric, and CV symptoms of unknown cause, a history of use or availability of antimalarial agents will be significant. Attempted abortion by quinine should be suspected in a pregnant patient with these complaints. Physical examination and evaluation of the vital signs, cardiac rhythm, auditory and visual acuity, pupillary size and reactions, funduscopic findings, visual-field testing, and cerebellar status are important. Studies to assist in the differential include determination of blood levels of quinine, quinidine, salicylate, electrolyte, glucose, liver enzymes, blood urea nitrogen, and creatinine along with a complete blood count. An ECG should also be obtained. If available, electroretinograms and visual evoked response testing may detect signs of retinal damage in quinine overdose.

ED MANAGEMENT

A suspected ingestion of antimalarials requires immediate attention to the vital signs, cardiac monitoring, and activated charcoal (AC). Prevention of absorption is most effective in the first hour and, if done early, may reduce peak plasma levels (6). The $t_{1/2}$ in healthy volunteers taking a therapeutic dose of quinine was reduced by 50% and, in overdoses, was shortened from more than 24 hours to 8 hours by repeated doses of AC. However, clinical outcome improvement has not been documented. AC may be problematic because of the rapid onset of central nervous system (CNS) depression, particularly with chloroquine overdose.

Hypotension usually responds to intravenous (IV) fluids but may require a vasopressor (e.g., dopamine or norepinephrine) and inotropes (e.g., dobutamine) (1,4). Hypotension, ventricular dysrhythmias, and cardiac conduction abnormalities often respond to serum alkalization to a pH of 7.5 (4). This may be accomplished by sodium bicarbonate administration, hyperventilation, or a combination. Lidocaine has been used but may potentiate the dysrhythmias. Class 1A and 1C antidysrhythmics should be avoided. Torsades de pointes is treated with IV magnesium and isoproterenol or overdrive pacing.

Benzodiazepines, combined with mechanical ventilation and inotropes, have improved chloroquine-overdosed patients (4). High doses of diazepam (0.5–3 mg/kg IV) may counteract the hemodynamic and ECG changes associated with chloroquine toxicity. Other sedating and anticonvulsant agents, such as barbiturates, have been suggested but may risk exacerbation of the hypotension seen in severe chloroquine toxicity (2). Because the cardiac toxicity seen is similar to hyperkalemia, aggressive potassium replacement is not advised unless it is severe (4).

Despite its theoretical potential for enhanced quinoline derivative elimination, acidification of the urine is unproven and may increase toxicity. Resin and charcoal hemoperfusion, hemodialysis, peritoneal dialysis, plasmapheresis, and exchange transfusion are ineffective because of protein binding and high volumes of distribution (1,4). Methylene blue should be given for methemoglobinemia (see Chapter 40, "Methemoglobinemia").

Attempts at reversal of retinal arteriolar vasospasm by stellate ganglion block, anterior chamber paracentesis, retrobulbar injections, and systemic vasodilators have not been effective and can produce significant complications (4). Hyperbaric oxygenation therapy has been promoted on the premise that retinal hypoxia secondary to arteriolar vasoconstriction contributes to visual loss. However, the reported benefit may represent natural recovery.

Recovery from quinoline overdose is usually gradual and complete, but visual defects from quinine may not completely resolve (4).

CRITICAL INTERVENTIONS

- Establish IV access, institute cardiac monitoring, and obtain an ECG.
- Protect the airway and assist ventilation in patients with seizures or significant CNS depression.
- Administer IV benzodiazepines and sodium bicarbonate to patients with severe chloroquine toxicity.
- Administer IV dopamine or norepinephrine to patients with hypotension unresponsive to IV fluids.

DISPOSITION

Patients suspected of ingesting a toxic amount of a quinoline derivative should be observed for 6 to 8 hours. Symptomatic patients and any with cardiac conduction abnormalities should be admitted to an intensive care unit. An ophthalmologist should be consulted in patients with visual symptoms.

COMMON PITFALLS

- Failure to obtain a history of antimalarial poisoning in patients with auditory, visual, cardiac, and neuropsychiatric abnormalities of unknown cause
- Failure to appreciate that rapid neurologic and CV deterioration can occur after chloroquine overdose
- Failure to appreciate that benzodiazepines can prevent dysrhythmias and seizures in patients with chloroquine overdose
- Failure to consider multiple-dose AC therapy
- Failure to appreciate that potassium replacement can exacerbate chloroquine-induced cardiac toxicity

ICD 9

961.4 Poisoning by antimalarials and drugs acting on other blood protozoa

REFERENCES

1. Bateman DN, Dyson EH. Quinine toxicity. *Adverse Drug React Toxicol Rev* 1986;5:215–233.
2. Clemessy JL, Taboulet P, Hoffman JR, et al. Treatment of acute chloroquine poisoning: a 5-year experience. *Crit Care Med* 1996;24:1189–1195.
3. Haile LG, Flaherty JF. Atovaquone: a review. *Ann Pharmacother* 1993;27:1488–1494.
4. Jaeger A, Sauder P, Kopferschmitt J, et al. Clinical features and management of poisoning due to antimalarial drugs. *Med Toxicol Adverse Drug Exp* 1987;2:242–273.
5. Lobel HO, Coyne PE, Rosenthal PJ. Drug overdoses with antimalarial agents: prescribing and dispensing errors. *JAMA* 1998;280:1483.
6. Neuvonen PJ, Kivisto KT, Laine L, et al. Prevention of chloroquine absorption by activated charcoal. *Hum Exp Toxicol* 1992;11:117–120.

CHAPTER 21

Herbicides

CLINICAL PRESENTATION

The toxicity of paraquat (1,1'-dimethyl-4,4'-bipyridilium) and diquat (1,1'-ethylene-2,2'-dipyridilium) depends on the dose and primarily the concentration involved (5,8,10). Exposure to dilute solutions (e.g., commercial concentrates that have been diluted for use) usually cause only local toxicity such as dermatitis, conjunctivitis, cough, sore throat, and burning in the mouth and throat. Concentrated solutions can cause dermal and corneal burns. Stomatitis, epistaxis, and bronchial irritation have been reported after inhalation. Ingestion causes oropharyngeal pain, dysphagia, substernal chest pain, abdominal cramps, diarrhea, and vomiting. Examination may reveal hemorrhagic mucositis and ulcerations of the mouth, larynx, trachea, esophagus, stomach, and small intestine. Paralytic ileus with third-spacing of fluid, esophageal perforation with mediastinitis, and hypovolemic shock may occur. Onset correlates with the dose and may be delayed with dilute solutions or small amounts of concentrate.

Systemic effects usually occur only after ingestion and include coma, seizures, pulmonary fibrosis (paraquat only), acute proximal renal tubular necrosis, centrilobular hepatic necrosis, myocarditis and necrosis, pancytopenia, and adrenal hemorrhage. In fulminant cases, corrosive effects are accompanied by multiorgan failure, with death occurring within hours to days from pulmonary edema (adult respiratory distress syndrome), seizures, and cardiogenic shock. Intracerebral hemorrhages have been reported in diquat poisoning.

Pulmonary dysfunction may result in dyspnea, chest pain, tachypnea, and cyanosis. The chest radiograph may demonstrate pulmonary infiltrates, atelectasis, pneumothorax, and pleural effusions. Pulmonary function testing may reveal low compliance and decreased lung volumes and diffusing capacity. Blood gas analysis reveals hypoxemia, with respiratory alkalosis and metabolic acidosis. Respiratory failure and pulmonary fibrosis from paraquat usually progress relentlessly. Renal involvement may result in uremia, proteinuria, and oliguria or anuria. Signs of hepatotoxicity include right upper quadrant tenderness and elevated serum bilirubin and transaminase levels. Those with cardiac involvement may have chest pain and electrocardiogram (ECG), serum cardiac enzyme, or imaging evidence of ischemia or myocarditis. Ventricular tachycardia and fibrillation can occur. Renal and hepatic toxicity are potentially reversible. An elevated serum creatinine, low serum potassium, and metabolic acidosis on presentation are associated with the development of renal failure and death within 48 hours. Coma, early-onset renal failure, abnormal urinalysis, elevated serum transaminases, ileus, pancreatitis, alveolar-arterial oxygen gradient, need for mechanical ventilation, oxygen requirement, cardiac dysrhythmias, and an Apache II score >20 are predictive of mortality.

The ingestion of concentrated chlorophenoxy acid herbicides may cause a burning sensation in the pharynx, chest, and abdomen (1,3,8,10). Vomiting occurs early and may be persistent. Within a few hours, agitation, confusion, headache, dizziness, lethargy, coma, and seizures may develop. Cyanosis, flushed skin, and diaphoresis are reported. Pupils tend to be small but reactive. Deep tendon reflexes and muscle tone may be increased, decreased, or normal. Opisthotonus, myoclonus, fasciculations, and muscle tenderness have been described. Dyspnea and tachypnea are often present. In severe cases, progressive tachycardia, hypotension, and hyperthermia may ensue. Early death may be as a result of ventricular fibrillation. Eye, skin, and respiratory tract irritation may follow exposure by these routes. Laboratory abnormalities include an increased anion gap metabolic acidosis, hypoxia, hyperkalemia, hypocalcemia, leukocytosis, evidence of rhabdomyolysis (increased creatine phosphokinase level and myoglobinuria), mildly elevated hepatic enzyme levels, and renal function disturbances (elevated blood urea nitrogen (BUN) and creatinine levels, proteinuria, and glycosuria). The ECG may show flat or inverted T waves. Although pulmonary edema and aspiration have been reported, the chest radiograph usually is normal. Nerve conduction and electromyographic studies may show evidence of peripheral neuropathy and myopathy.

In mild-to-moderate chlorophenoxy acid intoxication, recovery occurs within 2 to 3 days; in severe cases, it may take longer than 1 week. Coma and acidemia are poor prognostic signs (2). Neuritis and myopathy with limb pain, paresthesias, twitching, tenderness, and weakness may be delayed in onset and persist for several months (7).

The ingestion of concentrated solutions of organophosphorus-surfactant herbicides can cause acute gastrointestinal (GI) and pulmonary injury, delayed cardiovascular (CV) toxicity, and secondary hepatic and renal dysfunction (6,8,10). Glufosinate also causes neurologic toxicity, which can be delayed (4–36 h after ingestion) in onset and progressive (over 24–48 h) (9). Neurologic findings include ataxia, confusion, disconjugate gaze, nystagmus, tremors, central nervous system (CNS) depression ranging from drowsiness to coma with central hypoventilation and apnea, and seizures. Seizures are generalized, invariably preceded by coma, typically recurrent, and can last for several days. Complications include hyperthermia, acidosis, and rhabdomyolysis.

Signs and symptoms of GI, pulmonary, CV, hepatic, and renal toxicity are similar to those described for bipyridyl and chlorophenoxy acid herbicides. Hypovolemic shock may result from GI fluid losses and sequestration. Cardiogenic shock can occur subsequently. Severe GI injury, respiratory failure, and cardiogenic shock are associated with a fatal outcome. Patients with coma or seizures can have prolonged amnesia, encephalopathy, and myopathy, with recovery taking weeks. Exposure to organophosphorus-surfactant herbicides that have been diluted for use may cause eye, skin, and mucosal irritation, but systemic toxicity is unlikely.

DIFFERENTIAL DIAGNOSIS

Herbicide poisoning should be suspected in a patient with signs and symptoms of corrosive ingestion, cardiopulmonary toxicity, and hepatorenal dysfunction. The initial presentation may resemble that of other corrosive exposures (see Chapter 33, "Corrosives and Chemical Burns"). Paraquat poisoning is distinguished by progressive pulmonary failure. Diquat is more likely to cause acute renal failure and paralytic ileus (8). Colchicine, podophyllin, fluoride, iron, and heavy-metal ingestion can cause similar multisystem organ toxicity and corrosive GI effects. Except with glufosinate, the CNS depression caused by herbicides is not associated with respiratory depression. Other causes of CNS depression include trauma, infection, hypoglycemia, asphyxiant, opioid, and sedative–hypnotic poisoning.

Severe 2,4-D (2,4-dichlorophenoxyacetic acid) and glufosinate poisoning, with coma, seizures, tachycardia, hypotension, fever, rhabdomyolysis, and metabolic acidosis, may be confused with septic shock, diabetic ketoacidosis, severe stimulant poisoning (e.g., amphetamines, cocaine), and intoxication by methanol, ethylene glycol, and salicylates. Other uncouplers of oxidative phosphorylation, such as the dinitrocresol and dinitrophenol herbicides and the pentachlorophenol fungicides, may produce a similar clinical picture. Cresylic and phenolic herbicides may stain the skin yellow and cause dark-colored urine. Toxicologic analysis of the blood may be necessary for a definitive diagnosis.

ED EVALUATION

The history should include the concentration, amount, and route of herbicide exposure and the time of onset and nature of symptoms. Determining whether the product was diluted prior to exposure and estimating the exposure dose are particularly important. Commercial products containing concentrated herbicide (e.g., 15%–50% solutions) are highly toxic whereas significant poisoning is unlikely once these products have been diluted for use (typically by a factor of 100). Vital signs should include measurement of the oxygen saturation. The physical examination should include inspection of exposed surfaces for evidence of corrosive injury. Patients with eye exposures should have fluorescein and slit-lamp examinations. Patients with GI signs and symptoms should also have an ECG, chest radiograph, arterial blood gas analysis, pulmonary function tests, complete blood count, electrolytes, BUN, creatinine, glucose, amylase, liver function tests, cardiac enzymes, and urinalysis. Endoscopy is recommended for those with evidence of corrosive injury to the airway or upper GI tract. Nerve conduction studies and electromyography may be helpful in those with persistent paresthesias or weakness.

Toxicology screening tests are not helpful because herbicides are not detected by the methods used. The detection and quantitation of herbicides usually requires sending a blood specimen to a reference laboratory. Although results can confirm exposure, they will not be immediately available and, except for paraquat, they have no prognostic value and will not help with making treatment decisions. Plasma paraquat concentrations above 2.0, 0.9, 0.3, 0.16, and 0.10 g/mL at 4, 6, 10, 16, and 24 h after ingestion, respectively, are predictive of death (4), and a potentially lethal level may warrant the use of unproven but potentially beneficial therapies. Arrangements for a quantitative paraquat level can be made by calling Zeneca Ag Products (800-327-8633). A qualitative urine test detects paraquat concentrations >1 g/mL and confirms exposure but is not prognostic. It may be performed by adding 1 mL of a 1% solution of sodium dithionite in 2N sodium hydroxide to 10 mL of urine. A blue color indicates the presence of paraquat (4).

ED MANAGEMENT

Contaminated skin and eyes should be flushed with copious amounts of water. Immediate and aggressive GI decontamination is critical, even when small amounts have been ingested. Unless the risk of esophageal perforation is great (e.g., the patient is unable to swallow and many hours have passed since the time of ingestion), GI decontamination should be performed. Because the absorption of chlorophenoxy acids is slow, decontamination may be effective much longer after ingestion (possibly as long as 18 hours) than usual. Activated charcoal (AC) is the preferred method. Preceding AC by gastric aspiration or following it with gastric lavage and another dose of AC should be considered in those with potentially lethal ingestions. Multiple-dose activated charcoal therapy is also recommended.

In severe cases, endotracheal intubation and fluid resuscitation may be required. When intubating patients with chlorophenoxy acid poisoning, a nondepolarizing neuromuscular blocker (e.g., rocuronium) may be preferable to succinylcholine because the muscle effects of succinylcholine are similar to those caused by these herbicides. Benzodiazepines, muscle relaxants, or therapeutic paralysis should be used for agitation, fasciculations, myoclonus, or muscle rigidity, particularly those with hyperthermia or rhabdomyolysis. Propofol, which has antioxidant activity, should be considered for intubated patients with paraquat poisoning. Active external cooling measures may be necessary with hyperthermia. Avoid using salicylates that also cause uncoupling of oxidative phosphorylation. Urinary alkalinization and diuresis are helpful for rhabdomyolysis and also enhance the elimination of chlorophenoxy acid herbicides.

Supportive care should include monitoring for and treatment of hepatic, renal, cardiac, and pulmonary dysfunction and fluid and electrolyte abnormalities. With the exception of paraquat poisoning, standard therapies are employed. Because oxygen increases the pulmonary toxicity of paraquat, concentrations >21% should be used only when the Po_2 falls below 50 mm Hg. Positive end-expiratory pressure may improve arterial oxygenation.

Sodium bicarbonate is indicated to correct acidemia and enhance herbicide elimination in patients with chlorophenoxy acid poisoning (2,5). It also appears to improve survival (2). Chlorophenoxy acids have pKa values between 1.9 and 4.8, and increasing the pH increases the ionized fraction and traps these compounds in the blood and urine, thereby preventing their tissue distribution and enhancing their renal excretion. Sodium bicarbonate should be given as a bolus to correct acidemia and as a constant infusion to alkalinize the urine. Alkaline diuresis decreases the half-life of 2,4-D by about 50%. Urine pH must be increased to 8.0 to enhance excretion significantly. Extracorporeal elimination therapies are indicated for patients with severe paraquat, diquat, and chlorophenoxy acid poisoning or potentially lethal ingestions and progressive clinical toxicity. Charcoal or resin hemoperfusion are the procedure of choice for bipyridyls, although hemodialysis is preferred for chlorophenoxy acids. Early, prolonged hemoperfusion appears to be useful in removing paraquat and limiting systemic toxicity when started within 10 hours of ingestion (15–20 hours in the presence of renal failure) and performed 8 hours daily or continuously for 2 to 3 weeks. Hemodialysis and continuous arteriovenous hemofiltration also enhance the elimination of paraquat and may be useful if hemoperfusion is unavailable. Data are limited regarding the use of hemoperfusion in diquat poisoning. The efficacy of hemodialysis in enhancing 2,4-D elimination is about the same as inducing alkaline diuresis (1,3).

Free radicals scavengers and antioxidants have been used in an attempt to prevent pulmonary fibrosis paraquat poisoning, but their efficacy remains unproven (1,3,8). Given the lethality of this condition, however, the following treatments should be considered: corticosteroids, cyclophosphamide *N*-acetylcysteine, and vitamin E. *S*-carboxymethylcysteine, Loviscol, has been used when *N*-acetylcysteine is unavailable. Lung transplantation may be considered. Nitric oxide inhalation and extracorporeal membrane oxygenation might be useful as interim measures.

CRITICAL INTERVENTIONS

- Estimate the dose of herbicide before making treatment and disposition decisions.
- Obtain a serum paraquat level, administer oxygen only if absolutely necessary (e.g., pO_2 <50 mm Hg), arrange for hemoperfusion, and consider antioxidant therapy in patients with significant paraquat poisoning.
- Perform aggressive GI decontamination.
- Correct acidemia, institute alkaline diuresis, and consider hemodialysis in patients with chlorophenoxy acid herbicide poisoning.

DISPOSITION

The National Pesticide Telecommunications Network also provides 24-hour-a-day consultation services (800-858-7378). All patients with symptoms after herbicide ingestion and dermal burns from paraquat should be admitted. Unless the exposure is minor and the severity of poisoning is mild, transfer to a tertiary care center and admission to an intensive care unit are advised. Patients who remain or become asymptomatic after trivial ingestions or exposure by other routes can be discharged after evaluation and decontamination. Patients with ingestions should be observed for 4 to 6 hours (6–12 hours for chlorophenoxy acid herbicides) prior to discharge.

COMMON PITFALLS

- Underestimating the potential toxicity of herbicides, particularly with intentional ingestions of concentrated solutions
- Failure to appreciate that although concentrated herbicide formulations are highly toxic, the likelihood of serious toxicity is greatly diminished once they have been diluted for use
- Failure to appreciate that prolonged observation is necessary to rule out toxicity in patients with ingestions of dilute herbicide and with significant skin exposures to paraquat
- Failure to evaluate symptomatic patients for multisystem organ dysfunction, including metabolic disturbances and rhabdomyolysis
- Failure to appreciate that the pulmonary toxicity of paraquat is potentiated by oxygen and that the lowest possible concentration of supplemental oxygen should be administered
- Failure to appreciate that extracorporeal removal can enhance the elimination of paraquat, diquat, and chlorophenoxy acid herbicides

ICD 9

989.89 Toxic effect of other substance chiefly nonmedicinal as to source

REFERENCES

1. Bradberry SM, Watt BE, Proudfoot AT, Vale JA. Mechanisms of toxicity, clinical features, and management of acute chlorophenoxy herbicide poisoning: a review. *J Toxicol Clin Toxicol* 2000; 38(2):111–122.
2. Flanagan RJ, Meredith TJ, Ruprah M, et al. Alkaline diuresis for acute poisoning with chlorophenoxy herbicides and ioxynil. *Lancet* 1990;335:454.
3. Friesen EG, Jones GR, Vaughan D. Clinical presentation and management of acute 2,4-D oral ingestion. *Drug Saf* 1990;5:155.
4. Hart TB. A statistical approach to the prognostic significance of plasma paraquat concentrations. *Lancet* 1984;2:1222.
5. Jones GM, Vale JA. Mechanisms of toxicity, clinical features, and management of diquat poisoning: a review. *J Toxicol Clin Toxicol* 2000;38(2):123–128.
6. Lee HL, Chen KW, Chi CH. Clinical presentations and prognostic factors of a glyphosate-surfactant herbicide intoxication: a review of 131 cases. *Acad Emerg Med* 2000;7:906–910.
7. Lin Ja-Ling, Iwersen S, Dan-Tzu, LT, Chen KH, Huang. Repeated pulse of methylprednisolone and cyclophosphamide with continuous dexamethasone therapy for patients with severe paraquat poisoning. *Crit Care Med* 2006;34(2):368–373.
8. Schmoldt A, Iwersen S, Schluter W. Massive ingestion of the herbicide 2-methyl-4-chlorophenoxyacetic acid (MCPA). *J Toxicol Clin Toxicol* 1997;35(4):405–408.
9. Suntres ZE. Role of antioxidants in paraquat toxicity. *Toxicology* 2002;180:65–77.
10. Talbot AR, Shiaw MH, Huang JS. Acute poisoning with a glyphosate-surfactant herbicide ('Round-up'): a review of 93 cases. *Hum Exp Toxicol* 1991;10:1–8.

CHAPTER 22

Isoniazid

PRE-HOSPITAL CONSIDERATIONS
- Collect pills and pill bottles for identification in the emergency department.

CLINICAL PRESENTATION

Seizures may be seen after acute overdoses of isoniazid (isonicotinic acid hydrazide, INH), as low as 35 mg/kg in adults. Severe toxicity has been noted with ingestions of 5 to 7 g (80 to 150 mg/kg); death has occurred after the ingestion of as little as 3 g. Although ingestions of >12 g in an adult have a high fatality rate, survival has been reported after the ingestion of as much as 25 g (14). Poisoning is associated with an INH serum concentration >30 μg/mL, although such laboratory assays for INH are not routinely available.

The initial symptoms of acute poisoning, which may occur as soon as 30 to 120 minutes after ingestion, include nausea, vomiting, slurred speech, blurred vision, and disorientation. Anticholinergic signs (e.g., mydriasis, tachycardia, and urinary retention) and hyperreflexia or areflexia may also be prominent. In severe poisonings, seizures appear abruptly and precede the development of a profound metabolic acidosis and coma, the triad that forms the classic clinical picture. An arterial pH as low as 6.49 was recorded in an adolescent who survived INH poisoning with no sequelae. Other patients with INH-induced seizures and arterial pH <6.99 have survived with full recovery after receiving pyridoxine (1).

Multiple seizures over a short time period are the hallmark of INH poisoning. Other symptoms and signs include confusion or irritability, hallucinations, stupor, ataxia, garbled speech, hyperpyrexia, nausea and vomiting, and respiratory depression. Laboratory findings include lactic acidosis, ketosis, hyperglycemia, an increased anion gap, hyper- or hypokalemia, peripheral blood leukocytosis, cerebrospinal fluid pleocytosis, and renal defects (e.g., glycosuria, ketonuria, albuminuria, and oliguria). An elevated creatine phosphokinase (CPK-MM fraction) level as a result of rhabdomyolysis may precede myoglobinuria and renal failure. In one series of isoniazid poisoning, 60% had an elevated CPK-MM level, which correlated both with the dose of INH ingested and the frequency of seizures (8). An electroencephalogram (EEG) often demonstrates diffuse slowing or paroxysmal electrical activity compatible with subclinical seizures. A chest radiograph may reveal aspiration pneumonia. The clinical course of the untreated patient with a massive INH overdose is often unremitting seizures, resulting in death from acidosis and cardiovascular and respiratory collapse. Survivors may suffer from persistent neuropsychological sequelae, including personality changes, poor memory, learning problems, and/or motor skills deficits (7).

Hepatic damage, with elevated liver enzyme levels, has an incidence of 20 cases per 1,000 patients treated chronically with INH (3). Such hepatotoxicity appears transient in most cases, even with continued use of the drug (12,13). Patients rarely go on to develop acute liver necrosis, liver failure, and death (3,5,13). Toxic effects of chronic INH use also include euphoria, tinnitus, ataxia, impaired memory, encephalopathy, and optic neuritis. Progressive lethargy, garbled speech, confusion, and coma were described in a man who mistakenly treated his tuberculosis with 1,200 mg of INH daily for 6 weeks (9).

Allergic manifestations, such as rashes, eosinophilia, vasculitis, arthralgias, and a positive antinuclear antibody test, have also been described (6). By inhibiting P450 series cytochromes, INH can interfere with drug clearance and increase the toxicity of such agents as phenytoin, carbamazepine, theophylline, and warfarin (10). INH's action as a weak monoamine oxidase inhibitor may result in symptoms (e.g., headache, flushing, nausea, vomiting, palpitations) in patients consuming foods containing tyramine or histamine (10). Pure red cell aplasia occurred in two siblings on INH prophylaxis at 15 mg/kg/day for 6 months. Other hematological abnormalities such as neutropenia, thrombocytopenia, sideroblastic anemia, and autoimmune hemolytic anemia have also been described in association with exposure to INH.

Patients with underlying hepatic disease or impaired renal function do not metabolize INH well, have a prolonged serum half-life, and are at greater risk for intoxication. Those with a pre-existing seizure disorder are at higher risk for neurotoxic effects.

DIFFERENTIAL DIAGNOSIS

INH overdose should be strongly considered in the patient who presents with seizures refractory to conventional anticonvulsants and a high anion gap metabolic acidosis, especially within the context of a history of depression, suicidal ideation, and tuberculosis and with access to INH. A diagnostic clue to INH poisoning is the prompt termination of seizure activity after the administration of intravenous (IV) pyridoxine (vitamin B_6).

Agents that can cause a clinical picture similar to that of INH overdose include salicylates, cyanide, carbon monoxide, other hydrazines (e.g., monomethylhydrazine-containing mushrooms), anticholinergics, and sympathomimetics. Other pharmacological causes of status epilepticus include baclofen, carbamazepine, dimenhydrinate, and theophylline. Neurotoxins such as pesticides, camphor, lead, narcotics, strychnine, and tricyclic antidepressants should also be considered. Other medical conditions, such as bacterial meningitis with sepsis, diabetic ketoacidosis, uremia, other metabolic disorders, meningoencephalitis, and head trauma, should also be included in the differential of patients presenting with seizures, coma, and acidosis (4).

ED EVALUATION

The time, dose, and intent of ingestion; the time of onset, nature, and severity of symptoms; prehospital care; and medical and psychiatric history should be noted. The physical examination should focus on vital signs and neurologic status, including assessment for hyperreflexia, focal neurologic deficits, abnormal thought processes, and central nervous system (CNS) depression. Laboratory evaluation should include serum electrolytes, glucose, blood urea nitrogen, creatinine, and arterial pH and blood gases. In severe or chronic cases, creatine kinase and liver function tests should be obtained. A chest radiograph can diagnose aspiration, and an EEG may be helpful in patients with persistent coma.

ED MANAGEMENT

Advanced life-support measures should be instituted as necessary. Pyridoxine is the specific antidote for seizures; it should be given in gram-for-gram equivalency to the estimated total amount of INH ingested (11,14). If the total ingested dose of INH is unknown, 5 g of pyridoxine hydrochloride (IV injection solution available at a concentration of 100 mg/mL) can be given empirically by slow IV push (maximum 0.5 g per minute) and repeated in 20 minutes if there is no clinical response. Typically, the seizures abate and the patient's level of consciousness slowly improves. Diazepam (5–10 mg IV, preferably in a second IV site) may be of benefit as an adjunct to control seizures. Additional pyridoxine is sometimes necessary for the resolution of INH-induced coma.

The use of adequate doses of diazepam and pyridoxine has essentially eliminated the need for other treatment of INH overdose. Chronic pyridoxine overdosing can cause a peripheral sensory neuropathy and multiple large doses of pyridoxine should be avoided because of pyridoxine's neurotoxic potential; only gram-for-gram replacement is recommended in INH poisoning. Commercial IV pyridoxine is available in a solution using two different preservatives: chlorobutanol, which may cause mild sedation in high doses, and parabens, which has been implicated in hypersensitivity reactions (2).

Although severe metabolic acidosis should be treated with IV sodium bicarbonate, large doses are usually unnecessary, because the acidosis is secondary to seizures and resolves shortly after seizures have been controlled. Diuresis is not of benefit. After stabilization, instillation of activated charcoal should be given in early presenting, acute overdose patients to prevent further absorption of INH or other coingestants.

CRITICAL INTERVENTIONS

- Administer IV pyridoxine hydrochloride (gram for gram of INH ingested), along with benzodiazepines for INH-induced seizures.
- Obtain an arterial blood gas and administer IV sodium bicarbonate to patients with severe acidemia.

DISPOSITION

Asymptomatic or mildly symptomatic patients can be observed in the emergency department for 6 hours before discharge.

Moderately or severely symptomatic patients should be admitted to an intensive care unit. Patients with refractory seizures, severe respiratory depression, or renal failure should be transferred to a hospital with intensive care capabilities if they are not locally available.

COMMON PITFALLS

- Failure to consider INH poisoning in patients with seizures refractory to conventional anticonvulsants and a high anion gap metabolic acidosis
- Failure to appreciate that asymptomatic patients may rapidly deteriorate
- Failure to give pyridoxine early after a known overdose
- Administration of excessive doses of sodium bicarbonate for the treatment of metabolic acidosis, which spontaneously resolves when convulsions cease

ICD 9

961.8 Poisoning by other antimycobacterial drugs

REFERENCES

1. Alvarez FG, Guntupalli KK. Isoniazid overdose: four case reports and review of the literature. *Intensive Care Med* 1995;21:641.
2. Burda AM, Sigg T, Wahl M. Possible adverse reactions to preservatives in high-dose pyridoxine hydrochloride i.v. injection. *Am J Health-Syst Pharm* 2002;59:1886.
3. Centers for Disease Control. Severe isoniazid-associated hepatitis—New York 1991 to 1993. *MMWR* 1993;42:545.
4. Ehsan T, Malkoff MD. Acute isoniazid poisoning simulating meningoencephalitis. *Neurology* 1995; 45:1627.
5. Gal A, Klatt E. Fatal isoniazid hepatitis in a child. *Pediatr Infect Dis* 1986;5:490.
6. Goldman A, Braman S. Isoniazid: review with emphasis on adverse effects. *Chest* 1972;62:71.
7. McLay RN, Drake A, Rayner T. Persisting dementia after isoniazid overdose. *J Neuropsychiatr Clin Neurosci* 2005;17:256–257.
8. Panganiban LR, Makalinao IR, Cortes-Maramba NP. Rhabdomyolysis in isoniazid poisoning. *Clin Toxicol* 2001;39:143.
9. Salkind AR, Hewitt CC. Coma from long-term overingestion of isoniazid. *Arch Intern Med* 1997; 157:2518.
10. Self TH, Chrisman CR, Baciewicz AM, et al. Isoniazid drug and food interactions. *Am J Med Sci* 1999;317:304.
11. Shah BR, Santucci K, Sinert R, et al. Acute isoniazid neurotoxicity in an urban hospital. *Pediatrics* 1995;95:700.
12. Stuart RL, Grayson ML. A review of isoniazid-related hepatotoxicity during chemoprophylaxis. *Aust NZ J Med* 1999;29:362.
13. Stuart RL, Wilson J, Grayson ML. Isoniazid toxicity in health care workers. *Clin Infect Dis* 1999;28:895.
14. Wason S, Lacouture P, Lovejoy F. Single high-dose pyridoxine treatment for isoniazid overdose. *JAMA* 1981;246:1102.

CHAPTER 23

Organophosphate and Carbamate Insecticides

PRE-HOSPITAL CONSIDERATIONS

- Initiate decontamination procedures.
  - Think DABC: **d**econtaminate, **a**irway, **b**reathing, **c**irculation.
  - Remove all clothes and store as toxic waste (double bag).
- Protect health care workers (utmost importance).
  - Use impenetrable gloves (neoprene, nitrile).
  - Use gowns and eye protection.
- Decontaminate skin with gentle soap and water; a shower or gentle scrubbing is ideal before entering the emergency department (ED).
- Maintain airway and oxygenate.
- Provide intravenous access and place on cardiac monitor.

CLINICAL PRESENTATION

Acute Toxicity Patients with acute organophosphate (OP) poisoning are often critically ill. Cholinergic findings (Fig. 23.1) may be subtle or obvious, depending on the exposure. Vital signs may be unstable, including depressed respirations and heart rate. Respiratory failure may result from excess pulmonary and oropharyngeal secretions, central nervous system (CNS) depression, and neuromuscular weakness. CNS toxicity may include altered mental status, confusion, lethargy, seizures, and coma. Overstimulation of postsynaptic receptors at the neuromuscular junction results initially in fasciculations and then muscle fatigue and weakness. In the autonomic nervous system, parasympathetic effects predominate as muscarinic cholinergic nerve fibers are stimulated. The mnemonic DUMBBELS (see Fig. 23.1) is helpful in describing the cholinergic muscarinic findings as a result of parasympathetic stimulation of hollow viscous organs and glands. Sympathetic ganglia effects may result in hypertension and tachycardia. Diaphoresis occurs commonly as a result of direct cholinergic stimulation of sympathetic sweat glands. Pancreatitis and rhabdomyolysis are relatively common complications.

The severity and extent of cholinergic toxicity is dependent on dose, agent, and route of exposure. The onset of symptoms is generally most rapid after inhalation and most delayed after skin exposure. Highly fat-soluble agents such as fenthion may cause delayed or prolonged toxicity. Generally, toxicity is less with carbamate

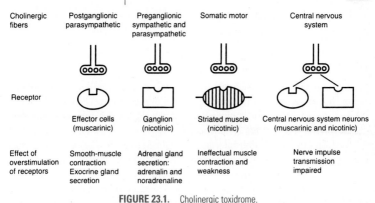

Cholinergic fibers	Postganglionic parasympathetic	Preganglionic sympathetic and parasympathetic	Somatic motor	Central nervous system
Receptor				
	Effector cells (muscarinic)	Ganglion (nicotinic)	Striated muscle (nicotinic)	Central nervous system neurons (muscarinic and nicotinic)
Effect of overstimulation of receptors	Smooth-muscle contraction Exocrine gland secretion	Adrenal gland secretion: adrenalin and noradrenaline	Ineffectual muscle contraction and weakness	Nerve impulse transmission impaired

FIGURE 23.1. Cholinergic toxidrome.

exposures. The OPs are a widely variable class, and some may produce protean cholinergic effects, whereas others may produce selected toxicity. The nerve gas agents (Sarin, Soman) typically produce more CNS effects and fewer peripheral signs of cholinergic toxicity. Therefore, muscarinic findings (DUMBBELS) may be absent in patients with significant nerve gas poisoning. The elderly are at especially high risk for complications, including aspiration and pneumonia, severe neurologic toxicity, and prolonged weakness. Patients with myasthenia gravis who intentionally or inadvertently develop toxicity from their own medications, such as pyridostigmine, may develop more severe cholinergic findings as a result of their compromised acetylcholine neurotransmission at baseline.

Intermediate Syndrome   In 1987, a syndrome of recrudescent OP neurotoxicity was described in a series of patients 1 to 4 days after acute OP poisoning (6). Although all had initially improved after therapy with atropine and pralidoxime, cranial nerve palsies and a progressive truncal and proximal limb weakness became evident; 40% of the affected patients required intubation. Symptoms lasted 5 to 15 days, and one patient died. Subsequent prospective studies have demonstrated that this syndrome occurs frequently after exposure to highly fat soluble OPs and is related to prolonged cholinesterase inhibition (2). It is proposed that redistribution of OPs from tissue reservoirs causes recrudescent toxicity at a time when atropine and oxime (pralidoxime) therapy have been completed (1).

Delayed Peripheral Neuropathy   A distinct polyneuropathy may occur 1 to 3 weeks after OP exposure. This syndrome was first described in 1930, when an estimated 40,000 persons became symptomatic as a result of contamination of an alcoholic beverage by tri-ortho-cresyl phosphate (4). The debilitating distal flaccid paresis resulting from the neuropathy was termed the *Jamaican ginger paralysis* after the contaminated beverage, a ginger extract imported from Jamaica. Patients with underlying medical problems such as alcoholism or nutritional deprivation may be at higher risk for developing delayed peripheral neuropathy. Recovery is incomplete in many cases, and motor symptoms are often persistent.

DIFFERENTIAL DIAGNOSIS

Similar cholinergic manifestations can be seen in patients poisoned with direct-acting cholinergic agonists such as bethanechol or pilocarpine. Digitalis, clonidine, calcium- or β-receptor antagonist poisoning, myocardial ischemia, or conduction disease should be considered in patients who present with altered mental status and bradycardia, without other obvious signs of cholinergic toxicity. Miosis, bradycardia, lethargy, and respiratory depression are also seen in opioid poisoning. Lethargy and prominent sialorrhea or salivation may occur with certain neuroleptic agents, such as clozapine and risperidone. OP-induced bronchorrhea and pulmonary edema may be difficult to distinguish from any other etiology of pulmonary edema. Patients with nicotine poisoning as a result of ingestion of tobacco products or harvesting wet tobacco may have similar findings, including vomiting, diarrhea, fasciculations, weakness, altered mental status, and autonomic instability.

ED EVALUATION

The history should document the amount, time, and route of exposure and the identity of the agent involved if known. A regional poison center can assist in product identification and characterization of anticipated toxicity. Continuous cardiac monitoring and pulse oximetry are crucial because of potential cardiac and respiratory toxicity. The physical examination should focus on the vital signs and assessment of cardiopulmonary and neuromuscular function, especially motor strength and respiratory effort. Cholinergic signs, particularly respiratory tract secretions, should be noted. Arterial blood gas (ABG) analysis and forced vital capacity (FVC) will help quantify respiratory dysfunction. An electrocardiograph (ECG), chest radiograph, and routine blood work, including complete blood count, electrolytes, blood urea nitrogen, creatinine, glucose, creatine phosphokinase, amylase, and liver function tests, should be obtained on symptomatic patients.

The diagnosis is confirmed by documenting decreased plasma or red blood cell (RBC) cholinesterase activity. RBC cholinesterase activity is more specific, but plasma (pseudo) cholinesterase activity tests are less expensive and more widely available. Although results are usually unavailable in a clinically relevant time frame, they can be helpful in cases in which the diagnosis is uncertain and in the evaluation of occupationally exposed patients. Specimens should be obtained prior to the administration of pralidoxime, because this antidote can increase measured enzyme activity. Interpretation of results may be difficult as a result of the variability in baseline values, which are subject to a variety of factors. In some cases (e.g., chronic or occupational exposures), serial activity levels, showing a return to baseline with time, may be necessary. Specific pesticides can also be identified by detecting certain compounds and metabolites in the urine.

ED MANAGEMENT

Health care providers should wear protective gear when treating patients with potential OP poisoning because significant dermal contamination may be present and can lead to secondary poisoning. Nitrile or neoprene gloves, impervious gowns, masks, and head and shoe covers are recommended. Self-contained breathing devises and chemical suits are necessary for rescuers responding to chemical spills and or nerve agent incidents.

Advanced life-support measures should be instituted as needed. This may require endotracheal intubation by emergency medical services in the field or soon after arrival in the ED. Atropine may be initiated prehospital in patients with bronchorrhea and/or bradycardia, because this may be effective in decreasing respiratory compromise. Skin decontamination should be undertaken as soon as the patient is stabilized. Activated charcoal is the preferred decontamination method for ingestions.

Patients who require intubation in the ED should undergo a rapid-sequence protocol. The duration of effect of succinylcholine may be much longer than usual as a result of the concomitant inhibition of cholinesterases that degrade succinylcholine (5). An alternative, short-acting, nondepolarizing neuromuscular blocking agent such as rocuronium may be preferable.

Patients with muscarinic findings, particularly excessive pulmonary secretions, should be given intravenous atropine (1–4 mg in adults and 0.02–0.05 mg/kg in children). Atropine, by competitively blocking acetylcholine at muscarinic receptors, acts to reverse the excessive parasympathetic stimulation. It is only partially effective in treating CNS symptoms and has a variable effect on seizures and altered mental status. It has no effect on nicotinic receptors and therefore does not reverse muscle weakness or sympathetic ganglionic effects. Repeated doses of atropine may be needed to decrease bronchorrhea and oropharyngeal secretions. Atropine should be titrated to the drying of secretions and not to irrelevant end points such as mydriasis or tachycardia. Tachycardia is often a result of respiratory insufficiency and inadequate atropine dosing. Atropine may be repeated every 5 to 15 minutes, with an atropine infusion (0.02–0.08 mg/kg/h) if frequent doses are needed. Atropine requirements are highly variable; patients with significant poisoning may require as much as 40 mg/d; one reported case describes a patient requiring 1,000 mg of atropine in a 24-hour period.

Any patient who requires treatment with atropine should also receive pralidoxime (2-PAM). Pralidoxime may be infused as a bolus therapy (1–2 g in saline and administered over 30 minutes in adults; 20–40 mg/kg to a maximum of 2 g loading dose in children), repeated in 1 to 2 hours if fasciculations are still present, and then given at 6- to 12-hour intervals for 24 to 48 hours. Alternatively, it may be administered as a continuous infusion of 500 mg/h (in adults). Pralidoxime initially binds to cholinesterase enzymes and then to the inhibitor. The inhibitor–pralidoxime complex detaches from the acetylcholinesterase enzyme, returning it to a functional state. Pralidoxime is effective in diminishing nicotinic effects, and it is synergistic with atropine at muscarinic receptors. Improvement in muscle strength is usually noted within 10 to 40 minutes. Although it is not thought to cross the blood–brain barrier, pralidoxime may reverse some CNS effects. Benzodiazepines may be needed for neurotoxic effects such as agitation and seizures.

Certain OPs have "aging" properties, which refer to their ability to bind permanently to acetylcholinesterase and not respond to pralidoxime. Although many OPs share this capability, aging occurs at different rates. Nerve gas chemical warfare agents age quickly, rapidly becoming resistant to any antidotal intervention (see Chapter 57, "Chemical Warfare Agents"). Because carbamates undergo spontaneous hydrolysis from the acetylcholinesterase enzyme, the need and safety of treating carbamate-poisoned patients with 2-PAM has been questioned. Recent data support treating any poisoned patient requiring atropine with 2-PAM, regardless of the anticholinesterase agent (3).

Therapy for the intermediate syndrome includes additional pralidoxime and, possibly, atropine, and supportive care. No specific therapy exists for peripheral neuropathy.

CRITICAL INTERVENTIONS

- Monitor oxygen saturation, evaluate airway patency, and obtain ABGs and FVC to assess oxygenation and ventilation.
- Monitor the cardiac rhythm and obtain an ECG.
- Administer atropine to patients with increased secretions and bronchospasm.
- Intubate early if inadequate improvement with atropine or if significant CNS depression.
- Administer pralidoxime to patients who require atropine.

DISPOSITION

Patients with an unintentional exposure who remain asymptomatic after at least 6 hours of observation may be discharged to home with a family member. Those requiring treatment with atropine or pralidoxime and those with evolving toxicity should be admitted to an intensive care unit (ICU) for close observation and monitoring. If the patient needs to be transferred to an ICU for admission, advanced cardiac life-support (ACLS) personnel should accompany the patient. Prophylactic intubation prior to initiating transport may be advisable in patients with borderline respiratory status. Even asymptomatic patients need follow-up with their family physician, because peripheral neuropathy can occur even in the absence of initial cholinergic manifestations.

COMMON PITFALLS

- Failure to decontaminate the skin of patients with dermal exposures and to take appropriate precautions to prevent secondary exposure to health care workers

- Failure to appreciate that tachycardia may be secondary to respiratory dysfunction and to give atropine to patients with tachycardia and dyspnea resulting from excessive respiratory tract secretions or bronchospasm
- Failure to appreciate that atropine should be titrated to drying of secretions rather than to heart rate or pupil size, and that doses far exceed standard ACLS recommendations
- Failure to treat all patients requiring atropine with pralidoxime to prevent "aging" of the cholinesterase inhibitor-enzyme complex and to decrease atropine requirements
- Failure to appreciate that highly fat-soluble OPs may cause delayed, prolonged, or recurrent toxicity

ICD 9

989.3 Toxic effect of organophosphate and carbamate

REFERENCES

1. Benson B, Tolo D, McIntire M. Is the intermediate syndrome in organophosphate poisoning the result of insufficient oxime therapy? [editorial]. *J Toxicol Clin Toxicol* 1992;30:347.
2. De Bleecker J, Van Den Neucker K, Colardyn F. Intermediate syndrome in organophosphorus poisoning: a prospective study. *Crit Care Med* 1993;21:1706–1711.
3. Mercurio-Zappala M, Hack J, Salvador A, et al. Carbaryl poisoning: 2-PAM or not 2-PAM [abstract]. *J Toxicol Clin Toxicol* 1998;36:428.
4. Morgan JP. The Jamaica ginger paralysis. *JAMA* 1982;248:1864–1867.
5. Selden BS, Curry SC. Prolonged succinylcholine-induced paralysis in organophosphate insecticide poisoning. *Ann Emerg Med* 1987;16:215–217.
6. Senanayake N, Karalliedde L. Neurotoxic effects of organophosphorus insecticides. An intermediate syndrome. *N Engl J Med* 1987;316:761–763.

CHAPTER 24

Nicotine, Pyrethrins, and Organochlorine Pesticides

CLINICAL PRESENTATION

Poisoning from nicotine can occur from (a) exposure to nicotine sulfate insecticides; (b) percutaneous absorption of nicotine in tobacco harvesters who pick and brush up against wet tobacco leaves (green tobacco sickness); (c) ingestion of tobacco products, such as cigarettes, snuff, chewing tobacco, and cigars; chewing or ingestion of nicotine chewing gum; and (d) improper use or ingestion of nicotine patches (10). Infants and young children are most susceptible to nicotine poisoning because of their small body size and the lack of tolerance. Similarly, tobacco harvesters are more likely to be symptomatic in the beginning of the harvesting season and workweek because of the lack of nicotine tolerance. Nonsmokers, lack of work experience, wet conditions, and the lack of protective clothing are risk factors for green tobacco sickness (5). Many nonsmoking tobacco harvesters resort to tobacco chewing as a means to develop nicotine tolerance. Overall, nicotine-related fatalities are rare because of its decreasing usage as a pesticide.

Onset of toxicity is rapid and can be seen within 15 minutes of exposure. Initial signs and symptoms include nausea, vomiting, salivation, bronchorrhea, abdominal pain, and diarrhea from parasympathetic stimulation and tachycardia, hypertension, and diaphoresis as result of sympathetic and adrenal stimulation. Early central nervous system (CNS) effects include dizziness, headache, confusion, agitation, incoordination, and seizures. Muscular fasciculations may result from neuromuscular junction stimulation.

As symptoms progress, hypotonia, muscle paralysis, respiratory failure, coma, bradycardia, and hypotension may ensue (6). Because of both stimulatory and inhibitory effects on multiple systems, the signs and symptoms vary by the time, dose, and route of exposure. In severe cases, such as nicotine pesticide poisoning, the progression from stimulation to inhibition of the various systems may be rapid (3).

In mild nicotine poisoning, symptoms can last for several hours. In severe cases, clinical toxicity can endure for 18 to 24 hours or more. Severe cases involve seizures and coma within 30 minutes, with respiratory arrest and death within 1 hour or less, especially with concentrated nicotine products. Patients who survive the first 4 hours usually recover fully. Radiographic and electrocardiographic (ECG) findings are nonspecific. Nicotine can be detected in the urine by chromatographic drug assays.

Direct toxicity from pyrethrins and pyrethroids is uncommon. When they occur, adverse effects are usually as a result of allergic hypersensitivity and include bronchospasm, vasomotor rhinitis, contact dermatitis, and, rarely, anaphylaxis (9). After inhalation, the most common presentation is a stuffy nose with clear discharge and a "scratchy" throat. In rare cases, sudden bronchospasm, swelling of the laryngeal mucosa, and shock (anaphylaxis) can occur. Patients allergic to ragweed have a higher risk of developing allergic reactions to pyrethrins. Natural pyrethrins are more likely to cause these reactions than are synthetic pyrethroids.

Direct dermal exposure to pyrethrins can produce a contact dermatitis consisting of redness, blisters, burning, stinging, and numbness. Transient paresthesia is related to the direct effects on cutaneous nerve endings and more commonly associated with type II pyrethroids. Ocular exposure to hydrocarbon propellants can cause eye irritation and corneal abrasions. Large exposures to type II pyrethroids can cause tremors, salivation, paresthesia, ataxia, choreoathetosis, and seizures. Similar exposure to type I agents can result in tremors, agitation, and hyperthermia (2).

The onset of symptoms after exposure to organochlorine insecticides may vary from minutes to hours, depending on the route and method of exposure and the physicochemical properties of the agent (1). Nausea, vomiting, and diarrhea can occur as soon as 45 minutes after acute ingestion. Initial CNS effects include apprehension, headache, dizziness, tremors, ataxia, and disorientation. Stupor, coma, and seizures with respiratory depression may be seen in severe cases. Dysrhythmias may result from increased myocardial sensitivity to catecholamines.

Aspiration of formulations containing a petroleum distillate can result in a chemical pneumonitis. CNS toxicity, including seizures, can also occur in children after prolonged or excessive topical lindane exposures during the treatment of lice or scabies (4). In severe cases, potential complications include lactic acidosis, rhabdomyolysis, and disseminated intravascular coagulation.

Chronic exposure to organochlorines can cause hepatomegaly. Extensive or prolonged dermal contact can result in skin irritation. Chronic ingestion of hexachlorobenzene has been associated with cutaneous porphyria. Leukemia has been associated with the use of chlordane or heptachlor to control termites in homes.

DIFFERENTIAL DIAGNOSIS

Without a history of exposure, there are no pathognomonic signs of nicotine poisoning. It could be confused with acetylcholinesterase inhibitor poisoning, such as organophosphate (OP) or carbamate insecticides, and carbamate drugs (edrophonium, physostigmine). In nicotine poisoning, however, there is no depression of the red blood cell cholinesterase.

Direct-acting cholinomimetic agents such as bethanechol, carbachol, methacholine, and pilocarpine can also produce cholinergic effects similar to those of nicotine. However, because these agents have minimal effects on nicotinic receptors (except for carbachol), they produce minimal or no sympathetic or muscular symptoms (8). Central and peripheral sympatholytics (α-adrenergic and β-adrenergic receptor blockers, clonidine, guanabenz, topical decongestant imidazoline derivatives, and calcium blockers) can mimic the later stages of nicotine poisoning. These agents will not produce any muscarinic symptoms or neuromuscular weakness. Tree tobacco (*Nicotiana glauca*), native to the temperate regions of America, contains the alkaloid anabasine, an isomer of nicotine that can cause similar symptoms. Other substances to consider are the insect repellent diethyltoluamide, *Veratrum* and sabadilla plants, *Clitocybe* and *Inocybe* mushroom species, and poison hemlock (*Conium maculatum*).

Pyrethrins and pyrethroids should be included in the differential diagnosis of patients who present with an apparent hypersensitivity reaction of the skin or respiratory system when exposed to flora, insecticides, or insect bites. Because almost all of the insecticides containing these compounds are in a hydrocarbon base, the risk of hydrocarbon pneumonitis must be considered in humans ingesting these products.

Acute organochlorine insecticide poisoning must be distinguished from any condition that produces "gastroenteritis" with an altered mental status, especially ataxia, tremors, and seizures. CNS disease, drug withdrawal, stimulant intoxication (e.g., from sympathomimetics, xanthenes, anticholinergics, hallucinogens, and isoniazid), and infectious etiologies should be considered.

ED EVALUATION

The history should document the time, agent, dose, route, intent, and duration of exposure and the nature and course of symptoms. The complete physical examination should pay particular attention to cardiovascular, respiratory, and neurologic function. Patients with vital sign abnormalities should have an ECG. Symptomatic patients should have cardiac and oxygen saturation monitoring. Chest radiographs, oxygen saturation measurement or arterial blood gas analysis, and pulmonary function tests can assess respiratory function and possible aspiration in patients with wheezing, dyspnea, cough, and fever. Blood chemistries and hematologic analysis should be obtained based on clinical severity.

No specific laboratory tests are diagnostic. The presence of nicotine in the urine of a nonsmoker is supportive. Plasma nicotine levels are not useful. Organochlorine insecticides can be measured in the serum by using gas chromatography/mass spectrometry, but levels are not useful for clinical management. However, in a patient with a suspicious exposure for DDT, a high DDT to DDE ratio confirms that the exposure was recent (7).

ED MANAGEMENT

Gastrointestinal (GI), skin, and eye decontamination should be performed. Activated charcoal (AC) is the preferred method of GI decontamination. Pyrethrins and pyrethroids are lipophilic, so milk, cream, or substances that contain animal or vegetable fats should not be administered. Except for recent ingestion (<1 hour) of large quantities of a nicotine pesticide, gastric aspiration or lavage would not likely provide additional benefit. Seizures and coma can occur rapidly, and emesis increases the risk of aspiration. If present, any transdermal patches should be removed.

Exposed skin areas should be washed with soap and water. Exposed eyes should be irrigated with copious amounts of water for 15 minutes. Powder contaminating the skin should first be vacuumed off. Contaminated clothing should be removed, and the skin, hair, and nails scrubbed.

The patient should be closely monitored for the first few hours after exposure. Supportive care, including oxygen, endotracheal intubation, and assisted ventilation, should be instituted as necessary. Intravenous (IV) access and cardiac monitoring are indicated for all but mild intoxications. Seizures should be treated with IV benzodiazepines such as diazepam (for adults, 5–10 mg initially, repeated every 5–10 minutes as necessary, up to 30 mg; for children, 0.25–0.4 mg/kg per dose) or lorazepam (0.05–0.1 mg/kg; may be repeated twice every 15 minutes as necessary). If seizures cannot be controlled with diazepam or lorazepam, a barbiturate (such as phenobarbital or pentobarbital) or propofol may be given. Phenytoin may be less effective than barbiturates and may actually increase the incidence of seizures in organochlorine insecticide poisoning.

Excess parasympathetic stimulation (e.g., marked bronchial secretions) from nicotine and type II pyrethroids can be controlled by atropine (adults, 0.5–1 mg IV, repeated every 5 minutes as necessary; children, 0.01–0.02 mg/kg IV). Hypotension should be treated with IV fluids; if it fails, dopamine or norepinephrine may be added. Oxygen and ventilation may be necessary. Mecamylamine (Inversine), an older antihypertensive agent, is a specific nicotine antagonist but is available only in tablets, however, and is not a practical therapy in a patient who is vomiting, seizing, or hypotensive. Anaphylaxis should be treated as usual. The management of hydrocarbon aspiration is supportive (see Chapter 36, "Hydrocarbons"). Respiratory distress as a result of bronchospasm is managed with inhaled bronchodilators and humidified oxygen. Parenteral administration of adrenergic amines (e.g., epinephrine) is not recommended in organochlorine insecticide poisoning because myocardial irritability may be enhanced. Contact dermatitis may be treated with topical corticosteroids.

Because organochlorine compounds have an extensive enterohepatic recirculation, multiple dose activated charcoal (MDAC) is recommended to enhance their elimination. Multiple doses of cholestyramine resin are also effective but is less well tolerated than charcoal. Extracorporeal procedures are not effective in enhancing organochlorine elimination. MDAC, hemodialysis and hemoperfusion have not been evaluated in nicotine and pyrethrin poisoning.

CRITICAL INTERVENTIONS

- Establish IV access and institute cardiac monitoring.
- Secure the airway and assist ventilation as necessary in patients with neurotoxicity.
- Administer benzodiazepines and, if necessary, barbiturates and propofol for seizures.
- Administer atropine to treat excess parasympathetic stimulation.
- Treat hypersensitivity reactions to pyrethrins/pyrethroids the same as any other allergic reaction.
- Administer MDAC for organochlorine insecticides ingestions.

DISPOSITION

Patients who remain or become asymptomatic after a 6-hour period of observation after an acute exposure may be discharged with appropriate follow-up. Patients with mild allergic reactions can be discharged after treatment. Chronic organochlorine insecticide exposures can generally be treated as outpatients. All others should be admitted to the hospital, observed, and treated supportively. Because the cardiorespiratory system requires monitoring, intensive care unit admission is advised. If such facilities are unavailable, the patient should be transferred with advanced life-support measures and anticonvulsants available. If necessary, consultation can be obtained from a regional poison center (1-800-222-1222) or the National Pesticide Telecommunications Network (1-800-858-7378). If the exposure occurred at the workplace, the proper health agency should be notified to prevent further occurrences.

COMMON PITFALLS

- Failure to discover a nicotine patch unintentionally stuck to the skin of an infant or toddler with altered mental status because they were not completely undressed
- Failure to properly decontaminate patients with dermal exposures
- Failure to diagnose and treat respiratory failure, the primary cause of death in nicotine poisoning
- Failure to appreciate that administering antacids for GI symptoms may increase the absorption of ingested nicotine
- Failure to consider the possibility of aspiration (hydrocarbon) pneumonitis in patients with respiratory symptoms after ingestion
- Mistaking organochlorine insecticides for OP insecticides (and vice versa), resulting in incorrect treatment

ICD9

989.84 Toxic effect of tobacco

REFERENCES

1. Chugh SN, Dhawan R, Agrawal N, et al. Endosulfan poisoning in Northern India: a report of 18 cases. *Int J Clin Pharmacol Ther* 1998;36:474.
2. Dorman DC, Beasley R. Neurotoxicology of pyrethrin and pyrethroid insecticides. *Vet Hum Toxicol* 1991;33:238.
3. Lavoie FW, Harris TM. Fatal nicotine ingestion. *J Emerg Med* 1991;9:133.
4. Lee B, Groth P. Scabies: transcutaneous poisoning during treatment. *Pediatrics* 1977;59:643.
5. McBride JS, Altman DG, Melissa-Klein WW. Green tobacco sickness. *Tob Control* 1998;7:294.
6. Mensch AR, Holden M. Nicotine overdose after a single piece of nicotine gum. *Chest* 1984;86:801.
7. Ray DE. Pesticides derived from plants and other organisms. In: Hayes WJ Jr, Law ER, eds. *Handbook of pesticide toxicology.* San Diego: Academic Press, 1991:585.
8. Taylor P. Agents acting at the neuromuscular junction and autonomic ganglia. In: Hardman JG, Limbird LE, Molinoff PB, et al, eds. *Goodman* & Gilman's: the pharmacological basis of therapeutics, 9th ed. New York: McGraw-Hill, 1996:192.
9. Wax PM, Hoffman RS. Fatality associated with inhalation of a pyrethrin shampoo. *J Toxicol Clin Toxicol* 1994;32:457.
10. Woolf A, Burkhart K, Caraccio T, et al. Childhood poisoning involving transdermal nicotine patches. *Pediatrics* 1997;99:E4.

CHAPTER 25

Rodenticides

CLINICAL PRESENTATION

The majority of rodenticide/oral anticoagulant exposures involve unintentional ingestions in children younger than 6 years of age (3). Acute, single, unintentional ingestions of conventional anticoagulants are unlikely to cause toxicity because of their low warfarin concentrations. Similarly, children who unintentionally ingest superwarfarins are unlikely to develop toxicity. In contrast, adults with intentional ingestions or children with repeated ingestions often develop a coagulopathy within 24 or, at the latest, 48 hours (3). If this goes untreated, bleeding complications may develop. The most common sites of bleeding are the gastrointestinal (GI) and genitourinary tracts (3).

Patients with acute ingestions of arsenic may have a garlic-like odor on their breath and present with severe vomiting and diarrhea, dehydration, ventricular dysrhythmias, and central nervous system and cardiovascular depression (see Chapter 31, "Arsenic and Mercury").

Cholinesterase inhibitor poisoning can occur by the oral, dermal, or inhalational routes. Signs and symptoms include salivation, lacrimation, urination, defecation, nausea, vomiting, GI cramping and/or pain, diarrhea, mental status change, seizures, muscle fasciculations, or weakness (see Chapter 23, "Organophosphate and Carbamate Insecticides") (6).

Red squill toxicity is similar to other cardiac glycoside poisoning such as digoxin; patients may have GI symptoms, cardiac dysrhythmias, and hyperkalemia (see Chapter 30, "Cardiac Glycosides").

Sodium monofluoroacetate (SMFA) toxicity can occur with inhalation; however, ingestion is the most common route of severe poisoning. Initial symptoms include nausea and apprehension, followed shortly by severe lactic acidosis, pulmonary edema, coma, hypokalemia, hypocalcemia, seizures, and dysrhythmias. A poor prognosis is associated with hypotension, the early onset of acidosis, and secondary renal insufficiency (4).

Strychnine toxicity is associated with opisthotonos, facial spasm (risus sardonicus), and decorticate posturing. Patients are often mistakenly described as having "seizures," but their mental status is usually normal. Prolonged muscle activity can lead to hyperthermia, rhabdomyolysis, lactic acidosis, and death, often from respiratory dysfunction (7).

Tetramine ingestion can cause rapid onset seizures that progress to status epilepticus. This toxin has a high fatality rate and may be associated with residual neurologic injury in survivors (1).

Thallium toxicity is associated with a 12 to 24 hour delay in symptom onset after ingestion. Initially, GI symptoms such as nausea, vomiting, diarrhea, constipation, and abdominal pain predominate. Characteristically, extremely painful paresthesias then develop in the extremities and are unique in their intensity. In severe cases, dysrhythmias occur and can cause death. Respiratory failure has also been described. Survival is characterized by a period of alopecia and neurologic findings such as neuropathies, paresis, ataxia, choreiform movements, and optic nerve atrophy (5).

Patients who ingest Vacor may develop rapid loss of glucose control and severe diabetic ketoacidosis (DKA). Along with DKA, patients often present with abdominal pain from acute pancreatitis, autonomic instability, and peripheral paresthesias (8). Survivors of Vacor exposure are characterized by brittle insulin-dependent diabetes and accelerated microvascular diabetic disease.

DIFFERENTIAL DIAGNOSIS

Exposure to an unknown rodenticide is common. In such cases, it is useful to classify rodenticides clinically, based on their time of onset and symptoms (Table 25.1). When the time of symptom onset and the nature of the symptoms are considered, a presumptive diagnosis can be established. Patients exposed to rodenticides with a rapid onset of action can be expected to manifest symptoms within 6 hours of ingestion. Those with exposure to rodenticides that have a delayed onset typically manifest symptoms beginning 12 hours or more after ingestion.

When symptoms are rapid in onset, cholinergic findings suggest organophosphate poisoning; muscular hyperactivity suggests strychnine; seizures, coma, and metabolic acidosis suggest SMFA or tetramine; severe GI symptoms suggest arsenic; hyperglycemia suggests Vacor; and GI symptoms with cardiac dysrhythmias suggest red squill.

Lack of symptoms during the first 6 hours after exposure to an unknown rodenticide suggests either a nontoxic exposure to a rapidly acting agent or a potentially toxic exposure to a rodenticide with a delayed onset of toxicity (e.g., an oral anticoagulant or thallium). The most common cause of delayed rodenticide poisoning is superwarfarin anticoagulants.

An additional diagnostic clue for suspected rodenticide exposure is odor. Arsenic and yellow phosphorus smell like garlic. Vacor smells like peanuts, and patients with Vacor-induced DKA may have the fruity odor of ketones on their breath.

ED EVALUATION

The history should include the amount and time of ingestion and the identity of the product involved. The most useful piece of information is the precise name

TABLE 25.1	Rodenticide by Time of Symptom Onset

Early onset
α—Naphthylthiourea
Arsenic
Barium
Bromethalin
Cholinesterase inhibitors
Norbormide
Red squill
Sodium monofluoroacetate
Strychnine
Tetramine
Thallium*
Yellow phosphorus
Zinc and aluminum phosphide

Late onset
Oral anticoagulants
Cholecalciferol
Salmonella
Thallium*
Vacor

*Symptoms can be early or delayed in onset.

and manufacturer of the ingested product. A family member should be asked to return to home and try to get this information if the product is not brought along with the patient. The actual container or list of active ingredients is preferred over the commercial name, because many commercial names have been used for several products with different active ingredients.

If this information is unavailable, the time of symptom onset and clinical manifestations may suggest the identity of the offending agent. While the diagnostic evaluation is proceeding, consideration and institution of therapy must occur simultaneously, as many of these poisons cause rapid and potentially fatal toxicity.

The initial assessment should address the airway, breathing, and circulation. Strychnine may cause respiratory failure secondary to tonic muscle contractions and inability to ventilate. Toxicity from several of the other rodenticides can evolve rapidly to produce cardiovascular collapse.

Vital signs should be obtained immediately and reassessed frequently. Life-threatening hyperthermia may occur as a result of increased muscle activity with strychnine poisoning. Clinical clues from the physical examination include specific odors associated with the different toxins and the quality and amount of emesis or diarrhea. Signs of bleeding in the GI or genitourinary tract may indicate oral anticoagulant exposure, although these findings would be delayed in onset.

Blood chemistries and a complete blood count are rarely useful in the absence of clinical findings. A low serum bicarbonate concentration might be found in symptomatic patients with SMFA, strychnine, tetramine, or Vacor exposures. An elevated serum glucose level, especially in association with a metabolic acidosis, suggests Vacor-induced DKA. A prothrombin time/international ratio (PT or INR) should be obtained in patients with remote (>24 hours) or repeated anticoagulant ingestions. If obtained shortly after a single ingestion, the PT/INR should be normal. In chronic anticoagulant exposures or in patients who present with active bleeding several days after exposure, an elevated PT/INR may be diagnostic.

The need for radiographic assessment should be guided by the toxin involved. Exposure to agents that produce pulmonary toxicity mandate a chest radiograph. Abdominal radiography may help detect opacities in the gut in recent ingestions of the metal toxins (arsenic or thallium). If a sample of an unidentified rodenticide is obtained, taking a radiograph of it may help determine its heavy-metal content (5).

ED MANAGEMENT

Treatment begins with stabilization of vital signs; advanced life-support measures are instituted, as appropriate. Once the patient is stable, gastric decontamination should be considered. For the asymptomatic patient who has ingested an unknown rodenticide, activated charcoal is the preferred method. Orogastric lavage may be used in any patient giving a history of recent ingestion (within 2–4 hours) of a highly toxic rodenticide such as arsenic, superwarfarin anticoagulants, sodium monofluoracetate, strychnine, tetramine, thallium, or Vacor. Although little data exist on the efficacy of orogastric lavage, this intervention seems justified given the severe potential toxicity and lack of effective antidotes for most of the compounds in this group. Activated charcoal should be given after lavage.

Management of asymptomatic patients with unknown ingestions involves daily follow-up with PT/INR testing to see whether anticoagulant toxicity has manifested. A normal PT/INR at 48 hours after ingestion excludes significant anticoagulant toxicity (1). Prophylactic treatment with vitamin K_1 is not recommended in these cases when there is a normal PT/INR. It is important to note that vitamin K_1 will not prevent toxicity, which might last for a month, and thus only delays detection (1).

The treatment of tetramine poisoning is entirely supportive. Management of arsenic poisoning also includes chelation therapy (see Chapter 31, "Arsenic and Mercury") and that for cholinesterase inhibitor poisoning also includes atropine and pralidoxime (see Chapter 23, "Organophosphate and Carbamate Insecticides"). Red squill poisoning is treated the same as cardiac glycoside toxicity from other causes; digoxin specific Fab fragments can be used (see Chapter 30, "Cardiac Glycosides").

Coagulopathy without significant bleeding is treated with vitamin K_1. It is important to note that not all vitamin K preparations are effective; phytonadione (AquaMEPHYTON, vitamin K_1) is the only antidote recommended for this purpose. The dose and the duration of treatment varies with the type and amount of anticoagulant ingested and the patient's rate of toxin metabolism. Obtaining serial levels of the toxin to determine its elimination curve may help guide the duration of treatment necessary (2). Doses of up to 100 mg/d of vitamin K_1 for as long as 10 months have been necessary for superwarfarin poisoning (1). In patients with life-threatening bleeding, fresh-frozen plasma should also be administered.

Suggested antidotal treatments for SMFA toxicity include glycerol monoacetate or ethanol, although neither approach has been well studied. Glycerol monoacetate is thought to work by bypassing the site of blockage in the Krebs cycle. Ethanol may inhibit the conversion of SMFA to fluorocitrate and allow for excretion of the nontoxic parent compound (3). Given the relative safety of ethanol administration and the severe toxicity of SMFA, treatment with ethanol appears warranted.

Treatment of muscle overactivity, the main problem that leads to the life-threatening complications in strychnine poisoning, includes high doses of benzodiazepines and, if necessary, neuromuscular paralysis. If the patient is hyperthermic, aggressive rapid cooling is critical.

Patients with thallium poisoning should be treated with prussian blue (ferric ferrocyanide) (5) and multiple-dose activated charcoal, with the addition of either hemodialysis or hemoperfusion in life-threatening cases. Prussian blue is given at a dose of 250 mg/kg/d with a cathartic in divided doses.

Niacinamide (nicotinamide) is an effective antidote for Vacor in experimental animals. In these studies the earlier the antidote was given after exposure, the better the outcome. Niacin is not an effective substitute. Niacinamide (500 mg initially, followed by 100–200 mg every 4 hours for 2 days) is recommended for all patients with Vacor ingestion. Because an intravenous formulation is not available, it should be given orally. Patients who develop DKA are managed like other diabetic patients.

CRITICAL INTERVENTIONS

- Positively identify the rodenticide's active ingredients.
- Arrange for a 48-hour follow-up PT/INR for asymptomatic superwarfarin or unknown rodenticide exposures.

DISPOSITION

For symptomatic patients exposed to a highly toxic rodenticide such as arsenic, superwarfarin anticoagulants, sodium monofluoracetate, strychnine, tetramine, thallium, or Vacor, hospital admission to a monitored setting is warranted. Because of the relative rarity of these exposures, consultation with a medical toxicologist or a regional poison center is recommended early in the presentation.

Patients with unintentional exposures who remain asymptomatic after 6 hours' observation can be discharged. For patients exposed to superwarfarin or long-acting oral anticoagulants, follow-up coagulation studies are needed at 48 hours after ingestion. These studies may be performed in the outpatient setting for patients with unintentional ingestions, provided there is adequate family and social support. All other patients, including those with intentional ingestions, are best managed as inpatients.

COMMON PITFALLS

- Failure to obtain a sample or container to identify the ingested agent
- Misidentification of the rodenticide because an identical or similar brand name or market name is used for more than one agent
- Failure to consider ingestion of an agent with delayed onset of action in a patient with an unknown rodenticide exposure who remains asymptomatic after a period of observation
- Using the wrong type of vitamin K to treat oral anticoagulant toxicity
- Beginning vitamin K treatment when the PT/INR is normal

ICD 9

989.89 Toxic effect of other substance chiefly nonmedicinal as to source

REFERENCES

1. Barrueto Jr F, Nelson LS, Hoffman RS, et al. From the Centers for Disease Control and Prevention. Poisoning by an illegally imported Chinese rodenticide containing tetramethylenedisulfotetramine—New York City, 2002. *JAMA* 289:2640.
2. Bruno GR, Howland MA, McMeeking A, et al. Long acting overdose: brodifacoum kinetics and optimal vitamin K dosing. *Ann Emerg Med* 2000;36:262.
3. Caravati EM, Erdman AR, Scharman EJ, et al. Long-acting anticoagulant rodenticide poisoning: an evidence-based consensus guideline for out-of-hospital management. *Clin Toxicol* 2007;45:1.
4. Chi CH, Chen KW, Chan SH, et al. Clinical presentation and prognostic factors in sodium monofluoroacetate intoxication. *J Toxicol Clin Toxicol* 1996;34:707.
5. Meggs WJ, Hoffman RS, Shih RD, et al. Malicious thallium poisoning: rapid diagnosis by x-ray, laboratory and clinical evaluation. *Vet Hum Toxicol* 1993;35:317.
6. Nelson LS, Perrone J, DeRoos F, et al. Aldicarb poisoning by an illicit rodenticide imported into the United States: tres pasitos. *J Toxicol Clin Toxicol* 2001;39:447.
7. Palatnick W, Meatherall R, Sitar D, et al. Toxicokinetics of acute strychnine poisoning. *J Toxicol Clin Toxicol* 1997;35:617.
8. Pont A, Rubino JM, Bishop D, et al. Diabetes mellitus and neuropathy following Vacor ingestion in man. *Arch Intern Med* 1979;139:185.

Cardiovascular Drugs

CHAPTER 26

Antidysrhythmic Drugs and Local Anesthetics

CLINICAL PRESENTATION

The onset of symptoms following acute oral antidysrhythmic overdose usually occurs within 4 hours and often occurs within 1 to 2 hours. However, drug absorption may continue for many hours following the ingestion of massive amounts, sustained-release preparations, or agents with anticholinergic effects. Delayed onset of toxicity is characteristic of amiodarone overdose (4).

Extracardiac manifestations of acute toxicity include dizziness, visual disturbances, psychosis, anticholinergic symptoms (disopyramide), hypoglycemia (disopyramide), hyperglycemia (encainide), hypokalemia, and hypersensitivity reactions (e.g., fever, rash, urticaria). Thrombocytopenia and a lupuslike syndrome (arthralgias, fever, myocarditis) with antinuclear antibodies have been well documented during chronic quinidine and procainamide therapy. The use of amiodarone is increasing despite the risk of numerous adverse effects, including corneal microdeposits, photosensitivity, hepatic dysfunction, myopathy, pulmonary fibrosis, hypo- or hyperthyroidism, and peripheral neuropathies.

Hypotension, bradycardia, central nervous system (CNS) depression, seizures, metabolic acidosis, and cardiovascular (CV) collapse can occur in severe poisoning. Seizures appear to be more prevalent with class IC drugs. Clinical effects associated with quinidine include seizures, immune-mediated hemolytic anemia, syncope, and cinchonism. Syncope is caused primarily by torsade de pointes but may also be associated with adrenergic blockade (orthostasis) or, rarely, idiosyncratic reactions. Cinchonism (see Chapter 20) is associated with chronic therapy and does not appear to be dose-related. Procainamide and quinidine predictably produce hypotension if given by too-rapid intravenous (IV) infusion. Death can result from refractory dysrhythmias or CV collapse.

Disturbances in cardiac conduction and rhythm are the electrocardiographic (ECG) hallmarks of antidysrhythmic poisoning. Excessive prolongation of the QT interval is almost always present in severe poisoning. With class IA agents, this results from prolongation of the QRS interval, whereas with class IC and class III agents, it is caused primarily by QRS and QT prolongation, respectively. In general, an increase of the QRS or QT interval by 25% is considered therapeutic, and widening by 50% or more suggests toxicity. The PR interval may also be prolonged, if there is sinus activity. Conduction disturbances and myocardial depression contribute to a host of supraventricular and ventricular dysrhythmias, including sinus bradycardia, atrioventricular dissociation, ventricular tachycardia (VT) or fibrillation, slow idioventricular rhythm, and asystole. Torsades de pointes is a triggered (early after depolarization) polymorphous VT resulting from excessive QT prolongation, most commonly associated with class IA and class III drugs (e.g., quinidine, amiodarone, dofetilide, ibutilide).

All antidysrhythmic drugs can aggravate existing dysrhythmias or induce new ones in patients being treated for supraventricular or ventricular dysrhythmias (i.e., antidysrhythmics may be proarrhythmic). The incidence of proarrhythmia is estimated at 5% to 20% and most often is associated with initiation of therapy or a dosage increase (6). The induction of dysrhythmias should always be suspected in patients on antidysrhythmic drugs who present with syncopal episodes.

The correlation of serum levels with clinical effects depends on previous exposure to the drug, the presence of heart disease, and the degree of absorption, metabolite formation, and elimination. In general, serum levels exceeding 7, 8, and 15 μg/mL for quinidine, disopyramide, and procainamide, respectively, should be considered toxic. Lower levels may result in toxicity in patients who ingest other CV agents. Patients on chronic therapy who take an acute overdose appear to be at greater risk for severe intoxication.

Although lidocaine toxicity can result from all routes of administration (1,7), it most frequently occurs during IV infusion (2,3). Manifestations involve the CNS and the CV system. CNS effects have been reported in up to 47% of patients receiving IV lidocaine. Initial symptoms, such as lightheadedness, dizziness, drowsiness, and euphoria, may occur at therapeutic concentrations. At higher concentrations, more serious symptoms include confusion, hearing loss, dysarthria, visual disturbances, ataxia, agitation, and muscle twitching, which may lead to seizures and coma. Seizures may be prolonged. CV toxicity is rare and usually occurs from rapidly administered IV infusions. When serum concentrations are >11 μg/mL, the refractory period is decreased, automaticity and myocardial contractility are depressed, and hypotension and bradycardia ensue. Conduction abnormalities include sinus bradycardia, atrioventricular block, complete heart block, and sinus arrest. Conduction defects are more common in patients with pre-existing bundle-branch abnormalities.

Mucosal absorption bypasses hepatic first-pass metabolism, making lidocaine more bioavailable than by intestinal absorption. Seizures have been reported several times in children following mucosal application of 2% to 4% viscous lidocaine (7). Therefore, topical or oral lidocaine for the treatment of painful oral lesions in children should be used cautiously, if at all.

Seizures have also occurred with lidocaine infiltration. During laceration repair, the total dose for infiltration of lidocaine without epinephrine should not exceed 4.5 mg/kg, nor should the dose exceed 7.0 mg/kg of lidocaine with epinephrine. The standard 1% lidocaine solutions contain 10 mg/mL of lidocaine; thus, the maximal volumes used for local infiltration in a 70-kg adult patient are roughly 30 mL without epinephrine and 50 mL with epinephrine. Fortunately, most wounds repaired in the emergency department (ED) only require small volumes of anesthetic.

The neurologic and cardiac toxicities of other local anesthetics are similar to that of lidocaine. For example, patients referred to the ED from dental offices often have CNS toxic effects as a result of injection of procaine or other local anesthetics for dental procedures. Several local anesthetics have also been reported to cause methemoglobinemia (see Chapter 40), especially benzocaine. Benzocaine is found in over-the-counter infant teething gels and adult oral anesthetics and is also used as a topical anesthetic to aid in endotracheal or gastric intubation and various endoscopic procedures.

DIFFERENTIAL DIAGNOSIS

Similar bradyarrhythmias may be caused by β-blockers, calcium antagonists, cholinergic agents (carbamate and organophosphate insecticides), digitalis, clonidine, lithium, and cyclic antidepressants. QRS and QT interval prolongation may result from poisoning with antihistamines, phenothiazines, cyclic antidepressants, lithium, magnesium, or potassium. Ventricular tachydysrhythmias may occur in poisoning with sympathomimetics.

Stimulants, hypoglycemia, hypoxia, and metabolic disturbances should be considered in the differential diagnosis of patients with CNS manifestations. Patients presenting with apprehension, anxiety, or other neurologic symptoms after very recent dental work, medical procedures on the upper aerodigestive tract, or wound repair would strongly suggest the possibility of local anesthetic toxicity. Methemoglobinemia should be considered in a patient who becomes cyanotic and is responding poorly to oxygen therapy after exposure to local anesthetics.

ED EVALUATION

The history should include the exact product, strength (immediate or sustained release), the amount ingested, the time ingested, and treatment before arrival. Any history of CV disease should be elucidated. Mechanisms for chronic toxicity, such as excessive dosing, exacerbation of congestive heart failure, or change in renal function, should be investigated.

The physical examination should focus on vital signs, with attention to CV stability and respiratory and neurologic status. A 12-lead ECG should be obtained as soon as possible to check for conduction blockade and dysrhythmias. In most patients with local anesthetic toxicity, an extensive metabolic workup will not be necessary. Patients suspected of having toxicity from antidysrhythmic drugs are often taking these agents therapeutically and often have significant underlying disease. For them, laboratory evaluation should include a blood glucose level; electrolyte analysis; blood urea nitrogen, creatinine, and magnesium measurement; liver function tests; and appropriate serum drug levels, if available. Chest radiography and arterial blood gas analysis are included for patients with depressed levels of consciousness or serious dysrhythmias. If suspected, venous or arterial blood should be sent for a methemoglobin level.

ED MANAGEMENT

Advanced life-support measures should be instituted as necessary. All patients suspected of antidysrhythmic drug toxicity should have an IV line, continuous cardiac monitoring, and pulse oximetry. Unstable patients must have close hemodynamic monitoring, supplemental oxygen, and airway management as indicated clinically. Acid-base, electrolyte, and magnesium derangements should be corrected. Potassium should be replaced cautiously, because hypokalemia may protect against cardiotoxicity as a result of quinidine (and possibly other agents). Seizures are treated with standard doses of IV benzodiazepines and barbiturates.

Hypotension is initially treated cautiously with IV normal saline. Infusions of sodium bicarbonate can reverse hypotension associated with class IA and IC drugs. Hypotension refractory to volume expansion may require the use of direct-acting vasopressors or inotropes (epinephrine, norepinephrine, dopamine), aortic balloon counterpulsation, or cardiopulmonary-bypass (CPB) pump support.

Sodium bicarbonate (2 mEq/kg IV bolus) should be given to patients with hypotension, prolonged QRS intervals, premature ventricular contractions (PVCs), and monomorphic VT if class I antidysrhythmic toxicity is suspected. Sodium bicarbonate has beneficial effects by increasing the serum-sodium level to help offset the sodium-channel antagonism, by increasing serum-protein binding (e.g., decreasing free drug) in a more alkalotic serum, and by driving drugs off the sodium channels. Symptomatic bradycardia or atrioventricular dissociation will probably require ventricular pacing, if there is inadequate response to atropine and sodium bicarbonate. Successful pacemaker capture may require concomitant epinephrine therapy (5).

After sodium bicarbonate, lidocaine is the drug of choice for ventricular ectopy (except, of course, for patients with lidocaine toxicity). Other antidysrhythmic drugs in the same class are contraindicated for treatment of dysrhythmias. Torsade de pointes usually responds to isoproterenol infusion (1–6 μg/min) and atrial or ventricular overdrive pacing; a heart rate of 150 beats/min is usually required. IV magnesium sulfate (1–4 g in several minutes to 1 hour, depending on the hemodynamic stability) may also be effective.

Once the patient has been stabilized, activated charcoal should be administered to decontaminate the gastrointestinal tract in patients with recent ingestions. Patients whose vital signs can be supported during endogenous drug elimination usually recover fully. Efforts to enhance elimination of these compounds have had variable success. Patients should be adequately hydrated to maintain renal perfusion. In the presence of renal failure, hemodialysis can increase the clearance of N-acetylprocainamide fourfold and that of procainamide twofold.

CRITICAL INTERVENTIONS

- Establish IV access, initiate cardiac monitoring, and obtain a 12-lead ECG on patients with potential toxicity from antidysrhythmic agents or local anesthetics.
- Administer sodium bicarbonate to patients with hypotension, prolonged QRS intervals, PVCs, and monomorphic VT as a result of class I antidysrhythmic poisoning.
- Administer magnesium sulfate IV and induce sinus tachycardia with isoproterenol or overdrive pacing in patients with torsade de pointes.

DISPOSITION

Patients with local anesthetic exposures can be discharged once free of neurologic and cardiac toxic effects, often within just a few hours. Those with persistent CNS symptoms or an abnormal ECG should be admitted to a monitored setting.

Patients who remain asymptomatic following antidysrhythmic agent ingestions and have a normal ECG after 6 hours of observation can usually be safely discharged. A 12-hour observation period is recommended if a sustained-release preparation is involved. Patients with amiodarone overdose should be admitted for prolonged observation. Patients who are symptomatic or exhibit ECG evidence of cardiotoxicity from either acute or chronic intoxication need admission to a monitored bed. Those patients with CV instability should be admitted to an intensive care unit. Patients with severe toxicity should be admitted to a facility with CPB and aortic balloon counterpulsation capabilities. Patients presenting after intentional overdose should undergo psychiatric evaluation before discharge.

COMMON PITFALLS

- Failure to appreciate that severe toxicity can result from therapeutic doses of antidysrhythmic agents
- Failure to consider the possibility of drug-induced dysrhythmias as a cause of syncope and weakness in patients taking antidysrhythmic agents
- Failure to appreciate that drug-induced dysrhythmias may resemble the ones for which the drug was prescribed; thus, drug levels should be checked before further drug treatment
- Failure to check the dose and concentration of local anesthetic solutions and to adhere to recommended dosing guidelines
- Failure to perform cardiac monitoring on patients receiving IV regional local anesthetics and large doses of local anesthetics by infiltration
- Failure to appreciate that local anesthetics can cause both CNS excitation and depression
- Failure to warn patients and parents of children that multiple doses of oral viscous lidocaine can be toxic and that the preparation should not be swallowed

ICD 9

968.2 Poisoning by surface (topical) and infiltration anesthetics
972.0 Poisoning by cardiac rhythm regulators

REFERENCES

1. Alfaro SN, Leicht MJ, Skiendzielewski JJ. Lidocaine toxicity following subcutaneous administration. *Ann Emerg Med* 1984;13:465.
2. Brown DL, Skiendzielewski JJ. Lidocaine toxicity. *Ann Emerg Med* 1980;9:627.
3. Bryant CA, Hoffman JR, Nichtes LS. Pitfalls and perils of intravenous lidocaine. *West J Med* 1983;139:528.
4. Goddard CJR, Whorwell PJ. Amiodarone overdose and its management. *Br J Clin Pharmacol* 1989;43:184.
5. Kerns W, English B, Ford M. Propafenone overdose. *Ann Emerg Med* 1994;24:98–103.
6. McCollam PL, Parker RB, Beckman KJ, et al. Proarrhythmia: a paradoxic response to antiarrhythmic agents. *Pharmacotherapy* 1989;9:144.
7. Mofenson HC, Caraccio TR, Miller H, et al. Lidocaine toxicity from topical mucosal application. *Clin Pediatr (Phila)* 1983;22:190.

CHAPTER 27

Centrally Acting Antihypertensive Agents

CLINICAL PRESENTATION

Signs and symptoms of toxicity of the centrally acting antihypertensive agents are similar, usually occur within 30 to 60 minutes after ingestion, and consist of bradycardia, respiratory depression, lethargy, coma, and miosis. Hypotension, hypothermia, and hyporeflexia are common symptoms of serious toxicity and may sometimes be delayed by several hours.

In adults, significant clinical toxicity can occur after the ingestion of 1 to 2 mg of clonidine. Children may develop serious toxicity after the ingestion of a single adult therapeutic dose of clonidine (0.1 to 0.3 mg) (8). Toxicity does not correlate well with the amount ingested, and a specific lethal dose has not been determined.

Intermittent apnea, responsive to physical or auditory stimuli, has been noted in children, and respiratory failure requiring mechanical ventilation has been reported. Clonidine interacts with other central nervous system (CNS) depressants, and the concomitant ingestion of these substances can aggravate CNS depression and contribute to coma.

Hypertension may be seen transiently in the initial phase of clonidine or methyldopa overdose. This elevation of blood pressure resolves spontaneously and is quickly and precipitously followed by hypotension. Hypertensive crisis, seizure, and anterior myocardial infarction occurred after an accidental administration of 12.24 mg of subcutaneous clonidine (3).

Adverse effects of maintenance therapy with clonidine include sedation and dry mouth, attributed to its relative affinity for central α_2-adrenergic receptors instead of imidazoline-I_1 receptors (7). Orthostatic hypotension, fatigue, sedation, constipation, sexual dysfunction, and dizziness can occur. In children, maintenance therapy has caused rare bradycardia and heart block (2), and alternative antihypertensive agents may be safer options in patients with sinus node or atrioventricular conduction abnormalities. Skin reactions including erythema, vesiculation, and induration have been associated with transdermal patch application.

The clonidine withdrawal syndrome is characterized by symptoms consistent with excessive sympathetic autonomic activity including rebound hypertension, tachycardia, tremulousness, insomnia, anxiety, sweating, and palpitations (5,6). Withdrawal can occur after the abrupt cessation of chronic clonidine therapy, especially after doses of >1.0 mg/d (5). A case report of abrupt clonidine withdrawal in an elderly female was associated with accelerated hypertension, tachycardia, and myocardial infarction within 24 hours (6).

Overdose with the other centrally acting antihypertensive agents is uncommon, but symptoms are similar to clonidine overdose, including early transient blood pressure elevations, drowsiness, miosis, respiratory depression, hypothermia, and hypotension (5).

Adverse effects of maintenance therapy with guanabenz and guanfacine are similar to those of clonidine. Adverse effects associated with methyldopa include drowsiness, neuropsychiatric abnormalities, dry mouth and nasal congestion. Depression occurs more frequently in association with methyldopa than with other antihypertensive agents, especially in patients with pre-existing depression (4). A positive direct Coombs test develops in 10% to 20% of patients taking methyldopa, but hemolysis is seldom a clinical problem. Hypersensitivity hepatitis occurs in 6% of patients using methyldopa (5). A rare parkinsonian syndrome has been associated with methyldopa use. Fatigue, sedation, and depression have been reported with reserpine therapy. Signs and symptoms of guanabenz, guanfacine, methyldopa, and reserpine withdrawal are similar to, but less pronounced than, those of clonidine withdrawal.

The adverse effect profiles of moxonidine and rilmenidine are similar to those of clonidine (dry mouth and dizziness), but the incidence of adverse effects is less, presumably because of their greater selectivity for central imidazoline-I_1 receptors compared to α_2-adrenergic receptors.

DIFFERENTIAL DIAGNOSIS

The presenting symptoms of poisoning with the centrally acting antihypertensive agents may be clinically indistinguishable from toxicity caused by other α_2-adrenergic and imidazoline-receptor agonists such as naphazoline, oxymetazoline, tetrahydrozoline, and xylometazoline. These imidazoline derivatives are common components of nasal-decongestant and topical ophthalmic preparations.

Because of the constellation of miosis, altered mental status, and respiratory depression, toxicity is often confused with that of opioid overdose. Centrally acting antihypertensive-agent toxicity may also resemble that caused by overdose of sedative-hypnotics, β-adrenergic antagonists, calcium-channel blockers, and digitalis. Hypoglycemia, sepsis, hypothermia, cerebrovascular accident, and head trauma should also be considered in the differential diagnosis.

ED EVALUATION

The evaluation of patients with known or suspected centrally acting antihypertensive- agent overdose includes continuous assessment of airway maintenance, ventilation and cardiovascular status, including continuous electrocardiographic monitoring, and an evaluation to rule out concomitant trauma or nondrug related medical abnormalities.

The diagnosis of poisoning is based on the history and clinical findings. There are no specific laboratory or clinical tests of diagnostic value. These agents are not detected on routine drugs of abuse screens. Quantitative drug levels are unavailable in the acute clinical setting and are of no value in management. Radiographic imaging, routine laboratory tests, and toxicologic analysis are useful only to rule out or confirm concomitant pathology.

ED MANAGEMENT

Prehospital care is supportive and consists of continuous electrocardiographic monitoring and maintenance of intravenous access. The routine administration of naloxone and evaluation or treatment for hypoglycemia are appropriate in symptomatic patients. Gastric lavage is of no benefit in this setting, and activated charcoal is the preferred method of gastrointestinal decontamination if warranted. In the case of clonidine transdermal patch ingestion, there may be a role for whole bowel irrigation.

Treatment of centrally acting antihypertensive agent overdose is primarily supportive and symptomatic. Respiratory depression and periodic apnea may require tracheal intubation and assisted ventilation. Bradycardia usually reverses with intravenous atropine, repeated based on heart rate and blood pressure response. Dopamine, epinephrine, and cardiac pacing are of theoretical benefit, but their use in clonidine poisoning has not been described. Hypotension usually responds to crystalloid infusion. Occasionally, vasopressors, such as dopamine and norepinephrine, are required. In the unusual case in which transient hypertension occurs, aggressive antihypertensive treatment should be avoided because of the potential for subsequent serious and prolonged hypotension (1). Elevated blood pressure usually requires only observation, although occasionally a short-acting titratable antihypertensive such as nitroprusside may be warranted. Hypothermia and coma are treated with supportive care. Clinical recovery is usually noted within 24 to 48 hours. Hemodialysis, charcoal hemoperfusion, and forced diuresis are of no proven value. Because clonidine is excreted unchanged in the urine, adequate urine output should be assured. Antacid therapy has been recommended to counter hyperchlorhydria during reserpine overdose.

There are no proven antidotes for centrally acting antihypertensive agent overdose. Naloxone has been used to reverse lethargy and respiratory depression associated with clonidine, but the response is inconsistent. The occasional anecdotal improvement in mental status and hemodynamic parameters has been explained by the association between central α_2-adrenergic receptors and opioid interneurons in the medulla. Naloxone's use is acceptable as a therapeutic trial in patients with depressed mental status. The optimal dose of naloxone in this setting is unknown, but doses similar to those used for opioid poisoning have been suggested. Both hypertension and hypotension have been temporally associated with the use of naloxone after clonidine overdose, so patients who are given naloxone should be closely observed for hemodynamic deterioration and recurrent respiratory depression.

Theoretically, α-adrenergic antagonists should reverse some of the toxicity associated with this overdose. Tolazoline's purported efficacy as an antidote is based on sporadic case reports, and it has potentially serious adverse effects (hypotension, tachycardia, and dysrhythmia). Tolazoline's use is not recommended. Yohimbine, a centrally acting α_2-adrenergic antagonist, has been suggested as a possible antidote for clonidine overdose, but there is little evidence and no clinical guidelines to support its use.

The acute symptoms of clonidine withdrawal have been treated with labetalol for control of elevated blood pressure and diazepam for tremor and agitation (6). The clonidine withdrawal syndrome is best treated by the reinstitution of clonidine therapy and tapering of the dose in 5 to 10 days. A similar approach can be used in the treatment of withdrawal from other similar agents.

CRITICAL INTERVENTIONS

- Establish intravenous access, and institute continuous respiratory and cardiac monitoring in patients with acute overdose or acute withdrawal.
- Keep advanced life-support airway equipment and cardiovascular drugs readily available.

DISPOSITION

Patients who remain asymptomatic 6 hours after an ingestion and who have normal vital signs may be discharged from the emergency department with appropriate psychiatric or social service follow-up. Symptomatic patients require admission to a medical unit capable of continuous cardiac and respiratory monitoring. There is no known cyclical nature to clonidine overdose, and improvement is not followed by relapse. Patients may be safely transferred to another facility with advanced life-support measures during transport.

COMMON PITFALLS

- Failure to appreciate that clonidine poisoning may result in severe CNS, respiratory, and cardiovascular depression
- Misdiagnosis of clonidine poisoning as narcotic overdose because of the constellation of miosis, altered mental status, and respiratory depression
- Overly aggressive treatment of early, transient hypertension, especially with long-acting agents
- Reliance on unproved antidotes rather than supportive care in the treatment of toxicity
- Failure to consider the possibility of child abuse or attempted homicide in children with overdose and to address psychiatric issues in patients with suicide attempts

ICD 9

Poisoning by other antihypertensive agents

REFERENCES

1. Campbell BC, Reid JL. Regimen for the control of blood pressure and symptoms during clonidine withdrawal. *Int J Clin Pharmacol Res* 1985;5:215.
2. Cantwell DP, Swanson J, Connor DF. Case study: adverse response to clonidine. *J Am Acad Child Adolesc Psychiatry* 1997;36(4):539–544.
3. Frye CB, Vance MA. Hypertensive crisis and myocardial infarction following massive clonidine overdose. *Ann Pharmacother* 2000;34(5):611–615.
4. Keller S, Frishman WH, Epstein J. Neuropsychiatric manifestations of cardiovascular drug therapy. *Heart Dis* 1999;1:241–254.
5. Sica DA. Centrally acting antihypertensive agents: an update. *J Clin Hypertens* 2007;9:399–405.
6. Simic J, Kishineff S, Goldberg R, et al. Acute myocardial infarction as a complication of clonidine withdrawal. *J Emerg Med* 2003;25:399–402.
7. Szabo B. Imidazoline antihypertensive drugs: a critical review on their mechanism of action. *Pharm Therap* 2002;93:1–35.
8. Wiley J, Wiley C, Torrey S, et al. Clonidine poisoning in young children. *J Pediatr* 1990;116:654.

Beta Blockers

PRE-HOSPITAL CONSIDERATIONS

- Transport pills and pill bottles when an overdose is suspected.

CLINICAL PRESENTATION

Most β-blocker overdoses are relatively minor and do not result in significant toxicity, particularly in the pediatric population (1,7); however, large doses or the combination of a β-blocker with another cardioactive medication (e.g., calcium channel blockers) can result in significant morbidity and mortality (7). Patients who remain asymptomatic for 6 hours from the time of ingestion are unlikely to develop toxicity (7,12) unless sotalol or an extended-release preparation was ingested. Sotalol has produced symptoms, QT prolongation, and other dysrhythmias up to 20 hours from the time of ingestion (3). With extended-release preparations, prolonged and erratic absorption may result in delayed toxicity.

Bradycardia and hypotension are the most common effects after overdose (1). Nausea and vomiting can occur. The skin may be pale and clammy. Lethargy and decreased mental status may result from hypoperfusion of the central nervous system. Hypoperfusion can lead to myocardial infarction, mesenteric ischemia, renal insufficiency, and stroke.

Highly lipophilic agents and those with membrane-stabilizing effects can cause altered mental status in the face of a normal blood pressure. Delirium, coma, and seizures may occur in severe poisoning.

The electrocardiogram (ECG) may reveal atrioventricular (AV) nodal dysfunction with PR interval prolongation and AV block (6). If the sinoatrial node is affected, sinus bradycardia may progress to sinus pauses or arrest. Negative inotropic effects add to cardiotoxicity, particularly with β-blockers that have membrane-stabilizing activity (MSA) (12). β-Blockers that have MSA can cause delayed depolarization with QRS prolongation and ventricular tachydysrhythmias (6,12). Sotalol is unique in that it also blocks delayed rectifier potassium channels, which results in delayed repolarization with QT prolongation, and can cause torsade de pointes (polymorphic) ventricular tachycardia and other lethal ventricular dysrhythmias (3).

In overdose, all β-blockers can cause β_2-antagonism, resulting in broncho-spasm. This scenario may be more prominent and dangerous in patients with a history of asthma or chronic obstructive pulmonary disease (1). Hypoglycemia and hyperkalemia are distinct metabolic derangements that result from β-receptor blockade, although they are usually mild and not clinically significant (1). Hypoglycemia may be more common in children.

DIFFERENTIAL DIAGNOSIS

Diseases that cause bradycardia include sick sinus syndrome, inferior wall myocardial infarction, hypothermia, severe sepsis, and carotid sinus hypersensitivity. Toxic causes include calcium channel blockers, cardiac glycosides, cholinergic agents, α_2-agonists, opioids, and sedative–hypnotics.

Like β-blockers, diltiazem and verapamil have strong negative inotropic and chronotropic effects. Dihydropyridine calcium channel blockers (e.g., nifedipine, nimodipine, and amlodipine) more typically cause reflex tachycardia in response to vasodilation and hypotension. In severe overdose, bradycardia is possible. Unlike β-blocker overdose, the mental status is often surprisingly normal. Also, in contrast to β-blockers, calcium channel blockers cause hyperglycemia rather than hypoglycemia.

Cardiac glycoside (e.g., digoxin) poisoning usually does not cause hypotension until a nonperfusable dysrhythmia occurs. Additionally, cardiac glycoside overdose induces characteristic ECG patterns different from β-blocker overdose. Vomiting is a more predominant feature in acute exposures. Like β blockers, cardiac glycosides can cause hyperkalemia, confusion, and lethargy.

Cholinergic agents (e.g., organophosphorus insecticides) cause diarrhea, lacrimation, urination, miosis, and vomiting along with bradycardia, bronchorrhea, and bronchoconstriction. Overdose with opioids, sedative hypnotics, and α_2-agonists may lead to mild bradycardia and hypotension associated with a depressed mental status, but cardiac conduction disturbances are not usually seen.

ED EVALUATION

The history should include the time and amount of drug(s) taken, treatment in the field (if any), the time of onset and nature of symptoms, known medical or psychiatric problems, and current drug therapy. Determining whether the β-blocker was a sustained-release preparation or whether there were any coingestants with cardiovascular effects is particularly important.

The physical examination should focus on the vital signs, cardiopulmonary system, and neurologic status. A 12-lead ECG should be a priority, along with continuous cardiac monitoring. A fingerstick or serum glucose concentration should be obtained, particularly in patients with an abnormal mental status. Arterial blood gases, chemistry panel, complete blood count, toxicology testing, and chest radiograph should be obtained when clinically indicated.

ED MANAGEMENT

Advanced cardiac life support measures should be instituted as needed. Once the airway, breathing, and circulation have been stabilized, gastrointestinal decontamination should be considered. Activated charcoal is the preferred method if ingestion occurred within 1 hour. If a sustained-release preparation has been ingested, activated charcoal or whole-bowel irrigation should be considered even later than an hour after ingestion. Precautions against aspiration must be considered with either method of gastrointestinal decontamination.

Should the patient become bradycardic and/or hypotensive, a stepwise approach is recommended, in which interventions, each employed to a maximal degree, are successively applied and the hemodynamic response assessed. In severely poisoned patients, multiple therapies must be instituted and maintained simultaneously. Patients with bradycardia need only close monitoring if the blood pressure is normal. Hypotension can initially be treated with intravenous fluids. If bradycardia is also present, atropine, 1 mg intravenously (0.02 mg/kg; minimum dose, 0.1 mg in children), repeated in 5 minutes as necessary, can be given with the expectation that this will be ineffective if the diagnosis is β-blocker overdose.

Glucagon (5 mg intravenously over 5 minutes; 50–100 μg/kg in children) may be effective for hypotension, even in the absence of bradycardia. If there is no effect after 10 to 15 minutes, the dose should be repeated. Patients who respond should be given an infusion of glucagon at a rate of 1 to 5 mg/h (50 μg/kg/h in children). Glucagon bypasses the β-blockade by activating a G protein bound to adenylate cyclase and activating the cascade indirectly to increase intracellular cAMP (Fig. 28-1). Glucagon often causes vomiting. Animal studies show that it has a positive chronotropic effect in β-blocker overdose but has minimal effect on mean arterial pressure (15). Although there are no human controlled trials, glucagon is widely accepted as effective in humans (1).

Intravenous calcium has been shown to assist with inotropy in animal β-blocker toxicity (8) and has been successful in reversing hypotension in humans (2,11). The dose is the same as for calcium channel blocker poisoning (see Chapter 29, "Calcium Channel Antagonists"). Vasopressors are often necessary. Although there are no human data to state whether one pressor is more efficacious than the other, theoretically isoproterenol would be the ideal agent. Unfortunately, this pressor can exacerbate hypotension and dysrhythmia, and there is minimal clinical experience with this agent. Dobutamine, epinephrine, and dopamine have all been used, but the dose is often much higher than what is traditionally used (1). If a vasopressor must be added to the treatment regimen, invasive cardiac monitoring or echocardiography should be performed to identify the agent that brings the appropriate response and to titrate to the desired effect, especially if the patient ingested other cardioactive drugs.

If the patient requires vasopressors, hyperinsulinemia-euglycemia (insulin and glucose) therapy should be considered and has been found anecdotally to be effective (5,10). The same protocol as in calcium channel blocker poisoning (see Chapter 29, "Calcium Channel Antagonists") should be used. In canine propranolol poisoning, this therapy was superior to glucagon and epinephrine (4). Hyperinsulinemia-euglycemia therapy may work by maximizing myocardial glucose utilization, augmentating cytosolic calcium concentrations, or possibly through a direct inotropic effect (4). The response may be delayed 15 to 60 minutes, so other therapies must be continued.

A phosphodiesterase inhibitor such as amrinone may also be effective (see Fig. 28-1) This drug has a propensity to cause vasodilation, is difficult to titrate, and often does not assist with the negative chronotropy seen in β-blocker exposure (15). Hence, it should be used only in conjunction with other treatments.

Should pharmacologic therapy be ineffective, invasive procedures such as cardiac pacing, artificial circulatory assistance, and extracorporeal drug removal should be considered. Intravenous cardiac pacing can be used to treat bradycardia; however, little improvement in cardiac output and difficulty with capture should be expected. Some authors have reported a decrease in blood pressure, which may be caused by loss of atrial contraction and/or impaired ventricular relaxation. Intra-aortic balloon pump counterpulsation and partial or complete cardiac bypass pump support have been utilized in severe poisoning (9). Hemodialysis has been used with apparent success in the treatment of atenolol and sotalol overdose; charcoal hemoperfusion might be effective for removing water-soluble

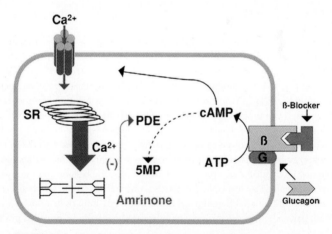

FIGURE 28.1.   The effects of amrinone and glucagon on cAMP. Extracellular Ca^{2+} influx will cause the SR (sarcoplasmic reticulum) to release Ca^{2+} exponentially to bind the excitation-contraction apparatus, made of actin and myosin filaments. cAMP increases intracellular Ca^{2+} and is created by an adenylate cyclase that is part of the β receptor and broken down by PDE (phosphodiesterase). Glucagon can activate the G protein, bypass the β receptor if blocked, and increase cAMP. Amrinone inhibits PDE, thus also increasing cAMP. (Figure by Walter Barrueto.)

β-blockers that have a low volume of distribution like atenolol and acebutolol (13,14). However, patients who would benefit from extracorporeal elimination measures are already hypotensive, making these procedures technically difficult and potentially hazardous. Continuous veno-venous hemodialysis is another alternative, but it has never been studied and is time consuming.

In patients with sotalol poisoning, hypokalemia and hypomagnesemia should be corrected. The treatment of recurrent torsade de pointes should include overdrive pacing and magnesium infusions (3). Bradycardia and hypotension are treated the same as with other β-blockers.

CRITICAL INTERVENTIONS

- Treat with intravenous fluids for hypotension and atropine for bradycardia.
- If hypotension and bradycardia persist, administer glucagon, calcium, vasopressors.
- Consider hyperinsulinemia-euglycemia therapy if the patient remains unstable.
- Consider invasive measures such as transvenous pacing, intra-aortic balloon pump counterpulsations, or extracorporeal circulatory support measures for patients who have not responded to other treatment modalities.
- Realize that certain β-blockers (e.g., atenolol, sotalol) are amenable to hemodialysis or hemoperfusion.

DISPOSITION

Patients with β-blocker ingestions who remain or become asymptomatic 6 hours after ingestion can be discharged or medically cleared for a psychiatric disposition. If sotalol or a sustained-release preparation was ingested, a 12- to 24-hour observation period is recommended. Patients with abnormal vital signs, mental status, or ECG findings require continuous cardiac monitoring and frequent vital signs to assess the progression of toxicity. This usually necessitates admission to an intensive care unit. The hospital's supply of glucagon should be ascertained, as many pharmacies are not prepared to administer the large doses required to treat β-blocker exposures. Transfer of the patient to a tertiary care facility should be considered in cases of severe poisoning where intraaortic balloon pump or other advanced therapies are available. Psychiatric consultation should be obtained for patients with intentional ingestions prior to discharge. Education in poison prevention, particularly in the pediatric population, should also be provided prior to discharge.

COMMON PITFALLS

- Failure to determine whether the drug ingested was an immediate- or extended-release formulation, potentially leading to inappropriate treatment and disposition decisions
- Failure to check a fingerstick blood glucose as β-blockers can cause hypoglycemia

- Lack of appreciation that β-blockers with membrane stabilizing activity can cause delayed depolarization, cardiac conduction disturbances (QRS prolongation), and ventricular tachyarrhythmias
- Failure to anticipate seizures with lipophilic β-blockers such as propranolol
- Failure to appreciate that sotalol has potassium channel-blocking effects and can cause a prolonged QT interval and torsades de pointes
- Failure to appreciate and plan for the fact that severe poisonings are likely to require invasive monitoring, multiple pharmacological treatments, and mechanical hemodynamic support

ICD 9

971.3 Poisoning by sympatholytics (antiadrenergics)

REFERENCES

1. Bailey B. Glucagon in β-blocker and calcium channel blocker overdoses: a systematic review. *J Toxicol Clin Toxicol* 2003;41:595–602.
2. Brimacombe JR, Scully M, Swainston R. Propranolol overdose: a dramatic response to calcium chloride. *Med J Aust* 1991;155:267–268.
3. Hohnloser SH, Woosley RL. Sotalol. *N Engl J Med* 1994;331:31–38.
4. Kerns W, Schroeder D, Williams C, et al. Insulin improves survival in a canine model of acute [beta]-blocker toxicity. *Ann Emerg Med* 1997;29:748–757.
5. Levine M, Boyer EW, Pozner CN, et al. Assessment of hyperglycemia after calcium channel blocker overdoses involving diltiazem or verapamil. *Crit Care Med* 2007;35(9):2071–2075.
6. Love JN, Enlow B, Howell JM, et al. Electrocardiographic changes associated with β-blocker toxicity. *Ann Emerg Med* 2002;40:603–610.
7. Love JN, Howell HM, Litovitz TL, et al. Acute beta blocker overdose: factors associated with the development of cardiovascular morbidity. *J Toxicol Clin Toxicol* 2000;38:275–281.
8. Love JN, Hanfling D, Howell JM. Hemodynamic effects of calcium chloride in a canine model of acute propranolol intoxication. *Ann Emerg Med* 1996;28:1–6.
9. McVey FK, Cork CF. Extracorporeal circulation in the management of massive propranolol overdose. *Anaesthesia* 1991;46:744–746.
10. Mégarbane B, Karyo S, Baud FJ. The role of insulin and glucose (hyperinsulinaemia/euglycaemia) therapy in acute calcium channel antagonist and beta-blocker poisoning. *Toxicol Rev* 2004;23(4):215–222.
11. Pertoldi F, D'Orlando L, Mercante WP. Electromechanical dissociation 48 hours after atenolol overdose: usefulness of calcium chloride. *Ann Emerg Med* 1998;31:777–781.
12. Reith DM, Dawson AH, Epid D, et al. Relative toxicity of beta blockers in overdose. *J Toxicol Clin Toxicol* 1996;34:273–278.
13. Rooney M, Massey KL, Jamali F, et al. Acebutolol overdose treated with hemodialysis and extracorporeal membrane oxygenation. *J Clin Pharmacol* 1996;36:760–763.
14. Saitz R, Williams BW, Farber HW. Atenolol-induced cardiovascular collapse treated with hemodialysis. *Crit Care Med* 1991;19:116–119.
15. Sato S, Tsuji MH, Okubo N, et al. Milrinone versus glucagon: comparative hemodynamic effects in canine propranolol poisoning. *J Toxicol Clin Toxicol* 1994;32:277–289.

CHAPTER 29

Calcium Channel Antagonists

PRE-HOSPITAL CONSIDERATIONS
- Transport pills and pill bottles to the emergency department.
- Administer calcium to bradycardic/unstable patients with confirmed calcium channel antagonist overdose.

CLINICAL PRESENTATION

Signs and symptoms of calcium channel antagonist (CCA) toxicity include hypotension, bradycardia, thready pulse, and peripheral cyanosis. Reflex tachycardia has been reported, especially with dihydropyridine ingestion. Inadequate perfusion may result in myocardial, cerebral, renal, and bowel ischemia or infarction. In severe cases, coma, seizures, and respiratory distress associated with cardiogenic and noncardiogenic pulmonary edema are described. The electrocardiogram (ECG) often shows decreased rate and first-, second-, or even third-degree atrioventricular (AV) block and may have changes indicative of ischemia or infarction (5; Fig. 29-1). QT-prolongation and torsades de pointes may be noted with bepridil ingestion. Chest radiography may show pulmonary edema. Laboratory abnormalities include metabolic acidosis and hyperglycemia. Serum drug levels are not readily available and are not useful in the management of these patients. Toxic effects typically last 24 to 36 hours but may be longer with bepridil, amlodipine, and sustained-release preparations.

DIFFERENTIAL DIAGNOSIS

Myocardial infarction and overdose of β-adrenergic antagonists, cardiac glycosides, clonidine, guanabenz, imidazolines, angiotensin converting enzyme inhibitors, cholinergic agents (nicotine, organophosphate and carbamate insecticides, and agents to treat myasthenia gravis), tricyclic antidepressants, alpha-methyldopa, and veratrum alkaloids may present similarly to those with CCA ingestion. β-adrenergic blocking agents are more likely to cause hypoglycemia, and CCAs are more likely to cause hyperglycemia. With cholinergic agents, salivation, nausea, vomiting, diarrhea, and weakness dominate the presentation. Tricyclic antidepressant (TCA) overdosage infrequently presents with heart block and bradycardia. Although both TCA and CCA ingestions may result in prolonged QRS complexes

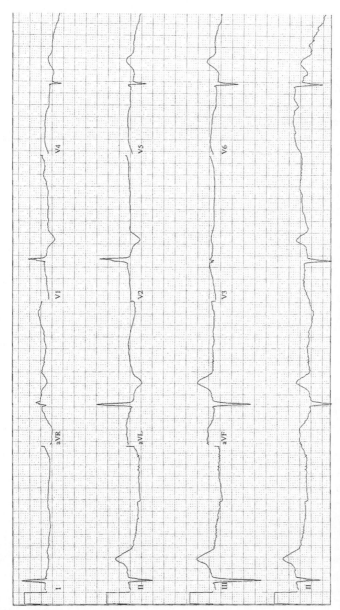

FIGURE 29.1. Initial electrocardiogram of a patient presenting after sustained-release verapamil ingestion. Findings include complete heart block with severe bradycardia and repolarization abnormalities.

(the latter as a result of ventricular escape rhythms), TCA-intoxicated patients often manifest evidence of antimuscarinic toxidrome and central nervous system (CNS) depression in normotensive or hypertensive patients.

ED EVALUATION

The history should include time of ingestion and identification of other substances ingested or available to the patient. Physical examination should focus on cardiopulmonary and CNS status. All patients should have cardiac monitoring, an ECG, and frequent monitoring of blood pressure. Those with symptoms, abnormal vital signs, or an abnormal ECG should have arterial blood gas analysis and determination of serum electrolytes, glucose, blood urea nitrogen, and creatinine. Continuous peripheral and pulmonary artery pressure monitoring may be necessary in patients with hemodynamic compromise.

ED MANAGEMENT

Supportive care, activated charcoal, and advanced life-support measures should be initiated as necessary. Intravenous access should be established in all patients, with whole-bowel irrigation recommended for ingestions of sustained-release preparations.

Mild hypotension may respond to a fluid challenge with 1 to 2 liters of saline solution (10–20 mL/kg in children). When bradycardia, with or without AV block, is also present, atropine (1.0 mg IV, 0.02 mg/kg in children) can be tried. Response is infrequent but may be improved after calcium administration (1,5). Patients with hypotension and concomitant symptomatic bradycardia or conduction defects should receive either calcium chloride (1 g IV slow push; 10–20 mg/kg in children) or calcium gluconate (3 g IV slow push; 30–60 mg/kg in children). This dose may be repeated every 5 to 15 minutes up to three times in patients who show incomplete, transient, or absent response (2). Calcium chloride extravasation can result in severe tissue damage, so limit calcium chloride use to central venous administration whenever possible. Owing to the short-lived effects of intravenous calcium, a continuous infusion at a rate of 0.2 to 0.4 cc/kg/h (10% calcium chloride) or 0.6 to 1.2 cc/kg/h (10% calcium gluconate) may be used to support heart rate and blood pressure in patients who respond to an initial bolus (6). Although calcium is frequently ineffective, proponents argue that this is a result of inadequate dosing. Doubling of serum calcium concentration was associated with significant hemodynamic improvement in both animal models and human cases. An ionized calcium of 2 mmol/L has been suggested as a target concentration (3). Calcium levels should be monitored in patients receiving more than two doses, but very high serum calcium levels are not a reason to discontinue treatment.

Patients who fail to respond to these therapies should receive early, aggressive hyperinsulinemia-euglycemia (HIE) therapy (see later discussion) and pressor therapy.

Insulin, used as part of HIE therapy, improves hemodynamics and survival and has reversed catecholamine-unresponsive shock in both animals and in case reports (6,7,9). Insulin has positive inotropic effects in conditions of myocardial stress without increasing myocardial oxygenation demand. During myocardial stress, the metabolism of myocardial cells is shifted away from fatty acid oxidation, toward carbohydrate dependence, improving the efficiency of energy biomechanics. In cases of severe CCA toxicity, hyperglycemia is frequently noted. The etiology is multifactorial, reflecting both impaired insulin release and peripheral resistance (4). The net result is that the CCA-intoxicated myocardium is further impaired secondary to limited cellular glucose uptake at a time of glucose dependence and subsequent transition back to less-desirable fatty acid metabolism. HIE is believed to reverse this impaired energy utilization state and improve myocardial glucose utilization. HIE also likely increases intracellular calcium concentrations, although this may cause only a small improvement. The failure of catecholamines and glucagon, despite initial transient improvement, may reflect catecholamine-induced increased myocardial oxygen demand and promotion of fatty acid metabolism and ketosis (7).

Although strong evidence-based data are lacking, most toxicologists advocate the early, aggressive use of HIE therapy in any patient who shows inadequate response after initial fluid resuscitation, atropine, and calcium administration. A bolus of 1.0 IU/kg regular insulin is recommended, followed by an infusion of 0.5 to 1.0 IU/kg/h, titrated to clinical effect (systolic blood pressure >90 mm Hg, heart rate >50/min). Patients with serum glucose levels <200 mg/dL should receive one 50-mL ampule of 50% dextrose (0.25 g/kg in children) followed by frequent glucose measurements and supplemental glucose as required. Owing to potential insulin-mediated effects on serum potassium, patients with serum potassium concentrations <2.5 mEq/L should receive 40 mEq of potassium (1 mEq/kg in children; maximum, 20–40 mEq/dose) as an oral supplement or IV potassium, 10 to 20 mEq (0.10–0.30 mEq/kg in children) administered over the course of 1 hour. Fluid and glucose support with D10½NS at 80% maintenance is recommended. Serum glucose should be checked every 20 minutes for the first hour and hourly thereafter. Serum potassium should be checked hourly during HIE therapy.

No single pressor agent has been consistently effective. Dopamine, dobutamine, norepinephrine, isoproterenol, alone or in combination, have been used with mixed success. Glucagon may also be of benefit for hypotension, but it should not be used until the effects of traditional pressors are optimized (1). Hemodynamically significant bradycardia or heart block unresponsive to atropine and calcium may respond to an infusion of glucagon or isoproterenol, but a pacemaker is often required (1,5). In a prospective study, electrical capture occurred in only 50% of patients (6; Fig. 29-2). Heart rate is improved more than blood pressure. Acidemia must be corrected, as it impairs the function of L-type voltage-operated calcium channels, enhances the toxic effects of some agents (e.g., verapamil), and decreases the efficacy of calcium. A swine

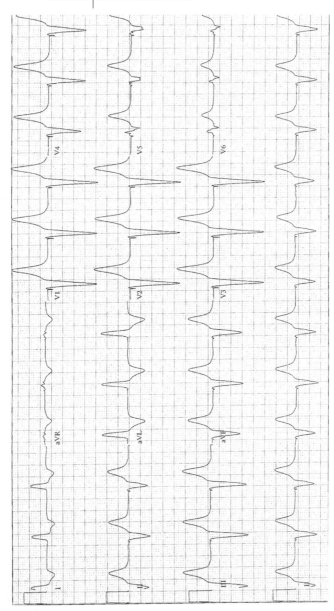

FIGURE 29.2. Follow-up electrocardiogram after emergent transvenous pacemaker placement. Note that electrical capture occurs in only 50% of patients and that blood pressure may not improve despite increased heart rate.

model of verapamil toxicity demonstrated improved myocardial contractility and cardiac output with sodium bicarbonate administration (8). In patients unresponsive to pharmacologic therapies, intra-aortic balloon counterpulsation and cardiopulmonary bypass have been successfully employed. The specific role of enhanced elimination, other than through gastrointestinal decontamination, has not been clearly defined. Based upon pharmacokinetic properties, extra-corporeal elimination would be expected to be of limited effectiveness. Full recovery can be expected unless prolonged shock has resulted in irreversible end-organ damage.

CRITICAL INTERVENTIONS

- Admit or observe asymptomatic patients with overdoses of sustained preparations for an extended period of time.
- Administer IV fluids, calcium, and atropine for hypotension and bradycardia.
- Initiate HIE therapy for hypotension unresponsive to fluids and calcium.
- Consider high doses of calcium, which may be needed for a clinical response.
- Consider early aggressive gastrointestinal decontamination, which is recommended owing to lack of consistently effective therapeutic interventions.

DISPOSITION

Asymptomatic patients should be observed for 4 to 6 hours after ingestion of standard formulations and 18 to 24 hours after ingestion of sustained-release ones. Those who remain asymptomatic may be discharged or referred for psychiatric evaluation. Symptomatic patients should be admitted to an intensive care unit. Transfer may be necessary if an intensive care unit bed is unavailable and should be arranged as soon as the ingestion is recognized, because CV performance may rapidly deteriorate. The patient should be transferred in an advanced life-support unit with an adequate supply of CV drugs on hand. A regional poison center or a toxicologist should be consulted if the physician is unfamiliar with the management of CCA overdose.

COMMON PITFALLS

- Failure to consider CCA poisoning in patients with hypotension, bradycardia, or AV block, particularly when hyperglycemia is present
- Failure to appreciate that ingestion of a single pill may be lethal in a toddler
- Failure to consider whole-bowel irrigation and multiple-dose charcoal for patients with overdoses of sustained preparations
- Failure to initiate aggressive HIE therapy in a timely manner

ICD9

972.4 Poisoning by coronary vasodilators

REFERENCES

1. Howarth DM, Dawson AH, Smith AJ, et al. Calcium channel blocking drug overdose: an Australian series. *Hum Exp Toxicol* 1994;13:161–166.
2. Isbister GK. Delayed asystolic cardiac arrest after diltiazem overdose: resuscitation with high dose intravenous calcium. *Emerg Med J* 2002;19:355–357.
3. Kline JA, Raymond RM, Schroeder JD, et al. The diabetogenic effects of acute verapamil poisoning. *Toxicol Appl Pharmacol* 1997;145:357–362.
4. Lam Y-M, Lau C. Continuous calcium chloride infusion for massive nifedipine overdose. *Chest* 2001; 119:1280–1282.
5. Ramoska EA, Spiller HA, Winter M, et al. A one-year evaluation of calcium channel blocker overdoses. Toxicity and treatment. *Ann Emerg Med* 1993;22:196–200.
6. Salhanick SD, Shannon MW. Management of calcium channel antagonist overdose. *Drug Saf* 2003; 26:65–79.
7. Shepherd G. Treatment of poisoning caused by β–adrenergic and calcium channel blockers. *Am J Health Syst Pharm* 2006;63:1828–1835.
8. Tanen DA, Ruha AM, Curry SC, et al. Hypertonic sodium bicarbonate is effective in the acute management of verapamil toxicity in a swine model. *Ann Emerg Med* 2000;36:547–553.
9. Yuan TH, Kerns WP II, Tomaszewski CA, et al. Insulin-glucose as adjunctive therapy for severe calcium channel antagonist poisoning. *J Toxicol Clin Toxicol* 1999;37:463–474.

CHAPTER 30

Cardiac Glycosides

CLINICAL PRESENTATION

Cardiac glycoside (CG) toxicity may occur in the acute or chronic setting. Acute toxicity occurs most often in a younger population as an accidental or intentional ingestion. In healthy adults, single acute doses of <5 mg of digoxin seldom cause toxicity. Fatal doses are almost always >10 mg. Chronic toxicity usually occurs in the elderly population. As a result of the narrow therapeutic range of digoxin, toxicity can occur with only two to three times the therapeutic dose in patients on chronic therapy.

Patients with acute digoxin toxicity will often present with nausea and vomiting. Chronic toxicity is more likely to present with central nervous system (CNS) findings, including confusion, lethargy, depression, fatigue, headache, paresthesias, weakness, scotomata, and disturbances of color vision, especially xanthopsia (yellow vision).

Virtually any dysrhythmia may develop as a result of toxicity, although rapid atrial fibrillation or atrial flutter are rare (Table 30.1). Premature ventricular contractions, either unifocal or multifocal, are most common. The three classically described dysrhythmias include paroxysmal atrial tachycardia with block (considered to be pathognomonic of digitalis toxicity), junctional (atrioventricular [AV]-nodal) tachycardia, and ventricular tachycardia (VT). The presence of any tachydysrhythmia with block (e.g., paroxysmal atrial tachycardia with block, atrial fibrillation with a regular ventricular response as a result of AV block with a junctional escape rhythm) is highly suggestive of CG toxicity. Any slowing of the ventricular response to atrial fibrillation in a patient on digoxin also suggests toxicity. AV-conduction blocks ranging from first degree to third degree may occur, although Mobitz type II is rare. Sinus bradycardia, from increased vagal tone, and other bradydysrhythmias are common. Hypotension suggests a hemodynamically significant dysrhythmia, loss of vasomotor regulation, or the presence of coingestant(s). Complications from inadequate perfusion include hypoxic seizures, encephalopathy, and acute renal tubular necrosis.

In 150 patients with acute ingestions, life-threatening complications were high-grade AV block (53%), refractory VT (46%), hyperkalemia (37%), and ventricular fibrillation (33%) (1). After acute overdose, the most common electrocardiographic (ECG) abnormalities are sinus bradycardia and varying degrees of AV

TABLE 30.1	**Common Digitalis-Induced Dysrhythmias**
Bradydysrhythmias	Tachydysrhythmias
Sinus exit block or sinus arrest	Atrial tachycardia with block
Sinus bradycardia	Junctional tachycardia
Atrioventricular nodal block first degree;	Ventricular premature beats
second degree type 1; third degree	Ventricular tachycardia, especially bidirectional
	Ventricular fibrillation

block; ventricular dysrhythmias are less frequently seen. Chronic intoxication is more commonly associated with ventricular dysrhythmias, atrial tachycardia, and junctional tachycardia. Hyperkalemia is common after acute overdose, whereas hypokalemia, probably related to concurrent diuretic use, is more common in chronic poisoning.

DIFFERENTIAL DIAGNOSIS

Intoxications that can cause CG-like bradydysrhythmias include those from class IB antidysrhythmics, baclofen, β-adrenergic blockers, calcium-channel antagonists, cholinergic agonists, cholinesterase inhibitors, clonidine, guanabenz, ingested imidazoline decongestants, and nicotine. CG-like tachydysrhythmias can be caused by poisoning with class IA, class IC, and class III antidysrhythmics, antihistamines, baclofen, cyclic antidepressants, fluoride, heavy metals, local anesthetics, meperidine, neuroleptics, propoxyphene, quinine and related antimalarials, and sympathomimetics. Plants causing similar cardiotoxicity include *Phoradendron tomentosum* (American mistletoe), *Remijia* sp, *Rhododendron* sp, *Schoenocaulon officinalis* (sabadilla), *Stylophorum diphyllun*, *Veratrum* sp (e.g., American hellebore), and *Zanthoxylum brachycanthum*. Worsening cardiomyopathy, congestive heart failure, CNS hemorrhage/ischemia, electrolyte abnormalities, myocardial ischemia/infarction, myocarditis, pericarditis, pheochromocytoma, pre-excitation syndromes, and thyroid dysfunction should also be considered in the differential diagnosis of CG-like cardiotoxicity.

Intoxications that can cause CG-like visual disturbances include carbon disulfide, ergot alkaloids, ethambutol, heavy metals, methanol, quinine and antimalarials, salicylates, and tamoxifen. The differential diagnosis of visual disturbances includes diseases such as cataracts, cerebrovascular disease, corneal disease, diabetes, glaucoma, macular degeneration, migraine, optic neuritis, retinal detachment, vasculitis, and vitreous hemorrhage.

ED EVALUATION

The history should include the amount, route, duration, and intent of exposure. Because CGs may be present in herbal supplements, the medication history should include herbal supplement use. The patient should be specifically examined for signs consistent with congestive heart failure and decreased peripheral perfusion. The patient should be placed on continuous cardiac monitoring, and a 12-lead ECG should be obtained. Routine laboratory studies include serum electrolytes, calcium, magnesium, blood urea nitrogen, and serum creatinine. Digoxin levels should be obtained, and serum levels can be checked every 3 to 4 hours after an acute ingestion. A chest radiograph should be obtained in patients with cardiac dysrhythmias, hypotension, underlying cardiac disease, or hypoxia. Patients with chronic intoxication should have liver function tests.

ED MANAGEMENT

Advanced cardiac life support (ACLS) measures should be instituted as necessary. Intubation should be considered in patients with an altered mental status. Acid-base abnormalities, hypoxia, fluid, and electrolyte imbalances should be corrected. Although hypokalemia can exacerbate digoxin toxicity, caution is advised when replacing potassium in the renal failure patient. Although intravenous (IV) calcium is commonly used to treat hyperkalemia, it should be avoided in the setting of digoxin toxicity, as hyperkalemia may be as a result of impaired intracellular pumping of potassium, in which case, cells are already relatively hypercalcemic. IV sodium bicarbonate, inhaled β-adrenergic agonists, insulin, and glucose can be used. Because hyperkalemia reflects transmembrane shifts, not total body overload, exchange resins that deplete potassium should be avoided. Digoxin Fab antibody fragments corrects the hyperkalemia from acute CG poisoning.

The preferred method of gastrointestinal decontamination following acute ingestion is activated charcoal. Repeat doses of activated charcoal can shorten the half life of digoxin and digitoxin and has been useful in the setting of yellow oleander toxicity (3). Only the first dose of activated charcoal should contain a cathartic, and the patient's production of stool and bowel sounds should be taken into consideration when giving additional doses of activated charcoal. Vagal effects associated with emesis and gastric lavage may worsen bradycardia and hypotension.

Antidigoxin Fab fragment antibodies are the treatment of choice for hemodynamically compromising or life-threatening bradydysrhythmias and tachydysrhythmias and for hyperkalemia (serum potassium ≥ 5.5 mEq/L) after an acute overdose (2). Although an elevated serum-digoxin level confirms an overdose, the degree of elevation should not guide the administration of Fab fragments. The use of prophylactic Fab therapy in the setting of non–life-threatening dysrhythmias and associated risk factors for toxicity remains to be proven (5).

Atropine (0.5 mg IV) can be given for bradydysrhythmias, but Fab fragments are more effective and safer than cardiac pacing (5). Irritation by the pacing wire in a digoxin poisoned heart can precipitate ventricular tachydysrhythmias, and pacing should not delay antibody therapy.

Standard therapy for CG-induced ventricular tachydysrhythmias includes IV phenytoin (25 mg/min until a desired effect is achieved or a total of 15 mg/kg has been given), lidocaine (1 mg/kg), and magnesium sulfate (2–3 g IV in 1 min). Such therapy may be necessary if digoxin Fab fragments are unavailable, while waiting for an effect, and when antibody therapy is unsuccessful. Refractory cardiac tachydysrhythmias induced by digoxin have responded to magnesium infusions (2 g/h for 4–5 hours) (4). Pulseless rhythms require defibrillation or cardioversion. Cardioversion may precipitate ventricular fibrillation. If possible, medical management should be used initially. When cardioversion is necessary, initial settings should be at reduced power settings (5–10 J).

Digoxin Fab fragments are prepared by immunizing sheep, purifying their antibodies, and cleaving off the Fc fragments with papain. Those patients with a history of allergy to sheep or papaya may be at risk for an allergic reaction. The two antibody preparations commercially available, Digibind (Glaxo Wellcome) and DigiFab (Protherics Inc.), are virtually identical therapeutically. Antibody fragments possess a greater affinity for digoxin than sodium potassium ATPase and lower the extracellular unbound digoxin concentration. Further equilibration of receptor-bound digoxin with the extracellular fluid leads to a rapid release of digoxin from its receptor sites (6). The drug-antibody complex is renally excreted, with a half-life of 16 hours in normal renal function and up to 4 days in patients with renal failure.

Digoxin Fab antibody fragments are given IV in 30 minutes unless the patient is in cardiac arrest, when it can be given as a bolus. If the quantity of digoxin ingested is known, the dose (in vials) of DigiBind or DigiFab can be calculated. The ingested dose in milligrams is divided by 0.6 mg/vial. Each vial of DigiBind contains 38 mg of Fab fragments, which will bind 0.5 mg of digoxin, although each vial of DigiFab contains 40 mg of Fab fragments. A typical dose for acute overdose is 5 to 10 vials. In chronic toxicity, the body load in milligrams can be estimated by multiplying the steady state serum concentration of digoxin by 5.6 times the patient's weight in kilograms divided by 1,000. The usual dose of Fab fragments in the setting of chronic toxicity is one to two vials. Resolution of the digoxin-induced dysrhythmias and hyperkalemia are usually noted within 30 minutes of Fab fragment administration, but it may take several hours for a maximal effect. In the setting of CG toxicity secondary to oleander or Bufo toad toxins, larger doses of Fab fragments may be required, because of weak crossreactivity.

Because serum digoxin assays measure both bound and unbound drug, after administration of antidigoxin Fab fragments, the serum digoxin level will rise as the drug is pulled from the tissues and is sequestered with the antibody in the serum. Free digoxin levels, measured by equilibrium dialysis or ultrafiltration, will be low if the proper amount of Fab-fragment drug is given. A rebound rise in serum digoxin levels within 24 hours of antibody administration is seen in patients with normal renal function and may be seen in up to 8 days in patients with renal failure. This rise is presumably as a result of metabolic degradation of the antigen-antibody complex. Recurrent clinical toxicity is rare.

CRITICAL INTERVENTIONS

- Administer digoxin Fab antibody fragments for hemodynamically compromising or potential lethal dysrhythmias and for hyperkalemia (K $>$5.5 mEq/L) after acute overdose.
- Avoid using calcium and exchange resins to treat hyperkalemia.
- Begin with low power settings when cardioverting tachydysrhythmias.

DISPOSITION

Intensive-care–unit admission is advised for patients with acute symptoms or who have elevated digoxin levels and dysrhythmias. Chronically poisoned patients that are hemodynamically stable and do not require active treatment may be admitted to a telemetry unit. If Fab fragments or pacemaker therapy are not available, the patient should be transferred by ACLS personnel to the nearest facility that has these modalities or the Fab fragments can be transported to the hospital.

COMMON PITFALLS

- Failure to consider plant products such as herbals or teas in the differential diagnosis of CG-like cardiotoxicity
- Failure to appreciate that toxicity is delayed up to 8 hours after acute ingestion
- Failure to appreciate that digoxin assays may not yield a measurable digoxin level with ingestions of CGs from plants or Bufo toads
- Failure to appreciate the differences between acute and chronic CG poisoning
- Failure to appreciate that pacemaker wires can irritate the myocardium and precipitate ventricular tachydysrhythmias in patients with CG poisoning

ICD 9

972.1 Poisoning by cardiotonic glycosides and drugs of similar action

REFERENCES

1. Bayer MJ. Recognition and management of digitalis intoxication: implications for emergency medicine. *Am J Emerg Med* 1991;9[Suppl]:29.
2. Bismuth C. Hyperkalemia in acute digitalis poisoning: prognostic implications and therapeutic implications. *J Toxicol Clin Toxicol* 1973;6:153.
3. De Silva HA, Fonseka MM, Pathmeswaran A, et al. Multiple-dose activated charcoal for treatment of yellow oleander poisoning: a single-blind, randomised, placebo-controlled trial. *Lancet* 2003; 361(9373):1935–1938.
4. Kinlay S, Buckley NA. Magnesium sulfate in the treatment of ventricular dysrhythmias due to digoxin toxicity. *J Toxicol Clin Toxicol* 1995;33(1):55–59.
5. Taboulet P, Baud FJ, Bismuth C. Clinical features and management of digitalis poisoning—rationale for immunotherapy. *J Toxicol Clin Toxicol* 1993;31(2):247.
6. Valdes R Jr, Jortani SA. Monitoring of unbound digoxin in patients treated with antidigoxin antigen-binding fragments: a model for the future? *Clin Chem* 1998;44(9):1883–1885.

Chemicals, Gases, and Metals

Arsenic and Mercury

PRE-HOSPITAL CONSIDERATIONS

- If possible to do so safely, bring containers in suspected cases of overdose/poisoning.
- Decontaminate the skin.
- Support airway, breathing, and circulation.
- Provide cardiac monitoring.
- For altered mental status, give dextrose, thiamine, naloxone, and oxygen.

CLINICAL PRESENTATION

Acute arsenic ingestion causes gastrointestinal (GI) symptoms such as nausea, vomiting, abdominal pain, and "rice water" diarrhea within 10 minutes to several hours after exposure. Patients may also develop shock and pulmonary edema owing to capillary leakage, toxic hepatitis, rhabdomyolysis, GI ulcerative lesions, acute tubular necrosis, delirium seizures, coma, and death (4). Arsenic toxicity may cause cardiovascular instability, hypotension, intravascular volume depletion, myocardial dysfunction, a prolonged QT interval, and dysrhythmias.

Subacute or chronic symptoms from arsenic poisoning include anemia, leukopenia, aplastic anemia, and sensory motor neuropathy. Arsenic-induced skin changes may include hyperpigmentation, hypopigmentation, hyperkeratosis, Bowen's disease, squamous cell cancers, basal cell cancers, or Blackfoot's disease (a form of arsenic-induced peripheral vascular disease resulting in gangrene). Mees lines (transverse white lines in the nails) occurs in a minority of arsenic toxic patients. Neurologic problems caused by arsenic toxicity include peripheral neuropathies, fatigue, central nervous system (CNS) depression, tremulousness, ataxia, and incoordination. Arsine gas is a colorless, nonirritating gas that causes a triad of abdominal pain, hematuria, and jaundice owing to massive hemolysis.

Subacute or chronic poisoning may present with CNS symptoms or GI or renal dysfunction. Symptoms include tremors, gingivitis, stomatitis, cheilitis, rash, headaches, choreoathetosis, weight loss, fatigue, and erethism, a syndrome that includes shyness, anxiety, emotional lability, irritability, and delirium.

Elemental mercury inhalation can cause symptoms within hours; these include cough, chills, fever, nausea, vomiting, diarrhea, interstitial pneumonitis, bronchitis, and lung fibrosis. Elemental mercury in the GI tract is unlikely to be absorbed

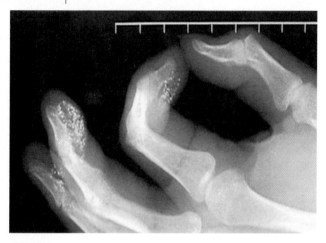

FIGURE 31.1. Multiple subcutaneous mercury deposits that were injected by a patient.

and does not cause systemic effects unless it becomes trapped in the gut by ileus or if there is GI perforation (2). Intravenous (IV) or subcutaneous injection of mercury may result in abscess or granuloma formation at the injection site and systemic symptoms (Fig. 31.1) (6).

Inorganic mercury salts such as those in mercury disc batteries, if ingested, causes irritant or caustic GI irritation, bloody diarrhea, abdominal pain, darkened and discolored oral mucosa, necrosis of the GI tract, hematochezia, hematemesis, circulatory collapse, acute tubular necrosis, and death. One to 4 grams of mercuric chloride may be fatal in adults (9). Mercuric stomatitis, gingivitis, loosening of the teeth, jaw necrosis, and acute renal failure may occur. Inorganic arsenic causes skin and mucous membrane irritation.

Ingestion of organic or alkyl mercury causes primarily CNS symptoms such as paresthesias, tremor, ataxia, dysarthria, dementia, and tunnel vision. Acrodynia or pinks disease was originally reported in children and results in erythema and induration of the palms and soles along with systemic symptoms.

Maternal organic mercury exposure may cause cerebral palsy, mental retardation, blindness, seizures, cataracts, hearing loss, and CNS abnormalities in the fetus. Organic mercury crosses the placenta and is secreted in breast milk. The US Environmental Protection Agency and the Food and Drug Administration (FDA) recommend that pregnant women, women who might become pregnant, nursing mothers, and young children to not eat shark, swordfish, king mackerel, or tilefish, but they can eat up to 12 ounces (2 average meals) a week of a variety of fish and shellfish that are lower in mercury (such as shrimp, canned light tuna, salmon) and check local advisories about the safety of fish caught by family or friends (8). Local fish may be tainted from nearby coal plants or incinerators.

DIFFERENTIAL DIAGNOSIS

Arsenic and mercury poisoning may present with GI symptoms and neurologic symptoms. Similar to other heavy metals such as iron, lead, and thallium, symptoms occur with other toxins such as botulism, viral or bacterial infections, mushrooms, and other toxic agents such as organophosphates, ricin, lithium, alcohol, theophylline, antimetabolites, and colchicine.

Infectious gastroenteritis mimics the GI symptoms, but neurologic symptoms and long-lasting unexplained symptoms warrant suspicion.

ED EVALUATION

The initial evaluation should identify specific symptoms and the route of exposure and specific chemical or product that the patient was exposed to. Physical examination should include vital signs, cardiovascular, respiratory, and neurologic evaluations. The mouth and oral mucosa may show corrosive injury. Elemental mercury inhalation and acute arsenic poisoning may cause acute respiratory distress, and a chest x-ray is therefore appropriate. Abdominal x-ray may identify retained mercury or arsenic densities. Electrocardiograph (ECG) monitoring to detect prolonged QT and dysrhythmias is appropriate for significant arsenic toxicity. Additional studies may be needed, including complete blood count (arsenic, arsine gas), arterial blood gas or oxygen saturation (elemental mercury, arsenic), serum electrolytes, blood urea nitrogen, creatinine, glucose, liver function tests, and creatine phosphokinase (severe mercury or arsenic poisoning).

Arsenic levels may be measured in blood, urine, hair, or nails. Blood arsenic is cleared within hours and is of little value. Urinary arsenic is the most reliable indicator of recent inorganic arsenic exposure (1). Twenty-four-hour urine arsenic is most commonly used but, if necessary, a spot urine arsenic corrected for creatinine concentration can be collected in the emergency department (ED) prior to chelation. Normal urine arsenic levels may vary from laboratory to laboratory but are usually <50 μg/L or <50 μg/g creatinine (1). Organic arsenic from seafood or shellfish ingestion may cause an elevated urine arsenic level for several days up to 2,000 μg/L, but it is relatively nontoxic and is rapidly cleared from the body. If organic arsenic is suspected, the laboratory can speciate the arsenic to determine whether the elevated level is due to organic or the more toxic inorganic arsenic. Urine arsenic elimination has three phases: First-phase half-life is 2 days (65% of dose), second-phase half-life is 10 days (30% of dose), and third-phase half-life is 40 days (4% of dose) (7). Arsenic levels may also be assessed in hair or nails, which may better reflect chronic arsenic toxicity. Hair levels, however, may reflect external contamination from water, sweat, or airborne arsenic and not internal contamination.

Normal whole blood mercury level is <10 μg/dL, but only a level >25 μg/dL requires treatment. Normal 24-hour urine mercury level is <20 μg/dL; levels >150 μg/dL require treatment. Urine mercury may correlate with inorganic mercury toxicity but may not be as useful for methylmercury or organic mercury toxicity. A blood mercury level is recommended for methylmercury or organic mercury toxicity. Elevated urine or blood mercury levels may occur after seafood or fish consumption. Mercury may also be measured in hair, but organic mercury is not detected in hair.

ED MANAGEMENT

Acute arsenic or mercury poisoning may be life-threatening, and advanced life-support measures may be required. The primary treatment for arsenic and mercury toxicity is supportive care and removal of the patient from further exposure. Urine arsenic levels or blood or urine mercury levels can be collected in the ED, but results are not available for several days. Aggressive IV fluid resuscitation may be needed with large ingestions of arsenic or inorganic mercury salts or arsine gas exposure. With arsenic, it is important to maintain potassium, magnesium, and calcium concentrations within normal ranges and to avoid use of drugs that would prolong the QT interval.

Acute inhalation of mercury vapor may result in life threatening respiratory failure, and ventilatory support may be needed. Patients exposed to arsine gas should have dermal decontamination. Both arsenic and mercury adsorb poorly to activated charcoal. Whole bowel irrigation can be helpful if abdominal x-rays show persistent radiopaque material in the GI tract.

If there are concerns about corrosive lesions or ulcers after inorganic mercury ingestion, upper GI endoscopy should be considered before lavage and whole bowel irrigation are performed. Inorganic mercury salt ingestion may result in severe gastroenteritis with third-spacing and cardiovascular collapse. As the most likely cause of death after ingestion of inorganic mercury salts is renal failure, aggressive fluid therapy to maintain renal perfusion may be helpful. Arsenic and mercury levels will usually fall to normal range within several weeks to months if the patient is removed from further exposure (5). Chelation therapy is recommended only for patients with significant symptoms or extremely high arsenic or mercury levels (3,6). Patients who are severely ill with known or high suspicion of acute arsenic or mercury poisoning can be chelated after a spot urine arsenic or spot urine mercury or blood mercury is collected. Dimercaprol or British anti-Lewisite (BAL) can be given as a 3- to 5-mg/kg intramuscular (IM) injection every 4 to 6 hours for severely arsenic-poisoned patients, but there is evidence from animal studies that BAL may shift arsenic or mercury into the brain (1). Patients with significant symptoms from inorganic mercury poisoning can be treated with BAL—5 mg/kg/dose every 4 hours IM for 48 hours, then 2.5 mg/kg every 6 hours for 48 hours, then 2.5 mg/kg every 12 hours for 7 days (6).

The oral chelator 2,3-dimercaptosuccinic acid (DMSA) is a more effective derivative of BAL if the patient can tolerate oral medication. Oral DMSA is the preferred chelator for organic mercury poisoning and for mercury poisoning if the patient has normal renal function and is not severely ill (6). BAL may be contraindicated with methylmercury (5). The usual dose for DMSA is 10 mg/kg TID for 5 days, then BID for 14 days. Use of DMSA is off-label as DMSA is approved by the FDA only for treatment of lead poisoning or mercury poisoning in children. Researchers have shown that 2,3 dimercaptopropanesulfonate sodium (DMPS) effectively chelates arsenic or mercury, but DMPS is not approved for clinical use by the FDA. Chelation with IM BAL is appropriate for patients with significant GI toxicity who are unable to take oral medications and may be started if there is a high level of clinical suspicion even before the blood or urine levels are available. BAL and DMSA are both renally excreted and should be used with caution in patients with renal impairment. Chelating agents should be used in pregnancy only if a patient is extremely ill.

Patients who have injected elemental mercury subcutaneously or intravenously should have x-rays of the affected sites. Large amounts of retained subcutaneous mercury should be surgically removed to prevent granulomas and skin necrosis (6). Hemolysis due to arsine gas exposure may respond to exchange transfusions or blood transfusions and does not respond to BAL chelation.

For spills of elemental mercury, appropriate clean-up measures include use of a high efficiency particulate air filter vacuum cleaner and a decontamination kit instead of sweeping. Usually the health department is notified to coordinate the clean-up.

CRITICAL INTERVENTIONS

- Keep in mind that (1) diagnosis of arsenic poisoning is based on appropriate symptoms and elevated urine arsenic level and that (2) diagnosis of mercury poisoning depends on appropriate symptoms and elevated blood or urine mercury level.
- Provide supportive care is appropriate such as IV fluids.
- Obtain blood mercury or urine mercury or urine arsenic level.
- Administer BAL or DMSA chelation for severe symptoms.
- If radiopaque material is present in the GI tract after a recent ingestion, consider whole-bowel irrigation, which may be appropriate.
- Avoid medication that will prolong the QT interval in arsenic poisoning.

DISPOSITION

Patients with significant symptoms from arsenic or mercury poisoning should be admitted to the hospital. Patients with moderate toxicity should be observed for 6 to 8 hours in the ED prior to discharge, particularly with acute arsenic ingestion (ECG monitoring), elemental mercury inhalation and arsine gas inhalation. Most patients with mild-to-moderate toxicity can be treated as outpatients and should have a follow-up visit set up 2 to 3 days after the ED visit. A psychiatric evaluation prior to discharge is appropriate for patients with intentional exposures or ingestions.

COMMON PITFALLS

- Failure to identify exposure source and preventing future exposure
- Inappropriate use of chelating agents in patients with mild toxicity who are asymptomatic.
- Failure to identify QT prolongation and dysrhythmias in toxicity or delayed pulmonary edema in severe inorganic arsenic poisoning, or hemolysis and renal failure after arsine gas exposure
- Failure to identify pulmonary effects from elemental mercury inhalation or severe neurologic and multisystem effects of organic mercury

ICD9

985.1 Toxic effect of arsenic and its compounds
985.0 Toxic effect of mercury and its compounds

REFERENCES

1. Ford MD. Arsenic. In: Goldfrank L, ed. *Goldfrank's Toxicologic Emergencies,* 7th ed. New York: McGraw-Hill; 2002:1183–1200.
2. Graeme KA, Pollack CV. Heavy metal toxicity: Part 1. Arsenic and mercury. *J Emerg Med* 1998;16(1):45–56.
3. Hughes MF. Biomarkers of exposure; a case study with inorganic arsenic. *Environ Health Perspect* 2006;114:17980–17986.
4. Hviid A, Stellfeld M, Wohlfahrt J, et al. Association between thimerosal-containing vaccine and autism. *JAMA* 2003;290:1763–1766.
5. Risher JF, Amler SN. Mercury exposure: evaluation and intervention: the inappropriate use of chelating agents in the diagnosis and treatment of putative mercury poisoning. *Neurotoxicology* 2005;26:691–699.
6. Sue YJ. Mercury. In: Goldfrank L et al., eds. *Goldfrank's Toxicologic Emergencies,* 7th ed. New York: McGraw-Hill, 2002:1334–1344.
7. Takagi Y, Matsuda S, Imai S, et al. Trace elements in human hair: an international comparison. *Bull Environ Contam Toxicol* 1986;36(6):793–800.
8. United States Environmental Protection Agency, US DHHS. What you need to know about mercury in fish and shellfish. Retrieved March, 2004 from www.cfsan.fda.gov
9. Von Burg R. Toxicology update: inorganic mercury. *J Appl Toxicol* 1995; 15(6):483–493.

CHAPTER 32

Carbon Monoxide

PRE-HOSPITAL CONSIDERATIONS
- Administer 100% oxygen.

CLINICAL PRESENTATION

The signs and symptoms of carbon monoxide (CO) poisoning are highly variable and nonspecific. At low levels, headache, dizziness, nausea, vomiting, and diarrhea are common. With higher levels, confusion, syncope, shortness of breath, and angina pectoris may occur. Severe poisoning may cause coma, seizures, hypotension, cardiac dysrhythmias, and death (1). Although the severity of intoxication usually parallels the CO-hemoglobin (CO-Hgb) level, there are reports of patients with severe intoxication at relatively low levels and of patients with high levels but minimal symptoms (3). Survivors of severe poisoning often have permanent neurologic injury, which may be gross (blindness, deafness, seizures, Parkinsonism, or vegetative state) or subtle (memory loss or personality changes) (1,4).

A cherry-red coloration of the skin, mucous membranes, and venous blood may occur inconsistently from the bright red color of the CO-Hgb complex. However, its presence or absence cannot be considered diagnostic; it is more likely to be noted at autopsy than in patients who survive. Neurologic examination usually reveals altered mental status, which may rapidly improve after the patient is removed from the poisoned atmosphere and given oxygen. Cerebellar ataxia has been found to be an important predictor of severity of intoxication (5). Arterial blood gas analysis and serum electrolyte levels often reveal metabolic acidosis caused by tissue hypoxia–ischemia. The arterial PO_2, and the calculated oxygen saturation are usually normal, because dissolved oxygen in the serum is not affected by CO. The oxygen saturation measured directly by co-oximetry is less than that calculated from the PO_2 (by an amount roughly equal to the percent CO–Hgb, but typically the oxygen saturation measured by pulse oximetry is falsely normal (6). Myocardial ischemia is frequently present on the electrocardiogram (ECG) and, occasionally, myocardial infarction (MI) occurs.

DIFFERENTIAL DIAGNOSIS

Other causes of coma and altered mental status should be sought, such as hypoglycemia, head trauma, stroke, meningitis, and drug or alcohol intoxication. Many suicidal patients ingest medications and alcohol as they poison themselves with CO. Other toxic gases should be considered in any patient with smoke inhalation. Cyanide, hydrogen sulfide, agents that cause methemoglobinemia, and other toxins may produce symptoms and signs of systemic hypoxia that are similar to those of CO (1).

ED EVALUATION

Immediate evaluation in the emergency department should include rapid neurologic assessment and determination of the specific CO-Hgb saturation (this may be performed on a venous or arterial blood sample). History that may be helpful in raising suspicion of CO poisoning includes being found in a car with the engine running, riding in the back of a pick-up truck, multiple victims found in a common room, smoke inhalation, and use of paint strippers or solvents that contain methylene chloride in a poorly ventilated area. Depending on severity, arterial blood gas analysis (using a co-oximeter), routine laboratory evaluation, ECG, and chest radiography may be indicated. Patients with suspected head trauma should have a computed tomography scan.

ED MANAGEMENT

Advanced life-support measures should be instituted as needed. Decontamination is performed by removing the victim from the toxic environment. Oxygen should be provided through a nonrebreather mask with an oxygen reservoir bag or by way of an endotracheal tube. Oxygen decreases the half-life of CO–Hgb: the higher the inspired oxygen concentration, the shorter the half-life. A nonrebreather mask with a reservoir delivers 60% oxygen at flow rates >10 L/min; 100% oxygen, which can be delivered only by endotracheal tube, decreases the CO-Hgb half-life to 40 to 80 minutes. If the patient is hypotensive, 1 to 2 L of crystalloid solution should be administered. ECG, arterial blood gases, and the carboxyhemoglobin level should be monitored. Mild-to-moderate metabolic acidosis (i.e., serum pH 7.2 to 7.3) should not be treated with sodium bicarbonate, because acidosis may facilitate oxygen delivery to the tissues by moving the oxygen-hemoglobin dissociation curve to the right.

Hyperbaric oxygen (HBO), 100% oxygen provided under pressures >1 atm, can further decrease the half-life of CO–Hgb to 20 minutes or less (1,5). Animal studies suggest a potential protective effect of HBO against CO-induced postischemic reperfusion injury, although this benefit may be nonspecific.

Controversy remains about which patients should receive HBO treatment. Most hospitals do not have ready access to a hyperbaric chamber, which means that unstable patients may require transport over long distances at a time when dysrhythmias and hypotension are more likely to occur. Because the half-life of

CO–Hgb in 100% oxygen at 1 atm is <1 hour, in most cases the level has already dropped to low levels by the time the HBO chamber is ready. Despite numerous case reports and uncontrolled case series supporting the use of HBO, its value has not been settled.

Recently, two double-blind, randomized, and placebo-controlled ("sham" HBO) studies were completed, with conflicting results (5,8). Both studies randomly assigned all patients regardless of severity. Scheinkestel found no benefit from HBO compared with normobaric oxygen (NBO), whereas Weaver (5) found a marginal but statistically significant benefit in a subset of neuropsychiatric tests. Weaver also reported that patients with cerebellar findings on admission were more likely to suffer neurological sequelae. Both studies had methodological flaws that have been highlighted by opposing sides in the debate (7).

Despite the lack of conclusive scientific data, HBO is often recommended for patients with coma (including a history of loss of consciousness or syncope), cardiovascular dysfunction (including ECG evidence of ischemia), significant acidosis, elevated CO-Hgb levels, symptoms that persist despite NBO therapy, or delayed-onset neuropsychiatric complaints. Weaver (5) recommends that HBO be considered for patients with any of the following: age >50 years; metabolic acidosis; history of loss of consciousness; or CO-Hgb level >25%.

Pregnant women and infants pose a special problem in CO poisoning, because fetal Hgb has a greater affinity for CO than does normal Hgb (2). Prolonged oxygen therapy and a lower threshold for HBO are often recommended, although, once again, studies are lacking.

The prognosis after severe CO poisoning is unpredictable but grim. As many as 40% of victims have permanent neurologic injury. Patients with an abnormal computed tomography, single-photon emission computed tomography scan, or magnetic resonance imaging scan on admission appear to be at higher risk for permanent sequelae (4).

CRITICAL INTERVENTIONS

- Administer oxygen at 10 to 15 L/min by nonrebreather mask with an oxygen reservoir bag or 100% by endotracheal tube to all patients with possible CO poisoning.
- Consult a poison center, toxicologist, or hyperbaric medicine specialist regarding HBO therapy for patients with a history of loss of consciousness or syncope, cerebellar findings, cardiovascular depression or ischemia, CO-Hgb fractions 25% to 40% or higher, significant acidemia, symptoms that persist despite NBO therapy, extremes of age, pregnancy, or delayed-onset neuropsychiatric complaints.

DISPOSITION

All patients with loss of consciousness, seizures, or evidence of MI or ischemia should be admitted to the hospital. Most authorities would also admit any patient with a CO-Hgb level >25%, regardless of symptoms.

A poison center or medical toxicologist may provide assistance with the decision to use HBO and may also know the location of nearby HBO chambers. If the patient is experiencing cardiac dysrhythmias or hypotension, a critical care nurse or physician should accompany the patient during transport to an HBO facility. Once the acute episode of poisoning has resolved, patients should be referred for follow-up neuropsychiatric evaluation. Those discharged from the emergency department should be instructed to return to the emergency department if any neurological symptoms develop.

COMMON PITFALLS

- Failure to consider the diagnosis of CO poisoning in patients presenting with headache, altered mental status, and symptoms of gastroenteritis or upper respiratory infection, particularly in cold climates or seasons
- Failure to consider the ingestion of alcohol or other drugs in patients with suicidal exposure to CO
- Failure to appreciate that the arterial blood gas PO_2, calculated oxygen saturation, and pulse oximetry oxygen saturation are usually normal despite severe CO poisoning
- Failure to appreciate that the severity of poisoning depends on the duration of exposure and that carboxyhemoglobin levels may not correlate with the severity of poisoning
- Failure to warn patients about the possibility of delayed neurological toxicity and to return if symptoms develop

ICD9

986 Toxic effect of carbon monoxide

REFERENCES

1. Weaver LK. Carbon monoxide poisoning. *Crit Care Clin* 1999;15(2):297–317, viii.
2. Greingor JL, Tosi JM, Ruhlmann S, Aussedat M. Acute carbon monoxide intoxication during pregnancy. One case report and review of the literature. *Emerg Med J* 2001;18(5):399–401.
3. Davis SM, Levy RC. High carboxyhemoglobin level without acute or chronic findings. *J Emerg Med* 1984;1:539.
4. Hopkins RO, Woon FL. Neuroimaging, cognitive, and neurobehavioral outcomes following carbon monoxide poisoning. *Behav Cogn Neurosci Rev* 2006;5(3):141–155.
5. Weaver LK, Hopkins RO, Chan KJ, et al. Hyperbaric oxygen for acute carbon monoxide poisoning. *N Engl J Med* 2002;347(14):1057–1067.
6. Vegfors M, Lennmarken C. Carboxyhaemoglobinaemia and pulse oximetry. *Br J Anaesth* 1991; 66(5):625.
7. Buckley NA, Isbister GK, Stokes B, Juurlink DN. Hyperbaric oxygen for carbon monoxide poisoning: a systematic review and critical analysis of the evidence. *Toxicol Rev* 2005;24(2):75–92.
8. Scheinkestel CD, Bailey M, Myles PS, et al. Hyperbaric or normobaric oxygen for acute carbon monoxide poisoning: a randomised controlled clinical trial. *Med J Aust* 1999;170(5):203–210.

CHAPTER 33

Corrosives and Chemical Burns

PRE-HOSPITAL CONSIDERATIONS

- Irrigate skin and ocular burns immediately and continue until arrival at the hospital.
- For oral burns or symptoms, rinse mouth liberally with water or milk.
- Give water or milk to patients who:
  ○ Are able to drink
  ○ Are not complaining of significant abdominal pain
  ○ Have no airway compromise or vomiting
- Establish patent airway. Early intubation is necessary for respiratory distress.
- Initiate intravenous fluid therapy.
- Institute pain relief.

CLINICAL PRESENTATION

Sites commonly affected by corrosive ingestion are the oropharynx, esophagus, and stomach, although injury may occur as far as the proximal jejunum (1,10).

Systemic toxicity may sometimes accompany severe gastrointestinal (GI) injuries and is usually secondary to tissue inflammation, necrosis, perforation, acidosis, and infection. Fluid and electrolyte shifts accompanying extensive burns can result in hypovolemic shock. Some corrosives also cause systemic toxicity when absorbed.

Patients usually present with oral, throat, chest, or abdominal pain. Dysphagia, drooling, and vomiting are common. Children may refuse to drink, cry excessively, or be unable to swallow their secretions. Stridor, hoarseness, hematemesis, and melena occur less frequently (5). Tachypnea can occur from aspiration of the corrosive with resultant pneumonitis or as a compensation for a metabolic acidosis. The metabolic acidosis may reflect tissue necrosis or the systemic absorption of ingested acids.

On inspection, superficial burns of the oropharynx are often covered with a pale membrane, and deeper burns are black, hemorrhagic, or friable. The presence or absence of burns in the oropharynx does not reliably predict more distal injuries (5,10). Full-thickness injuries to the esophagus or stomach are at risk for perforation and fistula formation into the trachea, mediastinum, or peritoneum (10). Mediastinitis presents with chest pain, respiratory distress, fever, subcutaneous emphysema, pleural rub, and Hamman sign (an audible crunch with each heart beat). Chest radiographic findings of mediastinitis may include mediastinal widening, pleural effusion (usually left-sided), pneumomediastinum, and pneumothorax.

The abdominal examination is also an unreliable indicator of the severity of the injury, but frank peritonitis is an ominous sign. Peritonitis may result from viscus perforation or the extension of severe gastric burns to surrounding abdominal organs. Patients with peritonitis may have marked third-spacing of fluids, resulting in abdominal distention and hypotension.

The late presentations after a corrosive ingestion include dysphagia, nausea, and vomiting as a result of the formation of strictures. Esophageal strictures develop in up to 70% of patients with deep esophageal ulcers and in nearly all patients with areas of necrosis (10). Ulceration superficial to the muscularis mucosa layer does not lead to stricture formation. Half of all esophageal strictures develop during the initial hospitalization, and 80% are evident within 2 months. Esophageal carcinoma, a late sequela of alkali ingestion, has been diagnosed after a latency period of about 40 years (9). This complication has been reported with acid burns in only a few cases.

Ocular injury most commonly results from splash exposures at home or in the work environment. The severity of these injuries ranges from transient irritation to severe disabling ocular damage and blindness. Manifestations include immediate eye pain, photophobia, blepharospasm, lacrimation, conjunctival injection or hemorrhage, and decreased visual acuity. The pupils may be nonreactive as a result of severe iritis. Intraocular pressure rises with damage to the trabecular meshwork, resulting in glaucoma. With more significant involvement, chemosis and corneal edema, opacification, sloughing, ulceration, and necrosis occur. Destruction of blood vessels may result in a very white sclera. Corneal ischemia and corneal opacification are both ominous signs. If penetration is deep enough, retinal damage occurs. Ultimately, inflammation leads to fibrosis, synechiae, and cataract formation.

Dermal exposure usually results in immediate pain at the affected site, but the onset of pain can sometimes be delayed for several hours. Petroleum distillates, weak sodium-hydroxide solutions, and cement typically do not produce burns unless allowed to remain in contact with the skin for prolonged periods. Such exposures may initially appear trivial but can progress to full-thickness burns. Chemical burns rarely blister, and the affected skin is usually dark, insensate, and firmly attached regardless of the burn depth. With time, the skin hardens and cracks, exposing the underlying dermis or subcutaneous tissue. Healing of chemical burns usually takes longer than for thermal burns.

DIFFERENTIAL DIAGNOSIS

With ingestions, it is important to exclude the coingestion of other agents. If shock or altered mental status are present soon after ingestion, other causes should be sought. The corrosive effects of ingested heavy metals and hydrocarbons can cause similar symptoms. Allergic reactions may present with some of the features of corrosive ingestion, if the hypopharynx or larynx is involved. Infections such as epiglottitis, croup, retropharyngeal abscess, and mucosal ulceration as a result of herpesvirus or coxsackievirus should be considered in children.

The differential diagnosis of corrosive injury to the eye includes traumatic corneal abrasion or ulceration, foreign body, allergic reactions, infectious processes such as viral or bacterial conjunctivitis, iritis, iridocyclitis, acute narrow-angle glaucoma, and exposure to fumes, vapors, and sensitizing agents.

Considerations in the differential diagnosis of chemical dermal injuries include thermal burns, radiation burns (including sunburns and from welding), mechanical irritation or trauma, allergic reactions and drug eruptions (such as Stevens-Johnson syndrome or toxic epidermal necrolysis), contact dermatitis, infections, and bacterial toxin-mediated conditions such as staphylococcal scalded skin syndrome or toxic shock syndrome.

ED EVALUATION

The identity, concentration, and amount of chemical or product involved and the time and circumstances of exposure should be determined. Product labels should be examined for ingredients and signal words. The signal words "caution," "warning," and "danger" identify a product as a weak irritant (to eyes, nose, and throat), strong irritant (to skin and mucous membranes), or corrosive (capable of causing permanent or fatal tissue damage), respectively. If a sample is available, the pH should be measured. A pH meter is more accurate than pH paper (e.g., pHydrion paper, which is also used for testing amniotic fluid) but is not generally available. A regional poison control center can assist with identification of the product and for advice on evaluation and management of the exposure.

In patients with corrosive ingestion, attention should initially be directed to airway patency, because obstruction may develop with progressive mucosal edema. In the absence of clinical indications for immediate endotracheal intubation, patients with respiratory symptoms should have the upper airway assessed by direct fiberoptic laryngoscopy. Patients suspected of having a significant corrosive injury should also have an electrocardiogram, arterial blood- as analysis, complete blood count, type and crossmatch, prothrombin time, electrolyte, glucose, liver function, and renal function tests. Radiologic studies should include an upright chest radiograph whenever the patient has respiratory symptoms and an acute abdominal series if perforation is suspected.

Endoscopy of the upper GI tract is the gold standard for the diagnosis of corrosive injury (7). Endoscopy should be performed in all symptomatic patients. A complete lack of symptoms or signs usually indicates that significant injuries are absent and that endoscopy is not necessary (5). Nevertheless, endoscopy should still be considered for apparently asymptomatic patients who have intentionally ingested a strong acid or alkali or if the history is unreliable. Endoscopy is optimally performed 12 to 24 hours after exposure (10). If undertaken earlier, the full extent of injury may not be apparent; if performed later, the risk of perforation may be increased by the procedure (1).

Esophageal and gastric burns are graded in a similar fashion as dermal burns. Grade 1 burns just have erythema of the mucosa (10). Grade 2 burns have partial thickness submucosal lesions, ulceration, and exudates. Some authors divide grade 2 burns into categories 2a and 2b. The 2a burns are noncircumferential, and the 2b are near circumferential. Grade 3 burns are deep, full thickness burns with ulcers and necrosis into the periesophageal tissues (5). Third-degree burns have an 85% incidence of stricture development. The best predictor for the development of strictures is the severity of the initial injury. Contrast esophagography is less sensitive than endoscopy in assessing burn injury, although it is useful for the detection of perforation. Importantly, a water-soluble contrast agent (Gastrografin) should be used whenever perforation is suspected. Cine-esophagography can detect esophageal motility disorders, which are also predictive of stricture formation.

The evaluation of patients with eye exposures should be deferred until after decontamination whenever significant pain is present. A complete eye examination including measurement of visual acuity, conjunctival pH, and a slit-lamp examination should be performed. If injury to the anterior chamber is suspected, the intraocular pressure should be measured.

The assessment of dermal injuries is similar to that for thermal burns. Location, size, color, texture, and neurovascular status should be noted. If the affected area is >5% of total body surface area or if systemic toxicity is possible, a more thorough physical examination and laboratory testing should be performed to assess for systemic involvement such as hypotension and metabolic acidosis.

ED MANAGEMENT

Any patient with evidence of significant upper airway obstruction such as severe respiratory distress, stridor, or inability to speak should undergo immediate endotracheal intubation. Delay in securing a definitive airway will only permit further development of airway edema and increase the difficulty with endotracheal intubation.

The efficacy of GI decontamination is limited. However, the mouth should be rinsed liberally with water in patients with oral burns. Emesis is contraindicated because it re-exposes the esophagus to the corrosive agent and increases the risk of aspiration. For this reason, antiemetics should be given to patients with persistent nausea or vomiting. A nasogastric tube for stomach emptying may be considered in recent, large-volume ingestions. Activated charcoal obscures the endoscopist's view, and most corrosives are not significantly adsorbed by charcoal. Dilution with oral fluids may be beneficial, although current evidence is inconclusive. If dilution is to be used, it should be within minutes of exposure in patients with a normal airway and mental status, without significant nausea, vomiting, or pain, and who are able to speak and co-operate. The amount swallowed should be limited to 5 mL/kg to avoid inducing emesis.

Although corticosteroids reduce the incidence and severity of esophageal strictures in animal studies, their value in humans is controversial. In human trials in which steroids were not given until up to 24 hours after exposure, there are conflicting conclusions and several points of general agreement. Patients with first-degree esophageal burns do not require steroids, because strictures do not develop in this group. Steroids do not appear to alter the development of esophageal strictures in patients with extensive areas of deep ulceration or necrosis (grade 3 burns) and may actually increase the rate of complications such as infection, hemorrhage, or perforation. For patients between these two extremes, whose injuries consist of circumferential or extensive superficial ulceration or small areas of deep ulceration or necrosis, steroids are of potential benefit. A recent pooled analysis of the available data did not show a statistically significant benefit of steroids for second-degree burns (4). The decision to use steroids should be based on the grading of the burns, which highlights the importance of early endoscopic evaluation.

Concomitant antibiotics are recommended whenever steroids are being used. The antibiotics of choice are penicillin, ampicillin, or clindamycin. Although they are of no proven benefit in promoting healing or reducing complications, antacids, sucralfate, H_2 blockers, and analgesics can provide symptomatic relief (1). Oral medications and feedings should be withheld until the results of endoscopy are known, and then they should be given only to patients with injuries limited to mucosal inflammation or small areas of superficial ulceration. These patients may be given oral fluids when they are able to swallow their own secretions. Those patients with more severe injuries should receive intravenous fluids and nothing by mouth.

Surgical exploration is indicated if perforation is confirmed by radiographs or endoscopy, when there is persistent hypotension, or in the presence of abdominal rigidity. Surgical exploration has also been recommended in patients who are at high risk for perforation, sepsis, necrosis, or hemorrhage. Because endoscopy cannot fully evaluate the depth of the burns (e.g., the status of the serosal surface), exploration has also been proposed for patients with grade 2 or 3 burns to overcome this limitation. In one study, a serum pH <7.22 and a base excess more than −12.0 were predictors of severe injury requiring an emergency salvage operation.

Immediate copious irrigation is the single most important intervention in the management of eye exposures (8). The severity of ocular damage at the time of presentation is a good predictor of the ultimate outcome, as are timeliness and adequacy of irrigation. Ideally, irrigation will have been performed immediately at the time of exposure in the home or workplace and continued en route to the hospital. If the patient has significant pain, irrigation must again be performed in the emergency department. Irrigation will be aided greatly by the application of topical anesthetic solution and the use of eyelid retractors. Intravenous analgesics or sedatives may also be required. Acceptable irrigation solutions include tap water, normal saline, Ringer lactate, or D5W. Initially, the eyelids should be everted, and any particulate matter should be removed with a cotton swab. Continuous irrigation of the eye is made easier with use of a scleral lens with inflow channel (Morgan Therapeutic Lens), or one can simply irrigate manually with intravenous tubing connected to irrigation solution beginning with 1 L and irrigating for at least 20 minutes. For highly corrosive substances, especially alkali exposures, initial irrigation should continue for at least an hour.

After irrigation, the pH of the inferior cul-de-sac should be tested with litmus or pH paper. If a neutral pH of 7 to 8 has not yet been achieved, continued irrigation is warranted. Once a neutral conjunctival pH is achieved, the pH should be checked every 30 minutes for 2 hours, because corrosive material may be slowly released from corneal tissue for several hours. A subsequent change in pH indicates the need for further irrigation.

Standard treatment for corneal injuries includes topical antibiotics, steroids, cycloplegics, and mydriatics. Topical timolol maleate and oral acetazolamide may be required, if intraocular pressure is elevated. Tetanus prophylaxis and analgesics should be administered if needed.

Initial management of dermal injuries is also directed at rapid decontamination. Copious irrigation of the skin surface with water is the decontamination method of choice for most exposures. Ideally, irrigation will have been initiated immediately at the scene and continued en route to the hospital (6). Delayed decontamination can result in increased tissue damage and deeper penetration of the offending agent. In industrial accidents, rescuers should wear appropriate protective gear such as gloves, gowns, masks, and eye shields. All contaminated clothing, footwear, jewelry, and contact lenses should be removed from the victim. In experimental alkali burns, irrigation of the skin with 5% acetic acid (household vinegar) decreases the severity of the injury, but clinical studies are needed to confirm this effect in humans. It must be emphasized that immediate irrigation with water should never be delayed to search for an alternative irrigation solution. Irrigation should continue for at least 20 minutes. A longer period of irrigation lasting up to several hours is required for alkalis and other serious exposures. Particulate material should be brushed away before irrigation is started. Adherent materials may be removed by gentle scrubbing with soapy water. Appropriate analgesia and tetanus prophylaxis should be provided, and wounds should be treated with topical antibiotic cream and protective dressings.

Irrigation should not be performed for burns caused by elemental forms of alkali metals such as sodium, potassium, lithium, cesium, and rubidium. These elements react with water to form hydroxides, strong bases that will significantly increase tissue damage. Furthermore, ignition or explosion occurs when water contacts pure magnesium, sulfur, strontium, titanium, uranium, yttrium, zinc, and zirconium. These two groups of substances should be covered with mineral oil to isolate them from water. Any solid particles that are removed from the victim must be stored in mineral oil to prevent further reactivity. These specific caustic agents are not readily available and are thus seldom encountered. Patients with such exposures may come to the emergency department with Material Safety Data

Sheets (MSDS) from their workplace. These data sheets provide specific information about the agent and the proper decontamination techniques.

CRITICAL INTERVENTIONS

- Evaluate the airway in patients with ingestions or facial-skin exposures, and perform immediate endotracheal intubation in patients with respiratory distress, stridor, or inability to speak.
- Begin irrigation immediately, and continue it for at least 20 minutes in symptomatic patients with eye and skin exposures.
- Consult a gastroenterologist for the endoscopic evaluation of all patients with GI symptoms or suicidal corrosive ingestion.
- Consult a surgeon for patients with radiographic evidence of perforation, endoscopic evidence of severe GI injury, peritoneal signs, hypotension, or metabolic acidosis after corrosive ingestion.
- Consult an ophthalmologist for patients who have evidence of corneal injury or persistent pain after eye exposure.
- Consult a regional burn center for patients with significant dermal injury.

DISPOSITION

Exposed patients who are asymptomatic or become asymptomatic after oral rinsing and dilution may be discharged from the emergency department after an observation period (9). It is generally agreed that patients who are asymptomatic after unintentional ingestions will have normal endoscopies (5). For patients with more significant exposures, endoscopy should be arranged, with transfer to an appropriate facility if necessary. All patients with confirmed or suspected suicidal ingestions require psychiatric evaluation. Importantly, the possibility of nonaccidental injury must be considered in all pediatric cases (9). Patients with no visible injury on endoscopy and those with injuries limited to mucosal inflammation or small areas of superficial ulceration may be medically discharged as long as they are able to tolerate oral fluids (2). Patients with persistent symptoms or inconclusive findings at endoscopy should be admitted for observation. If symptoms persist, endoscopy should be repeated.

Patients with mild chemical conjunctivitis can be referred to an ophthalmologist for follow-up the next day. Immediate ophthalmology consultation should be obtained for those with evidence of corneal injury or persistent pain. All patients with significant eye injuries should be admitted to the hospital for further irrigation, for assessment of injury progression and the need for surgical intervention, and to ensure initial compliance with the medical regimen.

Consultation with a general surgeon, plastic surgeon, or regional burn center is recommended for patients with significant dermal injuries. Patients with minor injuries may be discharged, if the patient is reliable and follow-up the next day can be arranged. Those patients with systemic toxicity; second- or third-degree burns; extensive first-degree burns (>5% of body surface area); burns to the face, eyes, ears, perineum, hands and feet; and high-risk patients such as those with significant pre-existing illness, the elderly, and psychiatric or otherwise noncompliant patients should be admitted (3).

COMMON PITFALLS

- Administering syrup of ipecac or unintentionally inducing vomiting by giving excessive amounts of oral fluid for dilution
- Giving activated charcoal, which is not indicated for acid or alkali ingestion and will obscure endoscopic evaluation
- Assuming that the absence of oropharyngeal burns precludes the presence of significant GI injury in symptomatic patients
- Failing to continue eye irrigation long enough, as determined by conjunctival pH testing
- Underestimating the severity of dermal exposures and failing to provide sufficient decontamination

ICD9

983.1 Toxic effect of acids
983.2 Toxic effect of caustic alkalis
983.9 Toxic effect of caustic, unspecified
989.9 Toxic effect of unspecified substance, chiefly nonmedicinal as to source

REFERENCES

1. De Jong AL, Macdonald R, Erin S, et al. Corrosive esophagitis in children: a 30-year review. *Int J Pediatr Otorhinolaryngol* 2001;57(3):203–211.
2. Estrera A, Taylor W, Mills LJ, et al. Corrosive burns of the esophagus and stomach: a recommendation for an aggressive surgical approach. *Ann Thorac Surg* 1986;41(3):276–283.
3. Fitzpatrick KT, Moylan JA. Emergency care of chemical burns. *Postgrad Med* 1985;78(5):189–194.
4. Fulton JA, Hoffman RS. Steroids in second degree caustic burns of the esophagus: a systematic pooled analysis of fifty years of human data: 1956–2006. *Clin Toxicol (Phila)* 2007;45(4):402–408.
5. Gorman RL, Khin-Maung-Gyi MT, Klein-Schwartz W. et al. Initial symptoms as predictors of esophageal injury in alkaline corrosive ingestions. *Am J Emerg Med* 1992;10(3):189–194.
6. Leonard LG, Scheulen JJ, Munster AM. Chemical burns: effect of prompt first aid. *J Trauma* 1982;22(5):420–423.
7. Rigo GP, Camellini L, Azzolini F, et al. What is the utility of selected clinical and endoscopic parameters in predicting the risk of death after caustic ingestion? *Endoscopy* 2002;34(4):304–310.
8. Saidinejad M, Burns MM. Ocular irrigant alternatives in pediatric emergency medicine. *Pediatr Emerg Care* 2005;21(1):23–26.
9. Wilsey MJ Jr , Scheimann AO, Gilger MA. The role of upper gastrointestinal endoscopy in the diagnosis and treatment of caustic ingestion, esophageal strictures, and achalasia in children. *Gastrointest Endosc Clin N Am* 2001;11(4):767–787, vii–viii.
10. Zargar SA, Kochhar R, Mehta S, et al. The role of fiberoptic endoscopy in the management of corrosive ingestion and modified endoscopic classification of burns. *Gastrointest Endosc* 1991; 37(2):165–169.

CHAPTER 34

Cyanide

PRE-HOSPITAL CONSIDERATIONS

- Remove source of cyanide (CN).
- Remove and bag all contaminated clothing and wash affected areas copiously with soap and water. For vapor contamination, removal of clothing may be all that is necessary.
- Prevent others, including self, from becoming contaminated.

CLINICAL PRESENTATION

Inhalation of high concentrations of hydrogen CN (HCN) may cause sudden loss of consciousness after only a few breaths. With ingestion of alkaline CN salts (calcium CN, potassium CN, sodium CN), life-threatening symptoms may occur in 30 minutes to 1 hour. In fatal cases, rapid progression to coma, seizures, dysrhythmias, intractable hypotension, apnea, and death is common.

Onset of symptoms may be delayed with exposure to cyanogens such as laetrile and cyanogenic glycosides from plant sources (up to 1.5 hours) or aliphatic nitrile compounds such as acetonitrile in artificial glue-on-nail removers (up to 6 to 12 hours) (5,6). Systemic poisoning may occur after dermal HCN exposure.

Tissues with the greatest oxygen demand (myocardium and brain) are most profoundly and rapidly affected by CN. Initial central nervous system (CNS) and cardiovascular (CV) stimulation is followed by depression. Initial signs and symptoms of CNS stimulation include giddiness, headache, and anxiety followed by confusion, seizure, and coma. The initial CV response may be characterized by a brief period of hypertension and bradycardia followed by hypotension and a reflex tachycardia. Ultimately there is hypotension and bradycardia.

Early in the clinical presentation, there may be CNS-mediated hyperpnea that is later followed by bradypnea. Both cardiogenic and noncardiogenic pulmonary edema (more correctly termed *acute lung injury*) are reported at autopsy. Gastrointestinal symptoms including nausea, vomiting, and abdominal pain may follow ingestion of CN salts and cyanogenic compounds.

Classically, CN poisoning is associated with a cherry-red skin color resulting from the inability of tissues to extract oxygen from the blood and the resulting increased oxygen saturation of venous hemoglobin. CN itself does not cause cyanosis; however, patients with apnea and circulatory collapse may exhibit cyanosis.

The smell of bitter almonds is classically associated with CN poisoning but is sporadically present, and even when present, only 60% of people are able to detect it.

CN poisoning resulting from iatrogenic exposure to sodium nitroprusside may present within hours to days of onset of therapy, typically in patients with renal failure. Manifestations include altered mental status and metabolic acidosis, particularly in the setting of tachyphylaxis to nitroprusside therapy. CN poisoning in this setting can be prevented by the concomitant administration of hydroxocobalamin or sodium thiosulfate (4).

DIFFERENTIAL DIAGNOSIS

Early symptoms may be confused with anxiety or hyperventilation, which are common after nontoxic exposures. Development of more serious clinical signs differentiates these benign conditions from true CN poisoning. Hydrogen sulfide and sodium azide poisoning may cause similar findings, and diabetic decompensation has been initially suspected in patients who were later found to have ingested CN.

The following laboratory values may suggest the diagnosis when no history is available: elevated plasma lactate level, elevated anion gap metabolic acidosis, relatively normal pO_2 in ventilating patients, and an elevated peripheral venous pO_2 (>40 mm Hg) or decreased arteriovenous O_2 saturation difference (central venous or mixed pulmonary artery O_2 saturation $>70\%$ with a relatively normal co-oximeter-measured arterial O_2 saturation), owing to decreased tissue oxygen extraction from the blood. Hydrogen sulfide and sodium azide poisoning can also cause this combination of laboratory findings. Patients exposed to hydrogen sulfide may have the odor of sulfur or "rotten eggs" on the body or clothes or in a freshly drawn tube of blood.

ED EVALUATION

Whenever possible, the history should include the specific compound involved, route of exposure, any decontamination measures already undertaken, possible dose, time since ingestion or exposure, and any pre-existing allergies or chronic medical conditions. Initial physical examination should focus on vital signs (monitored frequently and serially) and the respiratory system, CV system, and CNS. The cardiac rhythm should be continuously monitored.

Determination of serum electrolytes (with calculation of the anion gap), blood glucose levels, pulse oximetry, arterial blood gas analysis, chest radiography, and 12-lead electrocardiography should be done initially and monitored frequently if clinical signs or symptoms of CN poisoning are present. Whole blood CN levels can be measured, but results usually take hours or days to obtain and thus cannot be used to guide emergent diagnosis or treatment. They are useful only to document exposure. A more practical test is the plasma lactate concentration. In the right clinical setting, a lactate concentration >10 mmol/L that is refractory to ventilation, oxygenation, and perfusion is a marker of CN toxicity (2).

ED MANAGEMENT

Prehospital directives include the rapid, safe removal of victims from the scene by those with adequate training and protection. Start with airway management, 100% supplemental oxygen, cardiac monitoring, at least one large-bore intravenous line, and intravenous fluids if hypotension is present. Rescuers must not enter areas of potential CN gas exposure without a self-contained, positive-pressure breathing apparatus. Mouth-to-mouth resuscitation should be avoided, if possible. If it is unavoidable, rescuers must be careful not to inhale the victim's expired air. Exposed skin (particularly open wounds) and eyes should be decontaminated by copiously flushing with water. Contaminated clothing should be removed and isolated.

On arrival to the emergency department (ED), care again begins with the ABCs (airway, breathing, circulation), with the particular caveat that the significantly CN-poisoned patient may deteriorate rapidly. Pulse oximetry or arterial blood gases should be monitored, and metabolic acidosis should be corrected with adequate ventilation and sodium bicarbonate if appropriate. Pulse oximetry may be unreliable following administration of methemoglobin-inducing nitrite antidotes, and co-oximetry may be unreliable following administration of hydroxycobalamin. Once CN poisoning is suspected, either by history or by clinical presentation, specific antidotal therapy should be initiated. Antidotes for CN poisoning include all of the Cyanide Antidote Kit, thiosulfate alone, or the recently Food and Drug Administration–approved Cyanokit.

The Cyanide Antidote Kit, in use for decades in the United States, consists of amyl nitrite pearls, sodium nitrite 3% solution for intravenous administration, and sodium thiosulfate 25% solution. Until intravenous access is established, amyl nitrite pearls may be given by inhalation (broken in gauze and held close to the nose and mouth of spontaneously breathing patients or placed into the lips of the face mask or inside the ventilation bag in apneic patients) for 30 seconds out of each minute, using a fresh pearl every 3 to 4 minutes. Once intravenous access is obtained, sodium nitrate 3% solution is administered. The adult dose of sodium nitrite is one 10-mL ampule (300 mg) of the 3% solution. The pediatric dose ranges from 0.12 to 0.33 mL/kg (3.6–9.9 mg/kg). Sodium nitrite is a potent vasodilator; rapid administration may result in severe hypotension, which can be avoided by slow intravenous infusion over 5 minutes. Dilute the sodium nitrite in 50 to 100 mL of 5% dextrose in water. Start the infusion slowly, with frequent blood pressure monitoring, and then increase to the most rapid infusion rate not causing hypotension. The third component, sodium thiosulfate 25% solution, is also administered intravenously and is supplied in a 50 mL vial (adult dose: one entire vial. The pediatric dose is 1.65 mL/kg (up to 50 mL maximum). Second doses of sodium nitrite and sodium thiosulfate at one-half the initial amounts may be given 30 minutes later if there is incomplete clinical response. Continued metabolic release of CN from cyanogenic glycosides or aliphatic nitrile compounds may cause prolonged poisoning, necessitating multiple antidote doses (5). Repeated doses or a continuous infusion (1 g/h) of sodium thiosulfate (without further sodium nitrite) should be considered in such cases (5).

In addition to their vasodilatory effects, the amyl nitrite pearls and the sodium nitrite induce formation of methemoglobin, which binds CN to form cyanohemoglobin as part of the detoxification process. Methemoglobin levels should be monitored, especially if multiple doses of sodium nitrite are required, and should be kept to <30% of total hemoglobin. When oxygen transport is already compromised, as in a smoke inhalation patient with concomitant carbon monoxide poisoning, this induction of methemoglobinemia further impairs cellular hypoxia. (See Chapter 40.) A reasonable approach in the critically ill patient with suspected CN toxicity, particularly the seriously ill patient with a lactate level >10 mmol/L refractory to resuscitation with intravenous fluids and oxygen supplementation, is to administer only the usual dose of sodium thiosulfate. Sodium thiosulfate works indirectly to metabolize CN by supplying necessary sulfur atoms to catalyze the body's own conversion of CN to sodium thiocyanate, resulting in some delay in onset of antidotal effect.

The Cyanokit contains two 2.5 g vials of hydroxycobalamin. Hydroxycobalamin binds directly with CN to form cyanocobalamin (vitamin B_{12}), which is nontoxic and subsequently excreted in the urine. Additionally, hydroxycobalamin has been shown in human volunteers and in animal studies of CN poisoning to raise blood pressure (7). The main side effect of hydroxycobalamin is a clinically insignificant reddish-brown skin discoloration that resolves spontaneously. The adult dose is 5 g of hydroxycobalamin reconstituted in 100 mL 0.9% sodium chloride and given intravenously over 15 minutes; the pediatric dose is 70 mg/kg. A second dose may be repeated over 15 minutes to 2 hours in cases of severe poisoning.

Activated charcoal has decreased mortality in experimental CN poisoning (6), and 1 g may bind as much as 35 mg of CN (1). Consider administration of 1 g/kg activated charcoal in patients who have ingested CN.

Extracorporeal elimination procedures such as hemodialysis and hemoperfusion have no place in the treatment of acute CN poisoning. Hyperbaric oxygen will increase oxygen transport by increasing dissolved oxygen in the blood.

CRITICAL INTERVENTIONS

- Suspect CN poisoning in patients with rapid development of unexplained coma, seizures, elevated anion gap metabolic acidosis, and intractable hypotension.
- Administer sodium nitrite and sodium thiosulfate or hydroxycobalamin intravenously to comatose or persistently acidotic or seizing patients with possible CN exposure.
- Monitor methemoglobin levels in patients receiving sodium nitrite, especially in children or when multiple doses are given.
- Measure lactate and carboxyhemoglobin.

DISPOSITION

Asymptomatic CN-exposed patients should be observed in a controlled setting for 4 to 6 hours. Following ingestion of cyanogenic compounds or foods, the observation period should be extended to 12 hours (5). Mildly symptomatic patients can be observed in the ED until symptoms resolve. Those requiring antidote administration should be admitted to an intensive care unit until all symptoms have resolved or for a minimum of 24 hours.

Survivors of acute CN poisoning have developed parkinsonian-like states or more subtle neuropsychiatric deficits (3). Outpatient follow-up should be arranged for patients with significant acute toxicity to screen for these sequelae.

If transfer is necessary, the most rapid means available should be used. Accompanying personnel should be able to initiate intravenous access, perform endotracheal intubation and mechanical ventilation, and administer specific antidotes, sodium bicarbonate, anticonvulsants, and anti-arrhythmic medications.

COMMON PITFALLS

- Failure to stock an in-date CN antidote in the ED or other readily available location
- Failure to consider the diagnosis of CN poisoning in patients with smoke inhalation, sudden-onset coma, CV collapse, or lactic acidosis of unknown etiology
- Inappropriate antidote administration to a hemodynamically stable, conscious patient
- Administration of nitrites with concomitant carbon monoxide poisoning in a smoke-inhalation patient
- Rapid administration of sodium nitrite, resulting in hypotension
- Administration of adult doses of CN antidotes to children

ICD9

989.0 Toxic effect of hydrocyanic acid and cyanides

REFERENCES

1. Anderson AH. Experimental studies on the pharmacology of activated charcoal. *Acta Pharmacol* 1946;2:69–78.
2. Baud FJ, Barriot P, Toffis V, et al. Elevated blood cyanide concentrations in victims of smoke inhalation. *N Engl J Med* 1991;325:1761–1776.
3. Carella F, Grassi MP, Savoiardo M, et al. Dystonic parkinsonian syndrome after cyanide poisoning: clinical and MRI findings. *J Neurol Neurosurg Psychiatry* 1988;51:1345–1358.
4. Cottrell JE, Casthely P, Brodie JD, et al. Prevention of nitroprusside-induced cyanide toxicity with hydroxocobalamin. *N Engl J Med* 1978;298:809–811.
5. Geller RJ, Ekins BR, Iknoian RC. Cyanide toxicity from acetonitrile-containing false nail remover. *Am J Emerg Med* 1991;9:268–270.
6. Lambert RJ, Kindler BL, Schaeffer DJ. The efficacy of superactivated charcoal in treating rats exposed to a lethal oral dose of potassium cyanide. *Ann Emerg Med* 1988;17:595–598.
7. Riou B, Berdeaux A, Pussard E, et al. Comparison of the hemodynamic effects of hydroxocobalamin and cobalt edetate at equipotent cyanide antidotal doses in conscious dogs. *Intensive Care Med.* 1993;19:26–32.

35

Fluoride and Hydrofluoric Acid

PRE-HOSPITAL CONSIDERATIONS
- Irrigate skin and ocular burns with water immediately and continue until arrival at the hospital.
- Give water to patients who:
  - Are able to drink
  - Are not complaining of significant abdominal pain
  - Have no airway compromise or vomiting

CLINICAL PRESENTATION

Dermal hydrofluoric acid (HF) exposures are the most commonly encountered fluoride exposure in the emergency department. Exposure to other fluoride cleaning products (e.g., ammonium bifluoride) may cause similar effects. The main manifestation of these exposures is pain. At low concentrations (<20% HF), symptoms may be delayed more than 24 hours (4). Dermal findings may be minimal initially but can progress to full thickness injury. With lower concentration exposures, dermal findings range from normal skin to full thickness burns. In one series of low-concentration exposures, just over 50% of the patients had erythema and swelling, 5% developed blisters, and 23% had normal skin (4). Burns from high concentrations (>50% HF) may appear similar to other caustic injuries. Exposure of more than 1% of the body surface area to a 50% HF product may result in systemic poisoning. Ocular exposures to low-concentration products may result in eye pain and corneal injury, and animal models suggest that exposure to concentrations >20% will cause immediate corneal edema and opacification.

Patients with HF ingestions may have deceptively minimal or no findings suggestive of caustic exposure. Fatal fluoride intoxication has been reported without significant gastrointestinal (GI) symptoms (6). When present, GI symptoms include abdominal pain, vomiting, and hematemesis (6). Effects after HF inhalation may range from mild pulmonary irritation to hemorrhagic pulmonary edema and delayed multisystem organ failure. Systemic absorption of fluoride may occur after inhalational exposure. Manifestations of systemic fluoride poisoning include headache, paresthesias, visual complaints, and signs of hypocalcemia such as carpal-pedal spasm, positive Chvostek's and Trousseau's signs, hyperreflexia, tetany, and prolongation of the QT interval on the electrocardiogram. Coma, seizures, shock, dysrhythmias, and death may occur in severe cases. Lethal dysrhythmias include refractory ventricular tachycardia and ventricular fibrillation. Hypocalcemia is often severe (serum calcium level <5 mg/dl). Metabolic acidosis, hypomagnesemia, hyperkalemia, and coagulopathy can also occur.

DIFFERENTIAL DIAGNOSIS

HF acid exposure should be considered when a patient with a chemical exposure presents with severe pain and minimal dermal findings. Other diseases with similar findings would include other chemical burns, Raynaud's syndrome, local ischemia, or sensory neuropathy. Systemic fluoride poisoning should be considered for the patient who presents with cardiovascular (CV) instability and hypocalcemia. Other potential causes of this presentation would include acute hypoparathyroidism, hyperphosphatemia or poisoning from sodium ethylenediaminetetraacetic acid.

ED EVALUATION

Important factors in the history include the route of exposure, product involved, the use of protective equipment, and whether decontamination was performed. Signs and symptoms and their time of onset with respect to exposure should be noted. The physical examination should initially focus on the site of exposure. Patients with facial burns should have conjunctival pH determined and a full eye examination performed after any needed irrigation. Patients with limited (<5% body surface area) dermal exposures to HF products with a concentration <10% do not require any laboratory testing or monitoring. Patients with more extensive dermal exposures, dermal exposure to higher concentration products, or ingestion of HF products should have continuous cardiac monitoring, an electrocardiogram, and serum calcium determinations. Those with hypocalcemia should have a complete blood count, serum electrolytes, magnesium, blood urea nitrogen, and creatinine. Chest radiographs are indicated for symptomatic patients with inhalational exposure.

ED MANAGEMENT

The first step with dermal exposure is immediate irrigation, ideally at the scene, with water. In a series of more than 400 dermal exposures (most involving 40% HF) treated with immediate water irrigation, no patient developed deep tissue necrosis, and all recovered within days (3). Irrigation should be performed for a minimum of 20 minutes. If symptoms have not resolved, irrigation should be continued. Hexafluorine, a proprietary product that binds fluoride much more effectively than calcium, has been advocated. However, hexafluorine offers no clear advantage over water irrigation.

Patients who have continued pain despite irrigation or who present several hours out from exposure should be treated in a stepwise fashion. Topical calcium is the standard first-line therapy. The most effective way to deliver the calcium is to mix 10% calcium chloride with methylcellulose to form a gel with a final calcium concentration of 2.3 to 2.5%. If methylcellulose is not available, a water-based lubricant (e.g., KY jelly) may be used. The mixture is then applied topically to the affected area. Exposures involving the digits are best treated by having the patient wear a tight-fitting glove filled with the gel. The glove is worn for at least 30 minutes after the pain resolves. Fingernail removal is not advocated, and patients with exposure that involves the nail beds are best treated with regional perfusion (see further). Patients who have relief may be discharged with additional gel and told to apply the gel every 4 to 6 hours or sooner if needed, for the next 24 hours (2).

Patients who have continued pain despite topical calcium therapy should be treated with calcium injection or regional perfusion. Local subcutaneous injection of calcium gluconate is best suited for areas in which the tissue can expand to accommodate the fluid. The dose is 0.5 cc of 10% calcium gluconate per cm^2 of involved skin. Calcium chloride should not be used as it may cause tissue injury. The injection is performed with a small (27 g or smaller) needle. Successful treatment results in immediate improvement in symptoms (1). Use of a local anesthetic is not recommended as relief of pain is used as an indication of the success of therapy. Patients may be discharged with topical calcium gel therapy.

Often, the skin on the hand and foot cannot comfortably accommodate the volume of fluid injected during these injections. These areas are best treated by regional perfusion. This may be accomplished by either direct arterial injection or using intravenous injection with Bier's technique. Arterial perfusion requires placing an arterial catheter. After confirming intra-arterial placement by either waveform or arteriography, 100 cc of a 2.5% calcium gluconate solution is infused over 60 minutes (8). An alternative to arterial infusion is regional venous calcium infusion using a Bier block. With this technique, an intravenous catheter is placed in the hand or foot, and the extremity is exsanguinated by elevation (with or without application of an elastic bandage). A pneumatic tourniquet is applied proximal to the burn and inflated to 100 mm Hg above systolic blood pressure. Once the tourniquet is inflated, 10 cc of a 10% calcium gluconate diluted with 40 cc of saline is infused into the catheter in the affected extremity. After 15 to 25 minutes, the tourniquet is deflated slowly over 5 minutes (5). Most patients will require parenteral analgesia to tolerate the tourniquet.

Ocular exposures should be treated with immediate water irrigation. As with any caustic exposure to the eye, the ocular pH should be monitored. There is no evidence that irrigation with calcium or magnesium-containing solutions offers any advantage, and any delay that occurs while these solutions are obtained is likely to be detrimental. Although animal models suggest that severe injury is possible, reported cases have gone on to good recovery. One report suggested that calcium gluconate drops may be a useful adjunctive therapy after decontamination, but this is not routinely recommended.

Nebulized calcium gluconate has been used for inhalational exposures, but the evidence is anecdotal and limited, so this therapy cannot be considered standard.

Systemic fluoride poisoning may occur after exposure to many fluoride-containing products. The management of systemic fluoride poisoning does not vary depending on the type of fluoride or the route of exposure. Patients with ingestions of fluoride-containing products should rinse their mouth and drink 50 to 100 cc of water to dilute the caustic effects. Charcoal does not adsorb fluoride and should not be administered unless life-threatening co-ingestion is strongly suspected. Oral administration of calcium-containing solution is of unproven value. One animal model found a survival benefit but only when the ratio of calcium to fluoride exceeded a 1:1 equivalent ratio (7). This would translate to more than 3 g of calcium chloride for each gram of fluoride ingested. Accidental exposures to most nonprescription dental products that contain fluoride do not result in serious toxicity although patients may develop GI symptoms. Patients with small (suspect <30 cc ingested), accidental exposures to low-concentration HF products or dental sodium fluoride products almost always do well (6). Asymptomatic patients with small ingestions (e.g., a sip) should have venous access obtained and be placed on a cardiac monitor. Baseline calcium measurements should be obtained immediately. If the serum calcium is below the normal range, it is reasonable to administer 1 g of calcium gluconate over 30 minutes and then immediately repeat the calcium level. Persistent hypocalcemia suggests that there was a significant exposure, and the patient should be treated as if there were a deliberate exposure. Patients with deliberate ingestions (or accidental ingestions suspected to involve more than 30 cc) of low-concentration HF products or sodium fluoride may benefit from prophylactic treatment with intravenous calcium. Animal models suggest that such treatment improves survival. The author recommends that any patient who presents after deliberate ingestion of a HF product should be treated with prophylactic calcium gluconate (at a rate of 3 g/h) after baseline serum calcium is measured. Calcium chloride may be used, but it must be given through a well-functioning line, as extravasation may cause extensive tissue injury. If the initial serum calcium is normal, the infusion may be stopped, but serum calcium levels should be measured every 30 minutes for at least 3 hours and, if calcium levels are decreasing, the infusion should be restarted.

Patients who develop hypocalcemia or manifest CV effects must be treated very aggressively. Survival after cardiac arrest from fluoride poisoning has always been associated with very aggressive calcium therapy. One patient suffered cardiac arrest and survived after the administration of more than 110 mEq of calcium chloride (approximately 9 g) during a resuscitation (9). Although only suggestive, this case suggests that early administration may prevent CV collapse. Patients who have or develop hypocalcemia, hyperkalemia, cardiac dysrhythmias, hypotension, coma, or seizures should have central venous access obtained, and the calcium infusion should be changed from calcium gluconate to calcium chloride (which contains three times as much calcium per gram) and continued at the same rate using the central venous access. The serum calcium should be measured every 30 minutes and, if hypocalcemia persists, the calcium infusion rate should be doubled. Fluids should be administered for hypotension. Cardiac dysrhythmias and hyperkalemia do not respond to usual therapies. Magnesium and potassium levels should also be monitored, and magnesium should be administered to maintain a normal serum level. One should consider using sodium bicarbonate boluses and a sodium bicarbonate infusion to alkalinize critically ill patients to a serum pH of 7.45 to 7.50. Systemic alkalosis improves survival in animal models, but over-alkalinization may worsen hypocalcemia.

CRITICAL INTERVENTIONS

- Immediately irrigate dermal or ocular exposures with water or saline.
- Administer topical or subcutaneous calcium gluconate, followed by regional, intravenous, or intra-arterial calcium gluconate infusion, for patients who have skin findings or persistent pain after dermal exposure.
- Establish venous access, institute cardiac rhythm (and QT interval) monitoring, obtain a serum calcium level, and give prophylactic intravenous calcium gluconate to patients with intentional ingestions or large dermal, inhalational, or oral exposure.
- Establish central venous access and administer intravenous calcium chloride to patients with hypocalcemia or QT interval prolongation.

DISPOSITION

Patients who present with dermal exposures that have no symptoms after irrigation may be discharged with instructions to return or begin topical calcium therapy if pain develops. Similarly, patients who present with pain and respond well to topical or intradermal therapy in the emergency department may be discharged with topical therapy every 4 to 6 hours and a 24-hour follow-up. If visible burns are noted, a burn or hand surgeon should be consulted. Patients who require regional infusions are likely to require repeat therapy and should be admitted for 24-hour observation. Intra-arterial administration is an indication for intensive care unit admission (primarily for monitoring of the arterial line).

Patients who have no symptoms and a normal examination after irrigation for ocular exposures may be discharged with next day follow-up. An ophthalmologist should be consulted and see all patients with persistent symptoms or an abnormal ocular exam emergently. Patients with ingestions of HF products who have no symptoms and normal serum calcium levels after 6 hours may be discharged or referred for psychiatric evaluation. Those who require intravenous calcium should be admitted to an intensive care unit for ongoing monitoring and treatment. A poison center or toxicologist should be consulted if the physician is not familiar with the evaluation and management of fluoride and HF poisoning.

COMMON PITFALLS

- Failure to appreciate that patients with dermal HF injury may have pain without abnormal skin findings

- Failure to appreciate that systemic fluoride poisoning may occur in the absence of GI symptoms following ingestion
- Failure to appreciate that severe systemic fluoride poisoning may result from large dermal and inhalational exposures
- Failure to appreciate that large doses of calcium and magnesium may be required in patients with systemic fluoride poisoning

ICD9

983.1 Toxic effect of acids

REFERENCES

1. Anderson WJ, Anderson JR. Hydrofluoric acid burns of the hand: mechanism of injury and treatment. *J Hand Surg [Am]* 1988;13:52–57.
2. Chick LR, Borah G. Calcium carbonate gel therapy for hydrofluoric acid burns of the hand. *Plast Reconstr Surg* 1990;86:935–940.
3. Division of Industrial Hygiene, National Institute of Health. Hydrofluoric acid burns. *Ind Med* 1943; 12:634.
4. El Saadi MS, Hall AH, Hall PK, et al. Hydrofluoric acid dermal exposure. *Vet Hum Toxicol* 1989; 31:243–247.
5. Graudins A, Burns MJ, Aaron CK. Regional intravenous infusion of calcium gluconate for hydrofluoric acid burns of the upper extremity. *Ann Emerg Med* 1997;30:604–607.
6. Kao WF, Dar RC, Kuffner E, Bogdan G. Ingestion of low-concentration hydrofluoric acid: an insidious and potentially fatal poisoning. *Ann Emerg Med* 1999;34:35–41.
7. Kao WF, Deng JF, Chiang SC, et al. A simple, safe, and efficient way to treat severe fluoride poisoning—oral calcium or magnesium. *J Toxicol Clin Toxicol* 2004;42:33–40.
8. Siegel DC, Heard JM. Intra-arterial calcium infusion for hydrofluoric acid burns. *Aviat Space Environ Med* 1992;63:206–211.
9. Stremski ES, Grande GA, Ling LJ. Survival following hydrofluoric acid ingestion. *Ann Emerg Med* 1992;21:1396–1399.

CHAPTER 36

Hydrocarbons

PRE-HOSPITAL CONSIDERATIONS

- Decontaminate clothes, skin, and hair.
- Do *not* induce emesis.
- Do not give ipecac. It is contraindicated because of an increased risk of aspiration.
- Keep volatile-substance abusers calm and avoid interventions that cause anxiety or distress.

CLINICAL PRESENTATION

The nature of toxicity depends on multiple variables including the class of hydrocarbon (aromatic, halogenated, terpene or aliphatic), the route and duration of exposure, and the presence of other substances such as metals or pesticides in the hydrocarbon product. For example, inhalation of leaded gasoline has been associated with lead toxicity.

Acute hydrocarbon inhalation can cause euphoria, hallucinations, agitation, central nervous system (CNS) depression, and syncope. Coma can occur in severe cases. Chronic inhalation can lead to cognitive impairment, cerebellar ataxia, and oculomotor and corticospinal abnormalities. Dysrhythmias and "sudden sniffing death" syndrome are most often seen with chlorinated hydrocarbons and aromatic hydrocarbons (1). Victims are frequently noted to exhibit agitation and to have engaged in physical activity such as running prior to collapse.

Patients with chronic toluene exposure can have nausea, vomiting, dehydration, and weakness as a result of metabolic acidosis, hypokalemia, and hypophosphatemia resulting from distal renal tubular acidosis (i.e., bicarbonate wasting). Both increased anion gap metabolic acidosis and hyperchloremic normal anion gap metabolic acidosis can be seen. Rhabdomyolysis may also be present. Traumatic injury can result from impaired judgment, and burns may result from unintentional ignition of hydrocarbons.

Pulmonary toxicity occurs after inhalational exposure but more commonly results from aspiration during ingestion. Choking, coughing, or gagging suggests aspiration. Vomiting is common after hydrocarbon ingestion and is a risk factor for aspiration and pneumonia (3). Signs and symptoms of aspiration pneumonitis include dyspnea, tachypnea, nasal flaring, grunting, rhonchi, rales, and agitation (secondary to hypoxia). In the patient presenting after hydrocarbon exposure, lack of tachypnea has a high negative predictive value for aspiration (7). Symptoms usually begin within 30 minutes of exposure and typically worsen over the course of 1 to 5 days. Many of the children with aspiration pneumonia have an interstitial pneumonitis (3). Pulmonary edema, hemoptysis, pleural effusions, and pneumothorax can occur in severe cases. Radiographic abnormalities may lag behind clinical presentation. Other findings on chest radiograph include infiltrates, increased bronchovascular markings, pneumomediastinum, and pneumatoceles. Fever and leukocytosis are common with hydrocarbon pneumonitis (4).

Ingestion of petroleum distillates and most other hydrocarbons are associated with some degree of gastrointestinal (GI) symptoms. Oral mucosal irritation, nausea, vomiting and diarrhea are common. An abdominal radiograph may demonstrate a "double bubble" sign with hydrocarbon layering over stomach contents (2).

The ingestion of camphor and other terpenes can cause agitation, restlessness, and seizures and can occur as soon as 4 minutes after camphor ingestion (5).

Methylene chloride, found in many paint strippers, is metabolized by the liver to carbon monoxide so that ingestion or inhalation can cause carbon monoxide poisoning (see Chapter 32, "Carbon Monoxide") (6). Carbon tetrachloride can cause hepatic and renal toxicity that may not be evident until 2 to 3 days after ingestion. Naphthalene ingestion can cause methemoglobinemia and associated hemolytic anemia.

Intravenous injection of hydrocarbons, although rare, is associated with systemic and local effects. Local inflammation, sterile abscess formation, tissue necrosis, thrombophlebitis, myositis, and a pneumonitis are all reported after injection of various hydrocarbons.

DIFFERENTIAL DIAGNOSIS

The odor of a hydrocarbon or hydrocarbon product (e.g., that of pine oil) could assist in narrowing the differential diagnosis of hydrocarbon exposure. Intoxication by ethanol, carbon monoxide, gamma hydroxybutyrate, and other sedative-hypnotics, opiates and centrally acting pharmaceuticals such as phenothiazines, antihistamines and tricyclic antidepressants can affect the CNS similar to hydrocarbons. Changes in mental status can also mimic traumatic head injury or infection (either systemic or directly related to the CNS). Like camphor, isoniazid and tricyclic antidepressant can cause the rapid development of seizures after toxic exposure. Although petroleum distillates are poorly absorbed after ingestion, pulmonary aspiration and resultant hypoxia can lead to CNS depression.

Other etiologies of anion or nonanion gap metabolic acidosis include methanol, ethylene glycol, salicylates, and iron poisoning, which should be considered in the differential diagnosis of chronic aromatic hydrocarbon inhalation.

GI symptoms after hydrocarbon ingestions resemble a host of other etiologies, including other toxic ingestions (such as caustics) or more common entities, such as food-borne or infectious gastroenteritis.

The respiratory symptoms of hydrocarbon aspiration can mimic reactive airway disease, pulmonary infection, or pulmonary embolism. Pulmonary infiltrates, fever, and leukocytosis secondary to aspiration of hydrocarbons may mimic an infectious process. A delay in radiographic changes associated with the hydrocarbon aspiration frequently complicates the immediate diagnosis.

Tachydysrhythmias that result from aromatic and halogenated hydrocarbon inhalation can also be seen with electrolyte derangements, myocardial ischemia, or other toxic exposures (see Chapter 1, "General Considerations: Recognition, Initial Approach, and Early Management of the Poisoned Patient"). Pulmonary aspiration and resultant hypoxia from petroleum distillate ingestion can also lead to cardiovascular toxicity.

ED EVALUATION

Pertinent points of history include the name of product, identity of ingredients, manufacturer (if possible to assist poison control specialists in locating the product), time and route of exposure, time of onset, and nature of symptoms. If the substance could pose an inhalational or dermal hazard to the emergency department staff or other patients, the patient should be disrobed and decontaminated prior to entering the emergency department. The history should include a respiratory, neurologic, and GI review of symptoms. If the historian is a parent who suspects an ingestion in a child, he or she should be asked about the occurrence of vomiting, coughing, and other respiratory symptoms. The possibility of concomitant trauma should also be considered.

Oxygen saturation and cardiac monitoring should be initiated and an electrocardiogram obtained to evaluation for conduction abnormalities and tachydysrhythmias. Chest radiography is indicated for patients with respiratory symptoms or concern for development of respiratory effects, such as report of vomiting, gasping, or coughing immediately after a hydrocarbon ingestion. This should be done immediately in the symptomatic patient or delayed 6 hours after ingestion for the asymptomatic patient. Arterial blood gas should be considered in any patient with suspected aspiration with respiratory symptoms. Liver function tests should be obtained in those exposed to chlorinated hydrocarbons, such as carbon tetrachloride. Patients with altered mental status, weakness, dehydration, or chronic inhalational abuse should have serum electrolytes, creatinine, blood urea nitrogen, and creatine kinase and urinalysis ordered to screen for renal tubular acidosis and rhabdomyolysis. If necessary, the presence of alcohol or other centrally acting drugs of abuse can be confirmed by serum and urine toxic screens, although the results rarely change management. Patients with persistent neurologic dysfunction and a normal computed tomography scan should have a magnetic resonance imaging (MRI) of the brain, which is the best diagnostic tool for detecting CNS demyelination.

ED MANAGEMENT

Advanced cardiac life-support measures should be instituted as needed. If the stable patient presents a risk of contamination to the health care providers—for example, a patient with dermal hydrocarbon exposure containing a pesticide—decontamination with soap and water washing and rinsing should be performed prior to entering the emergency department. If this is not possible, health care providers should wear gloves and protective clothing. Flammability is also a potential hazard of many hydrocarbons, so again removal of clothing and decontamination are indicated.

Patients with respiratory symptoms should receive oxygen therapy. Consideration should be given to early endotracheal intubation, especially if the patient is to be transferred to another facility. Bronchodilators can be given for bronchospasm, and high-frequency jet ventilation, partial liquid ventilation, or extracorporeal membrane oxygenation should be considered in patients with refractory hypoxemia. Prophylactic antibiotics and steroids have not been found to be beneficial.

Seizures and agitation should be managed with benzodiazepines. Because tachydysrhythmias may be the result of sensitization of the myocardium to endogenous catecholamines, β-adrenergic blockers such as propranolol may be used. Lidocaine may also be used. Adrenergic agents, such as epinephrine, may be deleterious in such situations.

Gastric decontamination for ingested hydrocarbons is controversial. Because the risk of aspiration increases with maneuvers that manipulate the GI tract, gastric decontamination should be considered only when there has been an ingestion of potentially toxic amounts of agents with systemic toxicity (e.g. a pesticide or halogenated compound). Even in this situation, aspiration might pose a greater risk of morbidity to the patient. Finally, as most hydrocarbons are not well adsorbed by activated charcoal, this is reserved for co-ingestants and agents with systemic toxicity.

CRITICAL INTERVENTIONS

- Obtain a chest radiograph in patients with coughing, gagging, vomiting, tachypnea, abnormal pulmonary examination, or low oxygen saturation after hydrocarbon ingestion.
- Obtain serum electrolytes, creatinine, blood urea nitrogen, creatine kinase, and urinalysis in patients with altered mental status, weakness, dehydration, or chronic inhalational abuse.
- Admit patients with persistent tachypnea, hypoxemia, or abnormal pulmonary examination as a result of suspected hydrocarbon aspiration, even if the chest radiograph is normal.

DISPOSITION

Any patient presenting with known or suspected cardiac dysrhythmia should be admitted for cardiac monitoring. Patients with significant metabolic abnormalities, renal dysfunction, or potential hepatoxicity should also be admitted. Those with persistent neurologic signs should be considered for admission for further workup (neuropsychiatric testing, neurology evaluation, and MRI) or outpatient referral to an appropriate specialist.

Any patient with significant symptoms or radiographic abnormalities from hydrocarbon aspiration should be admitted and have continuous pulse oximetry. Those with severe aspiration should be admitted to an intensive care setting. Patients with hydrocarbon ingestion who are asymptomatic and have an initial radiograph that is unremarkable should be observed for 6 hours. If clinical and possible radiographic reexamination remain normal, the patient can be discharged. Those with suicidal ingestions require psychiatric evaluation prior to discharge.

COMMON PITFALLS

- Failure to consider the possibility of pulmonary aspiration in patients with hydrocarbon ingestion
- Performance of routine GI decontamination of patients with hydrocarbon ingestion—this is not warranted and may be harmful.
- Failure to recognize that radiographic findings of hydrocarbon aspiration can lag behind clinical toxicity
- Failure to consider the use of beta blockers in the treatment of tachydysrhythmias
- Failure to warn patients suspected of abusing volatile hydrocarbons of the dangers of this form of drug abuse

ICD9

987.0 Toxic effect of liquefied petroleum gases

REFERENCES

1. Bass M. Sudden sniffing death. *JAMA* 1970;212:2075.
2. Daffner RH, Jimenez JP. The double gastric fluid level in kerosene poisoning. *Pediatr Radiol* 1973;106:383–384.
3. Lishitz M, Sofer S, Gorodischer R. Hydrocarbon poisoning in children: a 5-year retrospective study. *Wilderness Environ Med* 2003;14:78.
4. Litovitz T, Green AE. Health implications of petroleum distillate ingestion. *Occup Med (Lond)* 1988;3:555.
5. Siegel E, Wason S. Camphor toxicity. *Pediatr Clin North Am* 1986;33:375
6. Truss CD, Killenberg PG. Treatment of carbon tetrachloride poisoning with hyperbaric oxygen. *Gastroenterology* 1982;82:767.
7. Wason S, Katona B. A review of symptoms, signs and laboratory findings predictive of hydrocarbon toxicity [abstract]. *Vet Hum Toxicol* 1987;29:492.

CHAPTER 37

Hydrogen Sulfide

PRE-HOSPITAL CONSIDERATIONS

- Remove source of hydrogen sulfide (H_2S).
- Wash affected areas copiously with soap and water.
- Prevent self-contamination with use of protective clothing or equipment (self-contained breathing apparatus).
- Prevent others from becoming contaminated.

CLINICAL PRESENTATION

Exposure to H_2S may cause local irritant or systemic effects. Keratoconjunctivitis was first described in petroleum industry workers, at levels of 50 to 100 ppm. Symptoms include eye pain, burning, lacrimation, and mucopurulent drainage (1). Blurred vision and colored halos around lights ("gas eyes") have been attributed to corneal edema and inflammation. Corneal ulceration occurs with severe exposure (1).

Prolonged exposure to H_2S at concentrations as low as 50 ppm results in respiratory mucosal irritation and inflammation. The upper and lower respiratory tracts are equally affected by exposure, resulting in pharyngitis, rhinitis, bronchitis, and pneumonitis. Symptoms include sore throat, nasal congestion and drainage, hoarseness, cough with occasional bloody sputum, and shortness of breath. Symptoms are more severe with longer duration of exposure. Pulmonary edema occurs after prolonged exposure to concentrations >250 ppm, may occur more rapidly at levels of 300 to 500 ppm, and occurs in 20% of cases (3). Physical examination findings include evidence of rhinitis or pharyngitis, including hyperemia and edema. Auscultation may reveal evidence of pneumonitis or pulmonary edema, including wheezes, rales, and rhonchi. Autopsy findings have noted hemorrhagic pulmonary edema and scattered pleural petechial hemorrhages.

Systemic effects of H_2S exposure predominantly reflect central nervous system (CNS) toxicity. At lower concentrations, CNS effects of H_2S intoxication are nonspecific and reflect progressive cellular hypoxia. Signs and symptoms include headache, anxiety, dizziness, ataxia, confusion, vertigo, seizures, lethargy, and coma. With acute, high level exposure, CNS effects predominate over the delayed local irritant and inflammatory effects. Levels >200 ppm are associated with CNS depression, and levels between 700 and 900 ppm are associated with rapid loss of consciousness ("knock down") and respiratory paralysis. Seventy-five percent of occupational exposures have loss of consciousness at the site of exposure (3).

Additional findings include early hyperpnea, cyanosis, hypertension or hypotension, sinus tachycardia or sinus bradycardia, nonspecific interventricular conduction delays, myocardial ischemia, and atrial fibrillation (1,6,9). The initial hyperpnea noted with systemic toxicity is a result of direct stimulation of carotid body chemoreceptors by the sulfide anion. Gastrointestinal complaints, including nausea, vomiting, diarrhea, and abdominal cramps, have been reported, particularly in cases of subacute intoxication.

In contrast to cyanide and carbon monoxide poisoning, cyanosis is frequently described in H_2S intoxication (5,9). Cyanosis in H_2S poisoning has historically been attributed to sulfhemoglobin (6) or the presence of an oxygen saturation gap (the difference between calculated and measured oxygen saturation), suggesting the presence of an unmeasured hemoglobin species (5). However, subsequent reports have discounted these explanations (1,8). Other theories suggest that the endogenous oxidative detoxification of H_2S is catalyzed by oxyhemoglobin, with subsequent deoxyhemoglobin production (1,2,8) or hypoxemia, from centrally mediated respiratory depression and ventilation-perfusion mismatch from pneumonitis or from pulmonary edema (8). The exact etiology remains unclear, however.

No analytic tests are available to confirm the diagnosis of H_2S poisoning (6). Laboratory abnormalities have included anion gap metabolic acidosis and elevated serum lactate levels reflecting the underlying cellular asphyxia and cerebral hypoxia. Oxygen saturation gaps have occasionally been observed, attributed to the presence of sulfhemoglobin.

Computed tomography imaging demonstrates basal ganglia ischemia and injury (4).

DIFFERENTIAL DIAGNOSIS

H_2S exposure is suspected from the rapid loss of consciousness (knock-down), and the odor of rotten eggs, which has been noted from clothing, blood, exhaled air, and gastric secretions (4). Blackening of copper and silver coins or jewelry after exposure to H_2S is another clue. The differential diagnosis includes other cellular asphyxiants (e.g., cyanide, carbon monoxide, sodium azide), simple asphyxiants (e.g., methane, carbon dioxide, helium, nitrogen), pulmonary irritants (e.g., ammonia, nitrogen dioxide), and acquired dyshemoglobinemias (e.g., methemoglobinemia). Other knock-down agents include carbon disulfide, organophosphates, acetylene, and carbonyl sulfide (6).

Other etiologies of syncope and collapse must be considered, including cardiovascular, neurologic, thromboembolic, and hypoglycemic causes. Concomitant occult traumatic injury must always be considered (3,4). In one review, 27% of H_2S intoxicated patients had associated trauma. The differential diagnosis of dermal irritation includes contact dermatitis, photosensitivity reactions, trauma, infection, and vasculitis. Other causes of a rotten egg odor include mercaptans, disulfiram, and sulfur dioxide.

ED EVALUATION

Despite loss of consciousness at the scene, patients may be asymptomatic or minimally symptomatic on arrival at the emergency department (3,4,8). Initial history is directed toward confirming H_2S exposure and the severity of symptoms prior to arrival. Important historical information includes location and actions preceding symptom onset, duration of exposure, time course of any alterations in level of consciousness, and any unusual odors noted. The possibility of coexistent trauma should also be addressed.

After evaluation of vital signs, the physical examination should focus on assessment for irritant (ocular, dermal, mucous membrane, pulmonary) and systemic (cardiovascular and neurologic) effects. An alert mental status does not preclude the existence of significant underlying CNS dysfunction. A thorough neurologic examination, including mental status testing and neuropsychiatric screening batteries, if available, should evaluate for subtle neurologic dysfunction. Patients with limited irritant symptoms, normal vital signs, and normal physical examinations require no laboratory assessment. Patients with evidence of systemic toxicity should have a chest radiograph, electrocardiogram, and arterial blood gas analysis for evaluation of oxygenation and acid-base status. Additional testing may include routine hematology and chemistry profiles. Patients with prolonged loss of consciousness, persistent alteration in level of consciousness, or focal neurologic deficits may require radiologic imaging to evaluate for cerebral ischemic insult and trauma.

ED MANAGEMENT

Initial management involves removing the patient from the source of exposure. Survivors frequently improve simply with this intervention (2,3). Rescuers should not attempt to enter the environment of exposure without wearing self-contained breathing apparatus. Numerous reports document the incapacitation of rescuers attempting to remove an isolated victim from high H_2S environments (3,5,8). As systemic toxicity does not result from dermal exposure, protective clothing is not required. However, decontamination should include removal of grossly contaminated clothing and cleansing with soap and water to limit local irritant effects. Ocular decontamination requires irrigation and the removal of contact lenses.

Supportive care is the mainstay of treatment for systemic toxicity, with specific attention to advanced life support modalities, and management of altered mental status, pulmonary edema, hypotension, acidosis, and concomitant trauma. Supplemental oxygen (100%) enhances oxygen delivery and increase endogenous sulfide metabolism (7). Laboratory studies demonstrate that endogenous sulfide detoxification is so rapid that minimal cytochrome-bound sulfide is expected by the time of patient arrival in the emergency department. As a result, specific data regarding antidotal therapy remain sparse and controversial.

Similarities with cyanide intoxication led to the use of sodium nitrite in severe H_2S intoxication. The resultant methemoglobinemia was thought to limit cytochrome-sulfide binding by acting as a sulfide scavenger and preferentially generating sulfide-methemoglobin complexes (sulfmethemoglobin) or by further catalyzing sulfide oxidation (1). Anecdotal reports and pretreatment animal models have demonstrated improvement with nitrite therapy (6,9); however, no convincing evidence exists that nitrite actually improves patient outcome or changes clinical course. In vitro time-course studies indicate that nitrite must be administered within minutes of exposure to be effective (2). Additionally, the induction of methemoglobinemia may further impair oxygen transport and worsen the clinical situation. Nitrite therapy remains recommended for patients with severe H_2S intoxication who do not rapidly improve on removal from the source, and the nitrite should be administered within 1 hour of exposure. The dose of sodium nitrite is identical to that used for cyanide (adults, 10 mL of 3% sodium nitrite intravenously over 5 minutes; children, 0.2 to 0.33 mL/kg, up to 10 mL). Sodium thiosulfate is not recommended, as rhodanese does not appear to be involved in H_2S detoxification. Improvement with hyperbaric oxygen (HBO) therapy has been reported, even in nitrite-refractory H_2S poisoning (6,7). HBO should be considered for severely intoxicated patients with persistent neurologic abnormalities, especially those patients unresponsive to supportive care or nitrite therapy, given the documented potential for delayed and persistent neuropsychiatric sequelae.

H_2S gas exposure may involve more than one victim. Consideration must be given to the load this may place on an emergency department. The "worried well" may present in large numbers. Given the lack of a direct test for exposure to H_2S, the emergency physician must work with prehospital personnel to determine areas of likely exposure as well as "safe zones." Variables such as vapor density, plume direction, temperature, humidity, and oxygen concentration can all be used to determine geographic areas of likely clinically significant exposure.

CRITICAL INTERVENTIONS

- Extricate the victim from the source rapidly.
- Provide aggressive supportive care; it is the mainstay of therapy.
- Search for concomitant trauma.
- Consider sodium nitrite or HBO in severely intoxicated patients.

DISPOSITION

Patients presenting after a minor H_2S exposure may be discharged after a 4- to 6-hour observation period. Patients with toxicity limited to dermal or ocular irritation may be managed as outpatients. Patients with significant exposure (including loss of consciousness) or local airway irritation should be monitored for at least

24 hours. Patients with abnormal vital signs and cardiopulmonary and neurologic examinations should be admitted to an intensive care unit. Patients with initial loss of consciousness should be followed up within 1 week for examination for delayed neuropsychiatric sequelae. Transfer of severely intoxicated patients should be considered if intensive care or nitrite therapy is indicated but unavailable.

COMMON PITFALLS

- Failure of the prehospital rescuer to wear self-contained breathing apparatus and becoming an additional victim
- Failure to consider the possibility of H_2S poisoning in otherwise healthy patients who suddenly collapse at work
- Failure to appreciate that the lack of an odor does not imply safety, as a result of olfactory paralysis at dangerous levels
- Failure to perform a scene search for possible other victims when an index case is found
- Failure to appreciate the potential for delayed pulmonary injury in the minimally symptomatic patient

ICD9

987.8 Toxic effect of other specified gases, fumes, or vapors

REFERENCES

1. Beauchamp RO Jr, Bus JS, Popp JA, et al. A critical review of the literature on H_2S toxicity. *Crit Rev Toxicol* 1984;13:25–97.
2. Beck JF, Bradbury CM, Connors AJ, et al. Nitrite as an antidote for acute H_2S intoxication? *Am Ind Hyg Assoc J* 1981;42:805–809.
3. Burnett WW, King EG, Grace M, et al. Hydrogen sulfide poisoning: review of 5 years' experience. *Can Med Assoc J* 1977;117:1277–1280.
4. Gabbay DS, De Roos F, Perrone J. Twenty-foot fall averts fatality from massive hydrogen sulfide exposure. *J Emerg Med* 2001;20:141–144.
5. Peters JW. Hydrogen sulfide poisoning in a hospital setting. *JAMA* 1981;246:1588–1589.
6. Policastro MA, Otten EJ. Case files of the University of Cincinnati fellowship in medical toxicology: two patients with acute lethal occupational exposure to hydrogen sulfide. *J Med Toxicol* 2007;3(2):73–79.
7. Smilkstein MJ, Bronstein AC, Pickett HM, et al. Hyperbaric oxygen therapy for severe hydrogen sulfide poisoning. *J Emerg Med* 1985;3:27–30.
8. Smith RP, Gosselin RE. Hydrogen sulfide poisoning. *J Occup Med* 1979;21:93–96.
9. Stine RJ, Slosberg B, Beacham BE. Hydrogen sulfide intoxication. *Ann Intern Med* 1976;85:756–758.

CHAPTER 38

Iron

PRE-HOSPITAL CONSIDERATIONS

- Collect pills and pill bottles for identification in the emergency department.

CLINICAL PRESENTATION

Clinical effects of iron poisoning are usually considered in stages (4). However, patients present at different times after ingestion, the time frame for staging is imprecise, and it can be difficult to distinguish between stages because of rapid progression and overlapping signs, symptoms, and laboratory manifestations. Patients can die in any stage of iron poisoning but for different reasons.

The first stage develops within the first few hours after ingestion, as a result of the direct corrosive effects of iron on the gastrointestinal (GI) tract, and is characterized by abdominal pain, vomiting, and diarrhea. Diarrhea may be the only manifestation in patients who ingest multiple vitamins with iron, particularly preparations intended for children. Hematemesis or melena may occur if there is significant GI bleeding. Patients with serious toxicity develop lethargy, shock, and metabolic acidosis as a result of hypovolemia, anemia, and tissue hypoperfusion. Serum iron concentrations may be normal or elevated.

With the second stage, GI symptoms resolve despite continued absorption of iron and increasing tissue iron burden. This stage may last until about 24 hours after ingestion. Patients frequently appear clinically improved, but this can be falsely reassuring. Laboratory studies are likely to show elevated serum iron levels and a progressive metabolic acidosis.

In the third stage, systemic iron poisoning becomes clinically evident. This may occur early in patients with severe poisoning (bypassing stage 2). Toxic amounts of iron have now moved from blood into tissues, disrupting cellular metabolism, causing third-spacing of fluids and producing venous pooling of blood. Shock and metabolic acidosis in this stage can result from hypovolemia, anemia, hepatic dysfunction, impaired oxidative phosphorylation, heart failure, and renal failure. Fulminant hepatic failure with hypoglycemia, hyperammonemia, and coagulopathy may occur, although significant hepatic injury is unusual if peak serum iron levels remain below 500 μg/dL.

The fourth stage is characterized by gastric outlet obstruction or small-bowel obstruction, which is an unusual occurrence but can develop as a result of scarring produced by iron's corrosive effects several weeks after the acute toxicity has resolved.

Elevated serum iron levels obtained near their peak, at 2 to 6 hours after ingestion, confirm the diagnosis of iron poisoning and may predict severity. Because iron in tissue produces systemic toxicity, a patient may be seriously ill but have a normal serum iron level many hours after ingestion. On the other hand, a serum iron level drawn early after ingestion may be misleadingly low if absorption is still occurring. Therefore, a normal serum iron concentration very early or many hours after ingestion does not exclude iron poisoning.

Although sometimes elevated, the white blood cell count (>15 k/mm^3) and serum glucose concentrations (>150 mg/dL) are not of sufficient sensitivity to assess the severity of acute iron poisoning (5). The "deferoxamine challenge" test, in which the presence of vin rosé–colored urine after giving a dose of deferoxamine was considered an indication for chelation therapy, is no longer recommended because this color change is unreliable (9). A kidney-ureter-bladder (KUB) radiograph may demonstrate radiopaque tablets in the GI tract, a finding often present in patients who develop serious poisoning. However, a normal KUB radiograph does not exclude the possibility of a significant ingestion. Even when iron tablets are noted initially, they are usually no longer visible at 24 hours.

DIFFERENTIAL DIAGNOSIS

The differential diagnosis of patients presenting with GI symptoms includes poisoning by acetaminophen, salicylate, hepatotoxic mushrooms, arsenic, caffeine and theophylline, caustics, copper salts, and mercurial salts. Infectious gastroenteritis, medical and surgical intra-abdominal conditions, or sepsis may cause vomiting, diarrhea, acidosis, and shock. Acute iron poisoning, however, is not accompanied by fever unless a complication such as aspiration or bowel infarction develops.

ED EVALUATION

The history should include the time and amount of ingestion, the identity of the iron preparation ingested, and the nature, severity, time of onset, and progression of symptoms. The physician should specifically ask about abdominal pain, vomiting, and diarrhea and whether blood was noted. The amount of elemental iron ingested, in milligrams per kilogram, should be calculated. The physical examination should focus on vital signs, overall appearance, and the abdomen.

Patients who have had only one or two episodes of vomiting or diarrhea and are subsequently asymptomatic should have a complete blood count (CBC) and measurement of serum electrolytes, glucose, blood urea nitrogen, creatinine, and iron levels. Those with more pronounced or persistent GI symptoms, evidence of hypovolemia, or lethargy should also have a prothrombin time, liver function studies, arterial blood gas analysis, and a KUB radiograph. Because laboratory methods to measure the total iron-binding capacity (TIBC) are inaccurate in the setting of iron overload (6), the TIBC is not helpful in the evaluation of iron toxicity and does not assist in the treatment decisions.

ED MANAGEMENT

Activated charcoal does not effectively bind iron, and its use should be limited to cases in which co-ingestion of other substances that bind to charcoal is known or suspected. If activated charcoal is administered, cathartics should be withheld, especially in patients who already have gastroenteritis, as this may exacerbate hypovolemia. Gastric lavage has not been shown to be of clinical benefit, possibly because most iron tablets are too large to evacuate by this method. Simulated overdose studies suggest that oral magnesium oxide (milk of magnesia, 60 mL/g of elemental iron ingested) (8) or a slurry of charcoal mixed with deferoxamine (1) can reduce iron absorption, but the utility of such treatments in actual overdose patients is unknown. If pills can be identified radiographically, whole-bowel irrigation with a polyethylene glycol-electrolyte solution has been used with good results, although controlled studies are lacking (7).

Patients who remain completely asymptomatic (including absence of lethargy) for 6 hours after ingestion and have a normal physical examination do not require treatment. Those who ingested >20 mg/kg of elemental iron but are seen within 6 hours might benefit from whole-bowel irrigation. If the serum iron concentration in an asymptomatic patient is <350 μg/dL and a repeat serum iron level shows no rise in the iron level, the patient can be released. Radiography demonstrating numerous tablets suggests that serum iron concentrations will be rising. Patients who have had only one or two episodes of emesis or diarrheal stool but who have remained asymptomatic for several hours and have a normal physical examination, KUB, and laboratory evaluation do not require further treatment.

Patients with more than two episodes of emesis or diarrhea or evidence of hypovolemia or exhibit lethargy require treatment with fluids and chelation therapy with deferoxamine mesylate. In patients with significant symptoms, treatment should not be delayed to wait for results of a serum iron determination, because the therapy is indicated regardless of the serum iron concentration. Iron ingestion can raise the serum iron level above the normal range, and an elevated iron level alone does not constitute an indication for deferoxamine or admission in the absence of clinical signs of toxicity.

With rare exceptions, all symptomatic patients are hypovolemic. Intravenous fluid challenges of 20 mL/kg of normal saline or lactated Ringer's are given to restore fluid volume and ensure a normal urine output. Patients commonly require maintenance infusions at twice normal rates to keep up with GI losses and third-spacing.

Deferoxamine mesylate can remove iron from tissues and nontransferrin-bound iron from plasma. Deferoxamine binds to iron to form ferrioxamine, which is excreted in the urine over days to weeks. Ferrioxamine occasionally imparts a vin rosé color to the urine, but this color change is inconsistent and should not be used to determine the need for additional treatment (4,9).

Deferoxamine mesylate can be mixed in any crystalloid and should be continuously infused intravenously at 15 mg/kg/h. Higher infusion rates can be tried in severe cases but are sometimes associated with hypotension (presumably from histamine release); this is rare with infusion rates below 45 mg/kg/h, however. Intramuscular deferoxamine is not recommended.

Many statements in the manufacturer's package insert for deferoxamine do not reflect currently accepted treatment practices. Deferoxamine is not contraindicated for the treatment of acute iron poisoning in pregnancy. Animal data and human experience strongly suggest that neither toxic amounts of maternally ingested iron nor deferoxamine or ferrioxamine cross into the fetal circulation (3). Fetal death, therefore, results from maternal demise, and a pregnant woman should be treated in the same way as any other patient. At 15 mg/kg/h, many patients receive well in excess of 6 g deferoxamine mesylate each day, which is safe for the short-term treatment of iron poisoning.

Deferoxamine causes falsely low serum iron concentrations (2), which should not be a cause for stopping chelation therapy. Intravenous deferoxamine should be continued until clinical toxicity has resolved, serum iron levels are normal or low, and vin rosé–colored urine (if ever present) disappears (4). Most patients require 12 to 24 hours of deferoxamine infusion, but occasional patients with very large overdoses require more prolonged therapy. The use of prochlorperazine (Compazine) and deferoxamine together has produced coma in humans and this drug combination should be avoided.

CRITICAL INTERVENTIONS

- Obtain a CBC, serum electrolytes, glucose, blood urea nitrogen, creatinine, and iron levels, prothrombin time, liver function studies, arterial blood gas analysis, and a KUB radiograph on patients with significant GI symptoms, hypotension, or lethargy.
- Administer intravenous normal saline and deferoxamine to patients with significant GI symptoms, hypotension, or lethargy.
- Consider whole-bowel irrigation when radiopaque tablets are seen on radiographs.

DISPOSITION

Patients who remain completely asymptomatic or those with a normal physical examination, KUB, and laboratory evaluation and only one or two episodes of emesis or diarrhea and then remain asymptomatic 6 hours after ingestion can be discharged.

Patients with mild symptoms should have repeat laboratory studies demonstrating no rise in the serum iron level and no evidence of metabolic acidosis before being cleared for discharge. Symptomatic patients should be admitted. The level of monitoring and treatment required usually necessitates admission to an intensive care unit. If serum iron levels or deferoxamine chelation therapy is not available, the patients should be transferred to a facility in which such services are available.

COMMON PITFALLS

- Failing to administer adequate amounts of intravenous fluids
- Waiting for the serum iron level before administering deferoxamine to a symptomatic patient
- Using the TIBC for evaluation and treatment decisions
- Sending patients home during the second stage of poisoning because they appear clinically improved
- Assuming that a normal iron level, serum glucose, white blood cell count, deferoxamine challenge, and KUB x-ray exclude significant iron poisoning
- Giving prochlorperazine (Compazine) and deferoxamine together
- Failing to appreciate that deferoxamine may falsely lower serum iron concentration

ICD9

964.0 Poisoning by iron and its compounds

REFERENCES

1. Gomez HF, McClafferty HH, Flory D, et al. Prevention of gastrointestinal iron absorption by chelation from an orally administered premixed deferoxamine/charcoal slurry. *Ann Emerg Med* 1997;30:587–592.
2. Helfer RE, Rodgerson DO. The effect of deferoxamine on the determination of serum iron and iron-binding capacity. *J Pediatr* 1966;68:804–806.
3. McElhatton PR, Roberts JC, Sullivan FM. The consequences of iron overdose and its treatment with desferrioxamine in pregnancy. *Hum Exp Toxicol* 1991;10:251–259.
4. Mills KC, Curry SC. Acute iron poisoning. *Emerg Med Clin North Am* 1994;12:397–413.
5. Palatnick W, Tenenbein M. Leukocytosis, hyperglycemia, vomiting, and positive x-rays are not indicators of severity of iron overdose in adults. *Am J Emerg Med* 1996;14:454–455.
6. Siff JE, Meldon SW, Tomassoni AJ. Usefulness of the total iron binding capacity in the evaluation and treatment of acute iron overdose. *Ann Emerg Med* 1999;33:73–76.
7. Tenenbein M. Whole bowel irrigation as a gastrointestinal decontamination procedure after acute poisoning. *Med Toxicol Adverse Drug* 1988;3:77–84.
8. Wallace KL, Curry SC, LoVecchio FL, et al. Effect of magnesium hydroxide on iron absorption following simulated mild iron overdose in human subjects. *Acad Emerg Med* 1998;5:961–965.
9. Yatscoff RW, Wayne EA, Tenenbein M. An objective criterion for the cessation of deferoxamine therapy in the acutely iron-poisoned patient. *J Toxicol Clin Toxicol* 1991;29:1–10.

CHAPTER 39

Lead

PRE-HOSPITAL CONSIDERATIONS

- Support airway, breathing, and circulation.
- Provide cardiac monitoring.
- Have seizure management protocols in place.
- If possible to do so safely, transport containers in cases of suspected overdose or poisoning.
- Decontaminate skin after obvious dermal exposure.

CLINICAL PRESENTATION

Patients with lead poisoning may present with such nonspecific symptoms as headache, fatigue, malaise, abdominal pain, constipation, and vomiting. The abdominal pain is usually colicky and not responsive to standard analgesics. There may be complaints of peripheral paresthesias or hypoesthesias and occasional frank neurologic symptoms (e.g., wrist or ankle drop). The classic wrist drop more common in the dominant arm is seen in painters. Muscle weakness may also be noted. Depression and other affective disorders have been reported in lead-poisoned adults. Hyperactivity, delayed development, or loss of recently acquired skills may be seen in children with coma and seizures in severe cases.

Physical examination is generally unrevealing, although the blood pressure may be elevated. Occasionally, in adults with poor dental care, a dark bluish black discoloration of the gingiva at the dental border (lead lines) may be present. This finding is seldom present in children or in adults with good dental hygiene. If increased intracranial pressure accompanies lead encephalopathy, examination of the optic fundi may show papilledema. Cardiac dysrhythmias such as premature ventricular contractions are reported.

An abdominal radiograph may reveal radiopaque foreign bodies in patients with pica or accidental lead ingestion. In developing children, long-bone radiographs may show an increased density of metaphyseal growth plates as a result of disordered calcium deposition resulting in "lead lines." This finding may persist into later childhood or adolescence but is seldom present in adults.

The laboratory usually reveals a hypochromic microcytic anemia. Lead may produce a nonautoimmune hemolytic anemia with increased red cell fragility and an elevated reticulocyte count. Basophilic stippling and eosinophilia are less often noted. Proteinuria, glycosuria, a Fanconi syndrome (with aminoaciduria and renal tubular acidosis), and increased blood urea nitrogen and creatinine levels may be seen in patients with lead nephropathy. Because lead reduces the excretion of uric acid, adults with lead toxicity are prone to develop gout.

The definitive diagnosis of lead poisoning depends on the measurement of whole-blood lead and free erythrocyte protoporphyrin (FEP). The former indicates exposure, and the latter is evidence that the lead has produced a biologic effect, that is, interference with heme synthesis. Lead levels as low as 5 μg/dL have been reported to produce biochemical abnormalities and, in children, may be associated with decreased intelligence and neurobehavioral problems (1). Lead levels above 10 μg/dL in children and above 40 μg/dL in adults are currently considered to be evidence of increased lead absorption serious enough to warrant intervention. Although the importance of FEP levels has been de-emphasized over the last decade, levels above 15 μg/dL are uncommon in healthy people and in the absence of iron deficiency suggest chronic lead exposure. Although FEP levels >20 μg/dL may be seen with either iron deficiency or lead poisoning, FEP levels >35 μg/dL usually indicate lead poisoning.

DIFFERENTIAL DIAGNOSIS

Lead poisoning shares symptoms with other heavy metal poisonings. The peripheral neuropathy from lead, more often seen in adults than children, tends to be more motor than sensory. Unlike arsenic, the peripheral neuropathy from lead is associated with decreased sensitivity; with arsenic, there are painful paresthesias. The "hallmark" of thallium poisoning is burning paresthesias and hair loss. Both lead and mercury poisoning are characterized by personality changes. Mercury intoxication is characterized by "erythrism" and rapid changes in affect, with outbursts of anger alternating with happiness. Lead poisoning is more often accompanied by depressive disorders. Urinary heavy metal analysis is usually necessary for differentiation.

ED EVALUATION

Patients who present to the emergency department with multisystem complaints, particularly chronic abdominal symptoms that have not responded to standard conservative therapy, should be suspected of having lead poisoning. The patient's occupation (3,6,10), hobbies, use of herbal or other folk remedies, or living conditions may suggest exposure to lead. Subtle changes in bowel habits, behavior, mood, and cognitive function and headaches, weakness, and paresthesias are nonspecific but provide supporting clues.

In addition to vital signs and a general physical examination, a detailed neurologic examination should be performed, including assessment for papilledema and gingival pigmentation. If recent lead ingestion is suspected, an abdominal radiograph showing a radiopaque specimen may be helpful. In children, long-bone radiographs (knee and wrist) may suggest chronic lead exposure. The laboratory evaluation should include a complete blood count, whole-blood lead and FEP levels, serum blood urea nitrogen and creatinine levels, and a urinalysis. Care must be taken to use lead-free collection techniques when measuring for lead.

Unless a patient is symptomatic with a high suspicion of lead poisoning, blood lead levels should be confirmed before initiating treatment. Conversely, a patient presenting with symptoms and signs consistent with lead poisoning and a history suggestive of lead exposure should begin on therapy immediately as any delay may have serious effects on survival.

In some cases, a patient is referred to the emergency department with a known exposure or a known elevated blood level of lead. These patients need a baseline assessment and a decision whether chelation is necessary. If children appear because parents are concerned about a possible exposure to lead contaminated toys, a blood level can be obtained and referral made for further management. If an acute ingestion is suspected, a plain film can be obtained to identify the need for whole-bowel irrigation.

ED MANAGEMENT

Cerebral edema should be treated by hyperventilation, elevation of the head, and restriction of fluids. Seizures should be controlled with pharmacologic agents such as benzodiazepines, barbiturates, and phenytoin. In patients with acute encephalopathy (with or without coma or seizures), chelation therapy should be initiated before obtaining confirmatory laboratory data, because the long-term outcome is related to the length of time the vital organs are exposed to elevated lead levels. Whole-bowel irrigation can be done if there is radiopaque material in the intestine, but decontamination should not delay parenteral chelation therapy. Because there is controversy that oral chelation may increase absorption of lead, it should not be done if there is lead within the intestinal lumen (4,5,7–9,11).

Although there are no randomized clinical trials reporting the use of chelation, it has been the standard of care since the late 1960s (2) to treat all children with elevated lead levels that might cause neurologic damage. That range has varied over time depending on prevailing data. Currently, chelation therapy is usually indicated for children with lead levels >45 μg/dL, for adults with levels >80 μg/dL, and for patients with lower levels who have a positive lead mobilization test or evidence of lead-associated symptoms or signs.

Dimercaprol (British antilewisite [BAL]) crosses the blood–brain barrier and forms a tight bond with lead; in patients with lead encephalopathy, it is the initial therapy of choice. An oil-based solution of dimercaprol is given IM in a usual dose of 3 to 5 mg/kg every 4 to 6 hours. Dimercaprol is painful when injected and foul-smelling, and it may produce adverse local and systemic reactions. Sterile abscesses may occur at the site of dimercaprol injection, and febrile responses are common. Many patients complain of a terrible taste in their mouths and of lightheadedness.

Calcium disodium ethylenediaminetetraacetic acid (EDTA: CaNa$_2$EDTA) is water-soluble and can be given IM or IV. The lead-EDTA bond is very strong and stable at a physiologic pH. However, in acid urine, the bond is less stable, and there is the potential for release of free lead into the renal tubule and subsequent renal tubular damage. The main side effects of EDTA are phlebitis (with concentrations >0.5 mg/mL) and potential renal toxicity. IV administration is preferred because IM injections are extremely irritating and produce elevations of creatine phosphokinase (2). If the IM route is used, procaine or lidocaine is usually added to produce an 0.5% concentration of the local anesthetic.

CaNa$_2$EDTA is given in a dose of 50 mg/kg/d. IV CaNa$_2$EDTA is given as a continuous drip. At a concentration of 0.5 mg/mL, a large amount of fluid must be infused. However, if the patient can tolerate the fluid load, the incidence of side effects, particularly renal dysfunction, may be decreased. IM CaNa$_2$EDTA is given in divided doses every 4 to 24 hours. Because the use of CaNa$_2$EDTA alone may liberate bone lead and transiently raise brain lead levels and increase symptoms, it is advisable to start with an initial dose of dimercaprol in all symptomatic patients and those with high blood lead levels (>55 μg/dL in children and 100 mg/dL in adults).

Oral chelation with dimercaptosuccinic acid or succimer (Chemet) is indicated for children with lead levels above 45 μg/dL and is as effective in clearing lead as the combination of dimercaprol and EDTA. The side-effect spectrum is minimal, with a small incidence of skin rash, transaminase elevations, and gastrointestinal (GI) discomfort. Although not officially licensed for use in adults, its effectiveness, combined with its low order of toxicity, argues for its use in this population. The published dosage in children may be used safely in adults—10 mg/kg/dose every 8 hours for 5 days, followed by 10 mg/kg per dose every 12 hours for an additional 14 days. Patients should be monitored for toxicity with weekly blood counts, chemistry profiles, and urinalysis. The presence of ketones in the urine may be used as a measure of compliance, because it is a very common accompaniment of successful treatment. A mild rash or mild transaminitis is usually not a reason to abandon therapy but requires closer observation, with more frequent laboratory investigation. It is important to ensure that no further exposure to lead occur while on oral chelation.

Another oral chelator, *d*-penicillamine, a derivative of penicillin, is given orally at a dosage of 30 mg/kg/d, with the average adult dose of about 1.0 to 1.5 g/d. It is usually used only for adults with mild or no symptoms but high lead levels. Side effects include diarrhea, renal toxicity, leukopenia and, occasionally, a rash. Penicillamine is less effective than dimercaprol or CaNa$_2$EDTA.

If renal toxicity develops as a result of antidotal therapy, fluid input should be increased in an attempt to dilute the lead content of the urine. Alkalinization of the urine may also be helpful.

Therapy should be continued until the lead level drops below 20 μg/dL in children and 40 μg/dL in adults. Maximum lead excretion occurs during the first 3 days of chelation therapy and falls off rapidly. After 5 days of therapy, it is unlikely that there will be further significant lead excretion without a rest period to allow lead to redistribute from tissue compartments to the blood. Hence, chelation therapy is usually limited to a 5-day course of parenteral drug, followed by a treatment-free interval of 2 to 7 days. Oral succimer therapy is usually discontinued after 19 total days of therapy. Additional courses of therapy are indicated if symptoms persist or blood lead levels remain elevated. Repeat lead levels should be evaluated, initially, at least weekly. Reinstitution of therapy, depending on the "rebound" in lead level, should be considered. Children with lead levels below 20 μg/dL and adults with levels below 40 μg/dL should be managed by preventing further exposure by environmental and by using educational interventions. Follow-up evaluation and periodic monitoring are required.

The vast majority of lead-poisoned patients survive although the final neurologic outcome may not be known for many weeks or months after treatment. Patients with cerebral edema have a poor prognosis.

CRITICAL INTERVENTIONS

- Consult a poison center or lead-poisoning expert for management advice in patients with suspected or confirmed lead poisoning.
- Admit patients with lead encephalopathy and administer dimercaprol (BAL) IM and calcium disodium EDTA IV.
- Obtain blood lead levels in children with suspected exposure and arrange for close follow-up.

DISPOSITION

All patients with evidence of encephalopathy should be admitted. Although chelation with CaNa$_2$EDTA, penicillamine, and succimer can be done on an outpatient basis, it is advisable to admit all patients who are symptomatic or who have markedly elevated lead levels (requiring dimercaprol therapy). However, because blood lead levels are not immediately available at the time of initial evaluation, patients who are not acutely ill can be discharged and admitted later if blood lead confirms the suspected diagnosis.

Further exposure to lead must be prevented. Environmental and occupational investigations should be performed to determine the most likely source of lead so that it can be eliminated. Involvement of the public health department, primarily in dealing with a child with lead poisoning, is imperative. The Occupational Safety and Health Administration may be helpful in investigating cases of occupational lead exposure. Many states also have active divisions of occupational and environmental health that may be helpful in the long-term treatment of patients.

Although chelation therapy is not difficult, some of the nuances are appreciated only after treating many patients. Hence, the physician unfamiliar with the evaluation and therapy of lead exposure and poisoning is advised to consult an experienced toxicologist, usually available through a regional poison control center (1-800-222-1222).

All patients should be seen within 2 weeks of chelation therapy for repeat lead and FEP levels, because lead will be mobilized from storage sites, and blood levels will rebound after treatment. However, without continued exposure to lead, it is rare for the lead level at 2 weeks after therapy to equal or exceed the initial level.

COMMON PITFALLS

- Failure to consider the diagnosis of lead poisoning in patients with cognitive dysfunction, neurologic symptoms, and GI complaints
- Failure to appreciate that elevated lead levels without coincidental elevations in FEP may be seen with recent exposures and to treat the patient with an extremely high lead level regardless of the FEP level
- Failure to appreciate that lead poisoning is a reportable illness in many states
- Failure to identify the source of lead and to prevent re-exposure

ICD9

984.0 Toxic effect of inorganic lead compounds
984.1 Toxic effect of organic lead compounds
984.8 Toxic effect of other lead compounds

REFERENCES

1. Canfield RL, Henderson CR Jr, Cory-Slechta DA, et al. Intellectual impairment in children with blood lead concentrations below 10 microg per deciliter. *N Engl J Med* 2003;348(16):1517–1526.
2. Chisolm JJ Jr. The use of chelating agents in the treatment of acute and chronic lead intoxication in childhood. *J Pediatr* 1968;73(1):1–9.
3. Cocco P, Hua F, Boffetta P, et al. Mortality of Italian lead smelter workers. *Scand J Work Environ Health* 1997;23(1):15–23.
4. Cory-Slechta DA, Weiss B, Cox C. Mobilization and redistribution of lead over the course of calcium disodium ethylenediamine tetraacetate chelation therapy. *J Pharmacol Exp Ther* 1987;243:804–813.
5. Cremin JD Jr, Luck ML, Laughlin NK, Smith DR. Oral succimer decreases the gastrointestinal absorption of lead in juvenile monkeys. *Environ Health Perspect* Jun 2001;109(6):613–619.
6. Osorio AM, Melius J. Lead poisoning in construction. *Occup Med* 1995;10(2):353–361.
7. Sanchez-Fructuoso AI, Cano M, Arroyo M, et al. Lead mobilization during calcium disodium ethylenediaminetetraacetate chelation therapy in treatment of chronic lead poisoning. *Am J Kidney Dis* 2002;40(1):51–58.
8. Seaton CL, Lasman J, Smith DR. The effects of CaNa(2)EDTA on brain lead mobilization in rodents determined using a stable lead isotope tracer. *Toxicol Appl Pharmacol* 1999;159(3):153–160.
9. Smith DR, Markowitz ME, Crick J, Rosen JF, Flegal AR. The effects of succimer on the absorption of lead in adults determined by using the stable isotope 204Pb. *Environ Res* 1994;67(1):39–53.
10. Sun JB, Wang JP. Recommended diagnostic criteria for occupational chronic lead poisoning. *Biomed Environ Sci* 1995;8(4):318–329.
11. Varnai VM, Piasek M, Blanusa M, Saric MM, Kostial K. Succimer treatment during ongoing lead exposure reduces tissue lead in suckling rats. *J Appl Toxicol* 2001;21(5):415–416.

CHAPTER 40

Methemoglobinemia

PRE-HOSPITAL CONSIDERATIONS

- Bring all substances the patient may have ingested to the hospital.
- Question witnesses and observe the scene for household products and other potential coingestants. Document and relay findings to emergency medical staff.
- At commercial or industrial sites:
  - Obtain relevant Material Safety Data Sheets (MSDSs) if available to identify commercial or chemical products.
  - Avoid dermal exposures.

CLINICAL PRESENTATION

Nonanemic patients with 10% to 20% methemoglobinemia usually present with unexplained cyanosis and no other symptoms. Headache, dyspnea on exertion, tachypnea, tachycardia, and mild hypertension usually are not noted until the methemoglobin levels reach 15% to 35%. Higher fractions can result in confusion, coma, seizures, apnea, ventricular dysrhythmias, bradydysrhythmias, hypotension, and lactic acidosis. Death is frequently seen with methemoglobin fractions above 70%.

Patients with underlying cardiovascular or cerebrovascular disease are more susceptible to the effects of hypoxia. Those with pre-existing anemia or with concomitant Heinz body hemolytic anemia suffer greater toxicity at a given methemoglobin level, because the remaining functional hemoglobin concentration is lower. Also, cyanosis may not be apparent in the anemic patient because a greater percentage of methemoglobin would be needed to reach the 1.5 g/dL threshold of cyanosis as compared to the nonanemic patient. Hence, anemic patients can suffer from significant methemoglobinemia without exhibiting cyanosis.

The cyanosis of methemoglobinemia is refractory to oxygen. The arterial PO_2 is normal or elevated. The oxygen saturation by pulse oximetry is falsely elevated with respect to the true value but less than the value calculated from the PO_2. Metabolic acidosis may be present in severe cases. Venous blood may have a brown hue. A low hemoglobin, bite cells on peripheral blood smear, Heinz bodies with this stain, and increased serum haptoglobin and pink plasma from hemoglobinemia occur in severe cases of hemolysis. The electrocardiogram (ECG) may reveal tachycardia, bradycardia, ventricular dysrhythmias, and myocardial ischemia.

DIFFERENTIAL DIAGNOSIS

Unlike cyanosis from hypoxia, the cyanosis of methemoglobinemia will have a normal PO_2 on blood gas analysis and is unresponsive to oxygen. Arterial blood gas reveals a normal PO_2 and a normal percentage of oxyhemoglobin (percentage saturation) because most blood gas instruments do not directly measure oxyhemoglobin fractions but, rather, calculate what the percentage hemoglobin saturation should be based on the oxygen tension. These calculations assume the absence of methemoglobin, carboxyhemoglobin, and sulfhemoglobin and further that there is no shift in the dissociation curve from changes in erythrocytic 2,3-diphosphoglycerate concentrations (5). A co-oximeter is required to directly measure the true percentage saturation, the total hemoglobin concentration, and percentages of oxyhemoglobin, methemoglobin, and carboxyhemoglobin. Sulfhemoglobin is usually recognized as methemoglobin by these instruments. The difference between the percentage of hemoglobin saturation calculated by the blood gas analyzer and the saturation measured by the co-oximeter is called the *oxygen saturation gap*. A large oxygen saturation gap in arterial blood is almost always as a result of carboxyhemoglobin or methemoglobin. To interpret blood gas reports accurately, the emergency physician must know whether reported percentage saturations on arterial blood gas samples are determined by co-oximetry.

Pulse oximeters (e.g., ear or finger oximeters) usually measure only oxyhemoglobin and deoxyhemoglobin and cannot account for methemoglobin or carboxyhemoglobin. As methemoglobin rises, the pulse oximetry reading approaches 84%. Therefore, a pulse oximeter can report a false hemoglobin oxygen saturation in the presence of methemoglobinemia or carboxyhemoglobinemia (5). Hyperlipidemia, seen after infusions of lipid emulsions or in patients with diabetes mellitus, interferes with the measurement of hemoglobin pigments by co-oximeters, resulting in falsely elevated methemoglobin concentrations (8). In these instances, the patient with a normal hemoglobin concentration and without cyanosis does not have serious methemoglobinemia.

A peculiar and poorly characterized cyanosis may also be seen in some cases of hydrogen sulfide. Sulfhemoglobinemia, a rare cause of cyanosis, causes noticeable discoloration at only 0.5 g/dL blood and can produce a saturation gap with a normal arterial PO_2. Most co-oximeters measure sulfhemoglobin as methemoglobin. Fortunately, sulfhemoglobin is rarely (if ever) severe enough to cause life-threatening symptoms. Generalized bluish discoloration from excessive administration of methylene blue may also be confused with cyanosis (4).

ED EVALUATION

A careful history should be taken from the patient and family regarding medications, occupational exposures to chemicals, family history of methemoglobinemia, recreational drug use and, in the case of children, any substances in the house that could have been ingested. The physical examination should focus on vital signs, skin color, and any evidence of cerebral or myocardial hypoxia.

Besides determining the methemoglobin fraction, the physician should seek evidence of hemolysis. Therefore, a hemoglobin-hematocrit, Heinz body stain, serum haptoglobin, and plasma-free hemoglobin concentration should be ordered if hemolysis is suspected. Additional evaluation should include a complete blood count, serum electrolytes, blood urea nitrogen, creatinine, and glucose, arterial blood gas analysis, urinalysis, and ECG.

A drop of the patient's blood can be placed on filter paper and allowed to dry. If the blood appears obviously brown, as compared with a drop of blood from a healthy person, a level of at least 15% methemoglobin is present, assuming a normal total hemoglobin concentration (3). Furthermore, venous blood from a healthy person becomes bright red when shaken in the air as oxyhemoglobin is formed whereas blood that contains elevated methemoglobin concentrations will remain dark brown.

ED MANAGEMENT

Patients with methemoglobinemia should be placed on oxygen to maximize the oxygen delivery of the residual normal hemoglobin. Intravenous access should be established, and the patient should be placed on a cardiac monitor.

Most patients with mild methemoglobinemia (<30%) are blue but asymptomatic and do not require treatment (1,3). Once exposure to the offending agent is terminated, methemoglobin levels usually return to normal within 12 to 36 hours. Patients with symptoms unrelieved by oxygen, with methemoglobin fractions above 30%, ECG changes, or a metabolic acidosis should receive antidotal therapy with methylene blue, provided there is no history of glucose-6-phosphate dehydrogenase (G6PD) deficiency. Methylene blue is usually available as a 1% solution (10 mg/mL) and should be given intravenously over 3 to 5 minutes at an initial dose of 2 mg/kg (0.2 mL/kg of a 1% solution) (3). A dramatic response with resolution of cyanosis is usually noted within 15 minutes. If the patient is seriously symptomatic and no response is noted within 15 minutes or if the patient remains moderately symptomatic after 15 to 30 minutes, repeat doses of 1 mg/kg (0.1 mL/kg of 1% solution) can be given. If methemoglobin levels are readily available, they should be performed before repeat doses of methylene blue are given, because large doses of methylene blue themselves might produce methemoglobinemia and can cause discoloration of skin (3,4). The total dose of methylene blue during the first 2 to 3 hours should not exceed 5 to 7 mg/kg (3).

Adverse effects of methylene blue include dysuria, substernal chest pain, and anxiety. Urine frequently turns blue and then green as the drug is excreted. Single doses of methylene blue as low as 5 mg/kg have been shown to induce methemoglobinemia in animals (6).

Methylene blue is contraindicated in patients with G6PD deficiency. These patients have low erythrocytic nicotinamide adenine dinucleotide phosphate (NADPH) concentrations, making augmentation of the NADPH-dependent, methemoglobin-reducing enzyme by methylene blue impossible. More important, methylene blue may trigger massive hemolysis in such patients, further compromising oxygen delivery to tissues (7). About 15% of African American males are thought to be deficient in G6PD; men and women of Mediterranean ancestry also have an increased incidence of this enzyme deficiency.

As soon as time allows, gastrointestinal and skin decontamination should be performed to limit continued absorption of the offending agent. This is particularly important after acute dermal exposures to chemicals or after intentional ingestions of toxic agents. Dermal decontamination can be performed with a triple wash (water rinse, soap scrub, water rinse). If the drug or chemical causing methemoglobinemia cannot be readily eliminated from the body (e.g., dapsone), methemoglobinemia may continually recur for hours or days despite successful initial treatment with methylene blue. In this instance, serial measurements of methemoglobin levels are required, and a constant intravenous infusion of methylene blue at a rate of 0.1 mg/kg/h has been used to maintain methemoglobin concentrations at a safe level (2). Repeated oral doses of activated charcoal may also enhance the elimination of dapsone. Additionally, high-dose cimetidine given intravenously has been shown to lessen dapsone-induced methemoglobin production. Renal failure is a relative contraindication to using a constant infusion or frequently repeated doses of methylene blue, because the drug is mainly renally excreted.

Treatment with hyperbaric oxygen (HBO) or exchange transfusions should be considered for patients with G6PD deficiency or for those who do not respond satisfactorily to methylene blue. HBO can provide enough dissolved oxygen to support life in the presence of severe methemoglobinemia. Symptomatic hemolytic anemia may require blood transfusions. Because massive hemolysis may cause hyperkalemia and acute renal failure, efforts should be made to maintain a good rate of urine flow.

Ascorbic acid also reduces methemoglobin to hemoglobin (nonenzymatically). A dose of 0.5 to 1.0 g ascorbic acid every 6 hours may be given intravenously or orally in conjunction with methylene blue. However, ascorbic acid works too slowly to be useful in the treatment of acute, acquired methemoglobinemia (3). Although *N*-acetylcysteine has been proposed as a possible adjunct, it has not been shown to reduce elevated methemoglobin levels in a human model of methemoglobinemia (9).

CRITICAL INTERVENTIONS

- Administer 100% oxygen to patients with suspected or diagnosed methemoglobinemia.
- Measure methemoglobin levels with a co-oximeter, if available.
- Obtain Heinz body blood stain, serum haptoglobin, and plasma-free hemoglobin concentration in patients with a low hemoglobin-hematocrit.
- Administer methylene blue to patients with signs of cardiac ischemia, dyspnea, metabolic acidosis, or methemoglobin levels >30%.

DISPOSITION

Patients with methemoglobinemia should be admitted after emergency department evaluation and management. Patients are best managed at a facility in which methemoglobin concentrations can be measured easily and quickly. If transfer is necessary, advanced life-support services should be provided and should include a supply of methylene blue. In the case of an accidental or intentional poisoning, the physician must evaluate and treat other toxic effects of methemoglobin-producing agents. All patients who receive methylene blue should be observed for recurrence of symptomatic methemoglobinemia and for adverse effects such as hemolysis.

An asymptomatic and otherwise healthy patient who has been cyanotic for several days does not require admission if the total hemoglobin concentration is normal, the methemoglobin level is below 20%, exposure to the offending agent is terminated, and reliable follow-up is available. Methemoglobin concentrations will return to normal in these patients as the offending drug is cleared from the body. A conservative approach would be to admit all young children and elderly patients for observation, serial methemoglobin concentrations and, when indicated, serial ECGs.

Any patient who unexpectedly develops methemoglobinemia should be referred to a hematologist for evaluation of possible NADH cytochrome-b5 reductase deficiency. Any patient with methemoglobinemia that is unresponsive to treatment with methylene blue should be evaluated, after full recovery, for G6PD deficiency or, much less commonly, NADPH methemoglobin reductase deficiency.

COMMON PITFALLS

- Failure to consider the diagnosis of methemoglobinemia in patients with cyanosis unresponsive to oxygen
- Failure to appreciate that a normal arterial PO_2 and normal oxygen saturation (as measured by pulse oximetry or calculated from arterial blood gases) do not rule out methemoglobinemia
- Failure to appreciate that resolution of cyanosis in a patient with methemoglobinemia may be as a result of accompanying hemolysis, with actual worsening of oxygen delivery to tissues
- Failure to appreciate that methylene blue is contraindicated in patients with G6PD deficiency

ICD9

289.7 Methemoglobinemia

REFERENCES

1. Ash-Bernal R, Wise R, Wright SM. Acquired methemoglobinemia: a retrospective series of 138 cases at 2 teaching hospitals. *Medicine* 2004;83:265–273.
2. Berlin G, Brodin B, Hilden J-O. Acute dapsone intoxication: a case treated with continuous infusion of methylene blue, forced diuresis, and plasma exchange. *J Toxicol Clin Toxicol* 1985;22:537.

3. Curry S. Methemoglobinemia. *Ann Emerg Med* 1982;11:214.
4. Goluboff N, Wheaton R. Methylene blue-induced cyanosis and acute hemolytic anemia complicating the treatment of methemoglobinemia. *J Pediatr* 1961;58:86.
5. Haymond S, Cariappa R, Eby CS, Scott MG. Laboratory assessment of oxygenation in Methemoglobinemia. *Clin Chem* 2005;51:434–444.
6. Lovejoy FH. Methemoglobinemia. *Clin Toxicol Rev* 1984;6:1.
7. Rosen PJ, Johnson C, McGehee WG, et al. Failure of methylene blue treatment in toxic methemoglobinemia; association with glucose-6-phosphate dehydrogenase deficiency. *Ann Intern Med* 1971;75:83.
8. Spurzem JR, Bonekat HW, Shigeoka JW. Factitious methemoglobinemia caused by hyperlipemia. *Chest* 1984;86:84.
9. Tanen DA, Lovecchio F, Curry SC. Failure of intravenous *N*-acetylcysteine to reduce methemoglobin produced by sodium nitrite in human volunteers: a randomized controlled trial. *Ann Emerg Med* 2000; 35:369.

CHAPTER 41

Pulmonary Inhalants

PRE-HOSPITAL CONSIDERATIONS
- Prevent self-contamination with use of protective clothing or equipment (self-contained breathing apparatus).

CLINICAL PRESENTATION

Inhalants with Immediate-Onset Symptoms. Agents that are intermediately or highly water-soluble generally produce immediate symptoms of mucous membrane irritation. The most commonly encountered agents in this category are chlorine gas, chloramines, and ammonia. Less commonly encountered agents include sulfur dioxide, formaldehyde, and chloropicrin.

Chlorine gas became infamous as a chemical warfare agent in World War I. It is heavy, dense, and greenish yellow in color. Exposure to chlorine gas may occur in several different settings. Industrially, it is used in water purification processes, as well as textile and paper bleaching processes (1). As the mixture of an acid (typically found in toilet bowl cleaners) with bleach liberates chlorine gas, household exposure is possible and occurs fairly frequently (2). Finally, exposure to concentrated chlorine gas has occurred from accidents and malfunctions in pool chlorination systems (3).

The mechanism of chlorine-induced injury involves its reaction with water on mucous membranes and the respiratory tract. When this occurs, hydrochloric acid (HCl) and hypochlorous acid (HOCl) are formed, leading to tissue injury. Furthermore, HOCl degrades to HCl and oxygen free radicals, which leads to oxidative cellular damage (1).

The clinical effects of chlorine gas exposure depend on the concentration and duration of exposure. Individuals with brief low-dose household exposure most commonly complain of cough followed by shortness of breath and throat irritation, and symptoms typically resolve within 6 hours (2). As the concentration and duration of exposure increase, the degree of mucous membrane and airway injury increases, ultimately leading to acute lung injury, adult respiratory distress syndrome, and even death with massive exposures (1).

Chloramines are produced when bleach is mixed with ammonia. On contact with mucous membranes and the respiratory tract, they degrade to ammonia,

HOCl, and oxygen free radicals. They cause an injury pattern similar to chlorine gas, and acute lung injury has occurred with household exposures (4,5).

Ammonia is a highly water-soluble gas that has a characteristic pungent odor. It is used as a component of agricultural fertilizer, in the manufacturing of plastics and explosives, and as a refrigerant and cleaning agent. On contact with water, it forms ammonium hydroxide, which causes a rapid onset of severe upper airway injury. Ammonia's strong odor and the rapid mucous membrane irritation it causes usually prevent ongoing exposure and further injury. However, individuals exposed to highly concentrated gas or those with prolonged exposure may develop lower respiratory tract injury and severe acute lung injury.

Sulfur dioxide (SO_2) is another highly water-soluble gas that has many industrial and occupational uses. It is a by-product in the smelting and oil refinery industries. It is also used as a preservative for fruits and vegetables, as a disinfectant in wineries and breweries, and as a bleaching agent in the textile and paper industries. In the presence of water, SO_2 is readily converted to sulfurous acid (H_2SO_3), which is largely responsible for producing the mucosal injury. Owing to its characteristic pungent "burning match" odor, potential victims tend to remove themselves from exposure before severe injury can develop, and effects are therefore most often limited to upper-airway and mucous membrane irritation. Higher concentrations, however, have been shown to cause morphologic changes consistent with acute lung injury, and indeed, individuals with large or prolonged exposure can develop acute pulmonary edema and die within hours of exposure (6).

Pure formaldehyde is a gas at room temperature. The majority of formaldehyde produced in the United States is used for plastics and resin manufacturing. It is highly water-soluble and produces mainly upper-respiratory mucous membrane irritation.

Chloropicrin is a fumigant that has been used for cereals and grains. Because it is a highly potent irritant and lacrimator, it is also added to structural fumigants as a warning agent. It causes mainly mucous membrane irritation, but lung injury may occur with a high dose or prolonged exposure.

Inhalants with Delayed-Onset Symptoms. In contrast to the agents with high and intermediate water solubility, gases with low water solubility tend not to cause immediate mucous membrane irritation. This may lead to prolonged exposure. Once poorly water-soluble gases are inhaled into the alveoli, their dissolution into the epithelial fluid occurs slowly over several hours, producing a delayed-onset pulmonary edema. Two important gases in this category are phosgene (carbonyl chloride) and nitrogen dioxide (NO_2).

Phosgene is a colorless gas with a smell often described as that of freshly mown hay. It was used as a chemical warfare agent in World War I and was estimated to cause more than 80% of all poisonous gas fatalities. Today, phosgene is used as an intermediate in the production of isocyanates, polyurethanes, pharmaceuticals, dyestuffs, and carbamate pesticides. In addition, it is formed on the combustion of chlorinated organic compounds (7).

Phosgene causes injury by two mechanisms: acylation and hydrolysis to hydrochloric acid. As phosgene reacts with sulfhydryl, hydroxyl, and amino groups, it acylates them, resulting in disruption of the cell membrane and various cellular enzymes and ultimately leading to pulmonary cellular death (8). Second, on contact with water, phosgene is slowly hydrolyzed to hydrochloric acid, resulting in mucosal and pulmonary injury.

Unless there is large exposure to concentrated gas, phosgene produces little to no immediate mucous membrane irritation. Although pulmonary injury may occur within an hour of exposure (18), the development of clinical symptoms may be delayed for 15 to 30 hours (8). The chest x-ray may appear normal or show only very subtle changes initially, but frank pulmonary edema may develop over 24 hours (7,8).

NO_2 is a reddish-brown gas with a pungent odor that may be encountered in several different scenarios. NO_2 can form in grain silos as the silage nitrates are fermented into nitrites, which subsequently combine with organic acids to form nitrous acid. Nitrous acid may then decompose to water and nitrogen oxides, which cause silo-filler's disease (9). Another potential route of exposure is through the exhaust of propane-powered ice cleaning machines in poorly ventilated ice skating rinks. Finally, nitrogen oxides may be generated by welding and as a by-product of the combustion of nitrocellulose, which is a major component of radiographic film.

Although NO_2 can directly oxidize cell membranes, it also forms reactive nitrogen species, particularly perioxynitrite (ONOO–). These reactive species cause inflammation and damage to bronchiolar and alveolar type I and II epithelial cells. In addition to generating reactive nitrogen species, NO_2 forms nitric acid upon contact with respiratory tract water, which further contributes to pulmonary injury (10). Owing to its poor water solubility, NO_2 causes little to no immediate mucous membrane irritation. The result is a relatively asymptomatic patient with a normal chest x-ray, who may go on to develop pulmonary edema and clinical symptoms within 24 hours of exposure.

Miscellaneous Irritants. Isocyanates are used in the production of urethane foams for insulation, packaging, and the sealing of electrical equipment. They are also used in many paints and finishes. Of the isocyanates, methyl isocyanate (MIC) is the most potent respiratory tract irritant, and its inadvertent release in 1984 in Bhopal, India, was responsible for more than 2,000 deaths. Today, MCI has largely been replaced by methylene diphenyl diisocyanate (MDI) and toluene diisocyanate (TDI). MDI is relatively safe because of its low volatility. However, TDI is volatile and can produce acute irritation of the mucous membranes and respiratory tract. It can also cause sensitization leading to the development of occupational asthma.

Pulmonary Inhalants with Systemic Toxicity. Arsine gas (AsH_3, arsenous hydride) is colorless with a garlic odor and may be generated when arsenic-containing materials contact water or acid (11). Common industrial processes that result in arsine formation include metal refining, smelting, and computer and fiberoptic chip manufacture. Arsine is generally a nonirritating gas, and exposures <0.5 ppm may not be readily apparent (12). Signs and symptoms may develop within two to 24 hours of exposure and include nausea, vomiting, abdominal pain, diarrhea, dizziness, and weakness (12). The most feared complication of arsine exposure is intravascular hemolysis, evidenced by "black" urine, jaundice, and acute renal failure secondary to both direct arsine toxicity and heme pigment-associated tubular necrosis. The classic presentation of arsine poisoning is the clinical triad of jaundice, abdominal pain, and hematuria. Other reported signs and symptoms include pulmonary edema, skin "bronzing," myalgias and delayed-onset peripheral neuropathy (13). Arsine-induced hemolysis may be related to disruption of red blood cell membrane ion gradients causing membrane instability and also direct heme release (12). Blood or spot urine arsenic measurements can aid in the initial diagnosis and can be followed up during treatment. Removal of the arsine hemoglobin complex and red blood cell fragments via early plasma exchange transfusion has been associated with clinical improvement and reduction in blood and urine arsenic levels (11). Chelation therapy has not been effective in arsine poisoning.

Ethylene oxide is a colorless gas with an ether-like odor commonly used as a sterilizing agent in hospitals. All of the following have been reported after acute ethylene oxide exposure: mucosal irritation, dermal burns, nausea, vomiting, chest tightness, cough, dyspnea, loss of consciousness, and seizures (14). After chronic exposure, ethylene oxide has been associated with contact dermatitis and peripheral neuropathy (14). Treatment is removal from the source and supportive.

Phosphine gas (PH_3) is generated from the contact of aluminum phosphide and water. Aluminum phosphide is a solid fumigant pesticide used to preserve grain. Unintentional exposure occurs from inhalation of or dermal exposure to phosphine generated from fumigated grains. Intentional phosphine poisoning, by ingestion of solid aluminum phosphide tablets that react with gastrointestinal mucosa to form phosphine, is a common form of suicide in countries such as India (15–17). Signs and symptoms include initial severe vomiting followed by coma, seizures, metabolic acidosis, and cardiovascular collapse. Survivors of ingestion may develop esophageal strictures. A characteristic fishy or garlic odor is commonly described with phosphine exposure and may be a helpful clue to diagnosis. "Off gassing" of phosphine from patients' vomitus or expired breath causing rescuer toxicity has not been demonstrated (15). Phosphine toxicity is believed to occur from free radical oxidant damage and cytochrome c oxidase inhibition (15). Treatment is removal from the source of exposure and provision of supportive care. There is no antidote for phosphine poisoning. Elevated blood and tissue phosphine levels have been reported after exposure (16). Treatment with immediate gastric lavage after ingestion, oral coconut oil, N-acetylcysteine, magnesium, and trimetazidine have all been reported, but none has been validated (15). Mortality has been reported as high as 60% (15).

Methyl bromide was used until the 1950s as a fire extinguisher but now primarily serves as a fumigant. It is a colorless and odorless gas even at high concentrations (17). Acute exposure is associated with early gastrointestinal upset, dizziness, and headache, which can be followed by progressive neurologic deterioration, including coma, myoclonus, seizures, and status epilepticus. Pulmonary edema and liver and renal insufficiency have also been associated with methyl bromide toxicity (17). Peripheral neuropathy and persistent psychiatric disturbances have been reported after large exposures (17). The mechanism of methyl bromide toxicity is unclear but may be related to direct alkylation of macromolecules (17). Plasma bromide levels may help confirm diagnosis (17). Treatment is removal from the source and supportive.

Ethylene dibromide (1,2-dibromomethane) is a colorless liquid with a chloroform odor sold in 3-mL ampules (18). It was commonly used as a fumigant in the United States until 1984, when its use was restricted; however, it is still used in countries such as India where it remains a common source of poisoning. Toxicity has been reported with ingestion, inhalation, and dermal exposure; death has been reported with ingestion of as little as one ampule (18). Clinical signs and symptoms include initial gastrointestinal and pulmonary disturbances, progressing to metabolic acidosis, liver and renal failure, and cardiovascular collapse (18). There is no antidote, and treatment is supportive.

Sulfuryl fluoride (Vikane) is a fumigant that is primarily an irritant, although limited data suggest potential systemic toxicity with enclosed exposures, including pulmonary edema, seizures, and death.

Polymer fume fever is a self-limited pulmonary process secondary to exposure to polytetrafluoroethylene (Teflon) pyrolysis products. Typically, heating of contaminated products, such as cigarettes or hairspray, causes inhalation of pyrolyzed fluorinated polymer fumes and development of fever, cough, and dyspnea but a normal chest radiograph. Resolution occurs over a 24- to 48-hour period and is treated supportively with bronchodilators, antipyretics, adequate ventilation, and education (19).

Metal fume fever ("Monday morning fever") is another self-limited respiratory illness secondary to metal oxide fume exposure, typically zinc. Similar to polymer fume fever, patients present with abrupt onset of fever, cough, dyspnea, myalgia, headache, and metallic taste. Chest radiographs are typically normal, and treatment is similar to that of polymer fume fever. Metal levels are not elevated. Interestingly, transient tolerance to oxide fumes is thought to occur, thus causing Monday morning fever on re-exposure at the beginning of the next work week (20).

DIFFERENTIAL DIAGNOSIS

Similar clinical presentations may be caused by cardiac, allergic, infectious, or intrinsic lung disease. Entities such as metal or polymer fume fever resemble influenza-like illness but are generally very rapid in onset and resolve relatively quickly compared to infectious diseases. As highly water-soluble gases generally cause acute mucous membrane and upper-airway irritation, prompt symptom resolution after removal from the exposure can help distinguish inhalant toxicity from other causes. Less water-soluble agents may cause delayed pulmonary toxicity and may mimic other causes of noncardiogenic pulmonary edema, such as opioid or salicylate poisoning. Unusual toxicities, such as arsine-induced hemolysis, could present similarly to other causes of intravascular hemolysis such as paroxysmal nocturnal hemoglobinuria. A detailed history from the patient, scene responders, family, or coworkers can be extremely helpful in differentiating an occupational exposure from an intrinsic medical cause. Unique odors may potentially be helpful, especially in cases of phosgene, phosphine, or arsine poisoning, for example.

ED EVALUATION

Because signs and symptoms after toxic pulmonary exposure may be nonspecific, an accurate exposure history and review of medical history are paramount.

The emergency department evaluation includes germane medical history and details of the presenting illness, such as the nature, timing, and severity of symptoms and antecedent recreational or occupational activity. Also, if several patients present with similar complaints, a common exposure to an irritant gas may be involved. The Material Safety Data Sheet (MSDS) should always be requested from work sites and carefully reviewed.

Vital sign abnormalities should be noted, especially decreased oxygen saturation, tachypnea, or fever. The physical examination should focus on any mucous membrane or skin involvement and abnormal cardiopulmonary findings. A chest radiograph should be performed in patients with significant respiratory distress or hypoxemia, especially when pulmonary edema is suspected. Routine laboratory testing is generally not needed unless it is to exclude other disorders. However, in cases of suspected arsine toxicity, diagnostic testing should include urine or blood arsenic levels, complete blood count, renal function, indirect bilirubin, haptoglobin, lactate dehydrogenase, and urinalysis. Likewise, for phosphine and bromide, appropriate blood samples may help confirm exposure.

ED MANAGEMENT

Removal from the exposure, rapid decontamination, and supportive care are the mainstays of prehospital treatment. A rescuer should never enter an area in which a pulmonary agent is potentially present without adequate protection. Along with provision of supplemental oxygen, thorough flushing of irritated surfaces with water may be required. Simple decontamination maneuvers include removal and containment of contaminated clothing and washing of skin with soap and water.

Respiratory therapy should include humidified oxygen, bronchodilators, and either noninvasive ventilation or endotracheal intubation with positive end-expiratory pressure (PEEP) as clinically indicated for bronchospasm or pulmonary edema. A course of high-dose corticosteroids to reduce inflammation may be theoretically beneficial and should be considered in patients with moderate, severe, or progressive symptoms. Regarding arsine-induced hemolysis, exchange transfusion may be needed. Supportive therapies may be indicated for additional toxicities, such as benzodiazepines or barbiturates for seizures, and hemodialysis for renal failure. Additionally, identification of sources of and reasons for exposure, especially in industrial settings, is also critical during emergency department evaluation so as to limit potential future poisoning.

CRITICAL INTERVENTIONS

- Measure oxygen saturation in all patients with irritant gas exposure.
- Administer oxygen and bronchodilators to patients with cough, dyspnea, or wheezing; consider corticosteroid therapy in those with severe or persistent symptoms.
- Administer PEEP or intubate and institute controlled ventilation in patients with pulmonary edema or severe respiratory distress unresponsive to supportive care.
- In cases of arsine toxicity, consult with nephrologist for early institution of plasma exchange.

DISPOSITION

The decision to admit or discharge depends primarily on the severity and progression of clinical and laboratory manifestations. Patients exposed to agents that do not cause delayed pulmonary edema and who are or become asymptomatic after 6 hours of emergency department observation and treatment may be discharged, with follow-up as necessary. Those with moderate, severe, or worsening symptoms, hypoxemia, or pulmonary edema should be admitted to the appropriate hospital unit. If delayed toxicity is possible, patients who have even minimal initial symptoms should be admitted and observed for 24 hours. In all cases, the MSDS should be reviewed, and the regional poison center and medical toxicologist should be consulted to help guide treatment and disposition. Patients who are discharged should be instructed to return if symptoms recur or worsen. Discharged patients should also be advised to avoid circumstances that resulted in exposure.

COMMON PITFALLS

- Failure to adequately decontaminate patients and to use proper protective equipment
- Failure to take an adequate environmental or occupational exposure history
- Failure to consider the possibility of delayed or systemic poisoning after gas exposure
- Failure to obtain the MSDS and call regional poison center for further information regarding specific agent
- Failure to instruct patients to avoid circumstances that led to exposure

ICD9

987.9 Toxic effect of unspecified gas, fume, or vapor

REFERENCES

1. Alter P, Grimm W, Maisch B. Lethal heart failure caused by aluminum phosphide poisoning. *Intensive Care Med* 2001;27:327.
2. Bogle RG, Theron P, Brooks P, et al. Aluminum phosphide poisoning. *Emerg Med J* 2006;23:e3.
3. Borak J, Diller W. Phosgene exposure: mechanisms of injury and treatment strategies. *J Occup Environ Med* 2000;43:110–119.
4. Brashear A, Unverzagt FW, Farber MO, et al. Ethylene oxide neurotoxicity: a cluster of 12 nurses with peripheral and central nervous system toxicity. *Neurology* 1996;46:992–998.
5. Charan NB, Myers CG, Lakshminarayan S, et al. Pulmonary injuries associated with acute sulfur dioxide inhalation. *Am Rev Resp Dis* 1979;119:555–560.
6. Danielson C, Houseworth J, Skipworth E, et al. Arsine toxicity treated with red blood cell and plasma exchanges. *Transfusion* 2006;46:1576–1579.
7. Fleetham JA, Munt PW, Tunnicliffe BW. Silo-filler's disease. *Can Med Assoc J* 1978;119(5):482–484.
8. Gapany-Gapanavicius M, Molho M, Tirosh M. Chloramine-induced pneumonitis from mixing household cleaning agents. *Br Med J* 1982;285:1086.
9. Garg PK, Jha D, Agarwal A, Jani UJ. Ethyelenedibromide poisoning. *J Assoc Physicians India* 2002;50:1063.
10. Hajela R, Janigan DT, Landrigan PL, Boudreau SF, et al. Fatal pulmonary edema due to nitric acid fume inhalation in three pulp-mill workers. *Chest* 1990;97(2):487–489.
11. Kaushik RM, Kaushik R, Mahajan SK. Subendocardial infarction in a young survivor of aluminum phosphide poisoning. *Hum Exp Toxicol* 2007;26:457–460.
12. Kaye P, Young H, O'Sullivan I. Metal fume fever: a case report and review of the literature. *Emerg Med J* 2002;19:268–269.
13. Mrvos R, Dean B, Krenzelok EP. Home exposures to chlorine/chlormaine gas: review of 216 cases. *South Med J* 1993;86(6):654–657.
14. Patel MM, Miller MA, Chomchai S. Polymer fume fever after use of a household product. *Am J Emerg Med* 2006;24:880–881.
15. Pauluhn J, Carson A, Costa DL, et al. Workshop summary: phosgene-induced pulmonary toxicity revisited: appraisal of early and late markers of pulmonary injury from animal models with emphasis on human significance. *Inhalat Toxicol* 2007;19:789–809.
16. Reisz GR, Gammon RS. Toxic pneumonitis from mixing household cleaners. *Chest* 1986;89:49–52.
17. Romeo L, Apostoli P, Kovacic M, et al. Acute arsine intoxication as a consequence of metal burnishing operations. *Am J Indust Med* 1997;32:211–216.
18. Snyder RW, Mishel HS, Christensen GC. Pulmonary toxicity following exposure to methylene chloride and its combustion product, phosgene. *Chest* 1992;101:860–861.
19. Song Y, Wang D, Li H, et al. Severe acute arsine poisoning treated by plasma exchange. *Clin Toxicol* 2007;45:721–727.
20. Winder C. The toxicology of chlorine. *Environ Res* 2001;85:105–114.

CHAPTER 42

Smoke Inhalation

PRE-HOSPITAL CONSIDERATIONS
- Give 100% oxygen by face mask.
- Intubate patients with agonal breathing. Advanced airway management may be necessary.
- Give albuterol by nebulizer for bronchospasm.

CLINICAL PRESENTATION

Respiratory signs and symptoms are the primary clinical manifestations of smoke inhalation toxicity. Clinical effects range from transient respiratory tract irritation to severe upper-airway compromise and respiratory failure. Cough is often the first symptom. Other initial responses include increased mucus secretion and sneezing. Upper-airway involvement results in hoarseness and stridor. Injury to the lower respiratory tract results in crackles and/or wheezing. Breath sounds may be inaudible in cases of severe bronchospasm. Important signs of potential inhalation injury include cough, dyspnea, hoarseness, soot in the oral cavity, singed nasal hair, edema of the posterior pharynx, burns to the face, and any major burn to the body.

Smoke inhalation may cause systemic manifestations as well. Examination of the eye may reveal the irritant effects of increased tearing, conjunctival injection, and blepharospasm. Progressive airway compromise and toxicity from agents with systemic effects, notably carbon monoxide, will produce signs and symptoms of hypoxia—tachycardia, tachypnea, dizziness, headache, nausea and vomiting, chest pain, and deteriorating mental status manifesting as agitation, confusion and ultimately seizures, coma, and death.

Laboratory evaluation may reveal hypoxemia, metabolic (lactic) acidosis, and elevated carboxyhemoglobin and methemoglobin fractions and whole-blood cyanide levels. The electrocardiogram (ECG) may reveal dysrhythmias or evidence of myocardial ischemia or infarction.

DIFFERENTIAL DIAGNOSIS

Patients with smoke inhalation may have concomitant dermal burns, traumatic injuries, or drug or alcohol intoxication and may be victims of arson, attempted murder, or attempted suicide. For patients presenting with coma and shock, head computed tomography scanning, whole-blood cyanide levels, toxicology screening tests, and invasive hemodynamic measurements (e.g., central venous and pulmonary artery pressures) may be necessary to define the etiology.

ED EVALUATION

Significant smoke inhalation injuries may be delayed after exposure. History of entrapment, fire within an enclosed space, and altered consciousness at the scene should all raise the suspicion of inhalation injury. Key risk factors associated with inhalation injury are in Table 42.1. The history should address the nature of burning material, presence of steam, evidence of trauma or suicidality and, for rescuers presenting as patients, the type of mask used.

Examination begins with obtaining vital signs and oxygen saturation. An important caveat is that transcutaneous pulse oximetry overestimates the true oxygen saturation in the presence of carboxyhemoglobin and methemoglobin (2,4). Co-oximetry directly measures an accurate oxygen saturation even in the presence of dyshemoglobinemias. A trauma survey with attention to signs associated with increased risk of smoke inhalation including facial burns, singed facial hair, soot in the nasal passages and airway, and burns involving extensive body surface area (>15%) should follow. The eyes should be examined with fluorescein staining to detect corneal burns and lacerations in comatose patients or those with eye complaints. Repeat examinations should focus on respiratory status and alterations in mental status.

Carboxyhemoglobin and methemoglobin should be measured by co-oximetry. An elevated carboxyhemoglobin fraction in a fire victim is an indicator of significant exposure to combustion products and is associated with a markedly increased risk of smoke inhalation injury and toxicity. A low or undetectable carboxyhemoglobin concentration does not rule out the possibility of developing even severe inhalation injury.

Obtaining whole blood cyanide levels does not affect the acute management because there is no timely confirmatory test. A more practical test is a plasma

TABLE 42.1	Risk Factors Associated with Inhalation Injury	
Initial Exposure	**Symptoms**	**Signs**
Entrapment	Cough	Soot in the oral cavity
Fire in an enclosed space	Shortness of breath	Singed nasal hair
Loss of consciousness at the scene	Hoarseness	Pharyngeal edema
Facial or neck burns; any major burn		Stridor
		Crackles/wheezing
		Altered mental status

lactate concentration. A level >10 mmol/L refractory to adequate ventilation, oxygenation, and perfusion is a surrogate marker of cyanide toxicity in the right clinical setting (1). Methemoglobin should be determined in symptomatic patients, particularly with cyanosis that does not improve with supplementary oxygen (see Chapter 34, "Cyanide," and Chapter 40, "Methemoglobinemia").

Arterial blood gas (ABG) measurements should be obtained to assess arterial oxygenation, alveolar ventilation, and the presence of metabolic acidosis. Initially, the ABG of even a significantly injured patient may be normal; serial measurements are recommended.

An ECG and chest radiograph are recommended in symptomatic patients, especially in those with pre-existing cardiovascular or pulmonary disease. Chest radiographs may appear normal early in the course of smoke inhalation and therefore lack sensitivity as indicators of inhalation injury. Early findings, if present, are subtle: perivascular cuffing, bronchial wall thickening, and subglottic edema (6). Serial chest radiographs, however, may be very useful in monitoring disease progression. Common complications that do not typically manifest radiographically until more than 24 hours after the initial insult include acute lung injury/acute respiratory distress syndrome, aspiration, volume overload, and infection.

ED MANAGEMENT

Prehospital directives include the rapid, safe removal of victims from the scene by those with adequate training and protection. Basic and advanced life support measures are instituted as indicated, and attention is given to cervical spine immobilization. Supplemental oxygen is indicated for all patients. The decision of whether a patient should be transported to a burn center, trauma center, or hyperbaric facility is determined by local practice guidelines. Intravenous access and cardiac monitoring may be established en route.

On arrival to the emergency department, upper airway patency must be determined immediately. Airway compromise may be present initially, rapidly ensue, or develop insidiously over the next few hours. Failure to appreciate the potential for rapid decline in airway status is the major pitfall in managing the smoke inhalation patient. The factors that best correlate with the need for intubation and edema of either the true or false vocal cords are soot in the oral cavity, facial burns, and/or body burns (7). Early endotracheal intubation, performed in a controlled setting before edema makes it impossible, may be life-saving and should be undertaken when these risks are present. In the patient with the edematous or difficult airway, fiberoptic laryngoscopy, flexible intubation guides, intubation laryngeal masks, retrograde intubation, transtracheal jet ventilation, and ultimately cricothyroidotomy may assist with establishing tracheal intubation. Aggressive rehydration of the burn victim may also cause airway edema requiring early intubation.

Early consultation for fiberoptic bronchoscopy, the gold standard for diagnosis and evaluation of inhalation injury, should be considered if there is suspicion of significant inhalation injury. It may also assist in clearing debris from the respiratory tract and permits fiberoptically assisted intubation if required.

β_2 adrenergic agonists may be useful in improving airflow. Corticosteroids are not indicated with smoke inhalation injury as they are associated with increased incidence of bacterial pneumonia and mortality and are not associated with improved pulmonary function (3). Prophylactic antibiotics also have no demonstrated benefit in the treatment of inhalation injury (5). Fever and leukocytosis that develop 2 days or more after injury do suggest infection, and empiric antibiotic treatment that covers *Staphylococcus aureus* and gram-negative organisms should be instituted until culture results become available. Progressive respiratory failure and the development of pneumonitis, acute lung injury/adult respiratory distress syndrome, or other complications may require mechanical ventilation, continuous positive airway pressure, positive end-expiratory pressure, and frequent suctioning of pulmonary secretions.

Trauma-related injuries as a result of falls or explosions and burns must be managed concurrently with inhalation injury. The patient with altered mental status and coma should receive dextrose, thiamine, and naloxone and consideration of other causes including drug and ethanol intoxication.

Carbon monoxide poisoning should be treated aggressively (see Chapter 32, "Carbon Monoxide"). Possible cyanide poisoning should be given an antidote (see Chapter 34, "Cyanide"). Hydroxocobalamin (Cyanokit) does not induce methemoglobinemia and may be safely administered to the smoke inhalation patient with suspected cyanide toxicity. Steps one and two of the Cyanide Antidote Kit induce methemoglobinemia. When oxygen transport is already compromised, as in a patient with concomitant carbon monoxide poisoning, further impairment by the inducement of methemoglobinemia may exacerbate cellular hypoxia. A reasonable approach in the smoke inhalation patient with suspected cyanide toxicity, particularly the seriously ill patient with a lactate level >10 mmol/L refractory to resuscitation, is to administer 12.5 g of sodium thiosulfate (50 mL of a 25% solution for adults; pediatric dose, 1.65 mL/kg).

Symptomatic methemoglobinemia and/or concentrations >20% to 30% should be treated with methylene blue (see Chapter 40, "Methemoglobinemia").

CRITICAL INTERVENTIONS

- Perform early endotracheal intubation in patients with oropharyngeal burns or edema, soot in the oral cavity, full-thickness circumferential neck burns, stridor, coma, or hypoxemia or respiratory distress unresponsive to oxygen administration.
- Obtain a carboxyhemoglobin level, ABG, chest radiograph, and ECG, and administer oxygen to patients with significant smoke exposure or respiratory symptoms.

TABLE 42.2	Indications for Admission after Smoke Inhalation

Facial or nasal burns
Persistent respiratory symptoms (including cough and chest tightness)
Crackles or wheezing on auscultation
Altered mental status
History of loss of consciousness
Abnormal ABG, CXR, or ECG
History of chronic cardiopulmonary disease
ABG, arterial blood gas; CXR, chest x-ray; ECG, electrocardiogram.

DISPOSITION

Indications for admission for observation and further treatment are listed in Table 42.2. Severity of illness and the presence of concomitant burns or traumatic injuries should guide the decision to admit to an intensive care unit, telemetry unit, or floor bed. Patients with carbon monoxide poisoning may require transfer for hyperbaric oxygen therapy (see Chapter 32, "Carbon Monoxide"), and those with significant surface burns or physical injuries may require transfer to a burn or trauma center. Advanced life-support capability should be available during transfer.

Patients in good general health who are asymptomatic (on arrival or after a short period of oxygen therapy) and have a normal physical examination including pulse oximetry, arterial blood gas results (while breathing room air), ECG, chest radiograph, and carboxyhemoglobin level may be discharged. These patients should be observed for at least 3 or 4 hours before discharge, and they should be instructed to return immediately if any respiratory symptoms develop. Scheduled follow-up at 24 hours may be prudent.

COMMON PITFALLS

- Failure to anticipate deterioration despite an initially normal initial physical examination, laboratory evaluation, and chest radiograph and failure to frequently re-evaluate the respiratory status
- Failure to evaluate and treat for coexisting carbon monoxide poisoning, drug or alcohol intoxication, traumatic injuries, and psychiatric problems
- Failure to give oxygen to all patients (including those with chronic obstructive pulmonary disease)
- Failure to fluid-resuscitate patients with trauma or surface burns for fear of exacerbating the edema of inhalation injury
- Failure to recognize the potential hazards of inappropriate corticosteroid, antibiotic, and cyanide antidote administration

ICD9

987.9 Toxic effect of unspecified gas, fume, or vapor

REFERENCES

1. Barker SJ, Tremper KK. The effect of carbon monoxide inhalation on pulse oximetry and transcutaneous PO2. *Anesthesiology* 1987;66:677–679.
2. Baud FJ, Barriot P, Toffis V, et al. Elevated blood cyanide concentrations in victims of smoke inhalation. *N Engl J Med* 1991;325:1761–1766.
3. Cha SI, Lee JH, Park JY, et al. Isolated smoke inhalation injuries: acute respiratory dysfunction, clinical outcomes, and short-term evolution of pulmonary functions with the effects of steroids. *Burns* 2007;33:200–208.
4. Eisencraft JB. Pulse oximeter desaturation due to methemoglobinemia. *Anesthesiology* 1988;68:279–282.
5. Herndon DN, Thompson PB, Traber DL. Pulmonary injury in burned patients. *Crit Care Med* 1985;1:79.
6. Lee MJ, O'Connell DJ. The plain chest radiograph after acute smoke inhalation. *Clin Radiol* 1988;39:33.
7. Madnani DD, Steele NP, de Vries E. Factors that predict the need for intubation in patients with smoke inhalation injury. *Ear Nose Throat J* 2006;85:278–280.

Psychotherapeutic Agents

43

Antipsychotic Agents

- Bring pills and pill bottles when transporting the patient to the hospital.

CLINICAL PRESENTATION

Although nausea and vomiting may develop soon after acute overdose of any neuroleptic, central nervous system (CNS) depression and cardiovascular (CV) effects dominate the clinical picture (1,3,4,9). Mild poisoning includes ataxia, confusion, lethargy, and slurred speech. Hypotension, both orthostatic and diastolic, may be caused by α-adrenergic blockade. Tachycardia may develop owing to antimuscarinic effects or as a reflex tachycardia. Miosis due to alpha blockade is common, but mydriasis due to antimuscarinic effects can also occur. Antimuscarinic signs and symptoms (Chapter 49, "Anticholinergic Agents") are often present, and patients may be hyperreflexic. Prolonged P-R and Q-T intervals and nonspecific ST-segment, T-wave, and U-wave abnormalities may be seen, particularly with sertindole, thioridazine, mesoridazine, and ziprasidone (6).

Moderate poisoning is characterized by sedation, with or without respiratory depression, and systolic hypotension accompanied by reflex tachycardia. Hyperthermia and hypothermia (less common) may be present. Paradoxical agitation, delirium, and tachypnea are reported but are likely antimuscarinic effects. Sialorrhea may be seen after clozapine overdose and at therapeutic doses.

In severe poisoning, deep coma with loss of brainstem and deep tendon reflexes, apnea, hypotension, tachycardia, and cardiac dysrhythmias (especially with thioridazine and mesoridazine) are seen. Tachydysrhythmias, rare bradydysrhythmias, and cardiac conduction delays (especially with thioridazine and mesoridazine) may occur. Q-T interval prolongation and torsades de pointes are reported after haloperidol, loxapine, phenothiazine, pimozide quetiapine, risperidone, sertindole, and ziprasidone overdose and during high-dose intravenous droperidol and haloperidol therapy (10). Noncardiogenic pulmonary edema can occur (7). Seizures are rare, except with chlorpromazine, loxapine, and clozapine (6).

The onset of symptoms of poisoning occurs within 1 to 2 hours of acute ingestion, with maximal severity usually apparent in 2 to 6 hours. Children appear more susceptible to toxicity than adults. Recovery can be expected within several hours to several days, depending on the severity and drug ingested. The mortality rate from acute poisoning is <1%.

Extrapyramidal symptoms (EPS) may occur early (within days), or late (after 3 months or more) after beginning neuroleptic therapy, increasing the dose, or changing the agent (2). Dyskinesia or acute dystonic reactions (see Chapter 45, "Dystonic Reactions"), akathisia, neuroleptic malignant syndrome (NMS), and parkinsonism occur early whereas tardive dyskinesia or dystonias occur late. These idiosyncratic reactions are most common with older high-potency agents. Akathisia, a subjective sensation of motor restlessness, occurs in about 20% of patients treated with traditional neuroleptics and is sometimes associated with severe parkinsonism. Transient akathisia has been observed in up to 50% of those treated with intravenous droperidol or prochlorperazine for headache, nausea, and vomiting. Women are affected more often than men. Patients complain of feeling restless, jittery, and tense; they cannot sit or stand still and when standing may shift their weight from foot to foot as if walking in place. Vital signs remain normal. Semipurposeful or purposeless limb movements (especially of the lower extremities), frequent shifting of body position, and tremors and myoclonic jerking may be noted. Focal perioral tremor, also known as *rabbit syndrome,* is a rhythmic motion of the mouth and lips, resembling the chewing movements of a rabbit. In contrast to oral tardive dyskinesia, tongue movements do not occur in rabbit syndrome.

NMS can be precipitated by concurrent illness, surgery, dehydration, heat stress, acute agitation and, very rarely, by acute overdose of neuroleptic agents (12). It is estimated to occur in <1% of patients treated with neuroleptics for psychiatric conditions and appears to be more common with parenteral therapy (6). NMS is characterized by elevated body temperature (>38°C or 100.4°F), altered mental status ranging from confusion and delirium to coma, autonomic dysfunction, increased motor activity, and laboratory abnormalities. Autonomic disturbances include hypertension (>150/100 mm Hg; diastolic or systolic blood pressure increased 20 or 30 mm Hg above baseline, respectively), tachycardia (heart rate >90–100 or increased by 30 beats per minute), increased respiratory rate (alternatively dyspnea, hypoxemia, or respiratory failure), diaphoresis (often profuse), sialorrhea and incontinence. Hypotension, rather than hypertension, sometimes occurs. Although "lead pipe" rigidity is the classic motor finding, lesser increases in muscle tone, akinesia, dystonia, dyskinesia, tremor, choreiform movements, opisthotonus, and parkinsonism (cogwheel rigidity) may be present. Hyperactivity of pharyngeal muscles may result in dysarthria, dysphagia, dysphonia, and trismus. Laboratory abnormalities include leukocytosis (white blood cells >14,000/mm^3 without a left shift), signs of rhabdomyolysis (creatine phosphokinase [CPK] >500 IU/mL or three times normal), and markedly elevated white blood cell count. Hyponatremia, hypernatremia, or hypokalemia may be present. Onset is typically insidious, and resolution occurs slowly, sometimes taking up to 2 weeks. Complications include aspiration pneumonia and other infections, coagulopathy, renal failure, and metabolic disturbances from rhabdomyolysis, myocardial infarction, heart failure, dysrhythmias, and venous thromboembolism. The mortality rate of NMS ranges from 12% to 20% and is primarily related to complications. Sequelae include dysarthria, dysphagia, myoclonus, and weakness.

DIFFERENTIAL DIAGNOSIS

Antidysrhythmic, tricyclic antidepressant, antimuscarinic, anticonvulsant, opioid, and sedative–hypnotic toxicity may all cause CNS or CV effects similar to those seen in neuroleptic poisoning. Urine drug immunoassays are unreliable because neuroleptics are most often undetectable, and false-positive tricyclic antidepressant immunoassay screens can result from the presence of typical phenothiazines or quetiapine (5). CNS infection, infarction, and trauma should also be considered in the differential diagnosis of neuroleptic poisoning.

EPS from neuroleptics may be misdiagnosed as anxiety or agitation related to an underlying psychiatric disorder. EPS can occur when beginning or increasing therapy with neuroleptic or nonneuroleptic dopamine antagonists (e.g., hydroxyzine, metoclopramide, reserpine), discontinuing or decreasing therapy with a dopamine agonist (e.g., amantadine, bromocriptine, carbidopa, levodopa, lithium, pergolide, pramipexole, ropinirole) or use of a catecholamine degradation inhibitor (e.g., catechol-o-methyltransferase inhibitors such as entacapone and tolcapone). The differential diagnosis of NMS also includes dystonic reactions, lithium, monoamine oxidase inhibitor, salicylate, stimulant, and strychnine poisoning, heat stroke, malignant catatonia, malignant hyperthermia (MH), encephalitis, meningitis, pheochromocytoma, serotonin syndrome (SS), tetanus, thyrotoxicosis, and withdrawal states.

Distinguishing NMS from MH or SS (see Chapter 48, "Serotonin Reuptake Inhibitors and the Serotonin Syndrome") is difficult as clinical features overlap. The correct diagnosis relies primarily on the drug exposure history. Onset after general anesthesia or ketamine administration strongly suggests MH. Use of proserotonin drugs is suggestive of SS. SS also begins more abruptly and resolves more quickly than NMS (over hours rather than days). Myoclonus, hyperreflexia, and shivering are rare in NMS but common in SS.

Although specific criteria have been proposed for the diagnosis of NMS, the required elements are not universally agreed on, and patients can have NMS without manifesting a classic or characteristic feature (e.g., fever or rigidity). Diagnosing patients with attenuated forms of NMS relies primarily on the clinical settings and history of drug exposure.

ED EVALUATION

A complete history should always be obtained from the patient and, when possible, corroborated with the person who found or brought the patient to the emergency department. The name, quantity, and time of ingestion should be determined. In patients taking neuroleptics for therapeutic purposes, a history of a recent medication or dosage change, illness, or surgery is important.

The physical examination should focus on the vital signs, CV system, and neurologic function. An initial rhythm strip and subsequent 12-lead electrocardiogram (ECG) should be evaluated for prolonged QRS or QTc intervals or other dysrhythmias. Pulse oximetry can monitor respiratory status. Because phenothiazines can be radiopaque, abdominal radiographs may be useful to quantify or verify an ingestion. However, the lack of x-ray visualization does not rule out ingestion or imply successful gastric decontamination. Routine laboratory evaluation should include a complete blood count and measurements of electrolytes, blood urea nitrogen, creatinine, and glucose to rule out concomitant abnormalities. Other laboratory tests should include urinalysis to check for myoglobin, and serum CPK to evaluate for rhabdomyolysis. In patients with hyperthermia, liver function tests and coagulation profiles are useful to determine hepatic injury or disseminated intravascular coagulation. Lumbar puncture should be considered as meningitis may present in a similar manner as NMS. In seriously ill patients, toxicologic analysis of the urine and serum may confirm the identity of the agent, but results will often not be readily available. Quantitative drug levels are not helpful in predicting clinical toxicity or in guiding treatment. Although neither sensitive nor specific, the Forest, Mason, and Phenistix colorimetric urine tests may be positive with phenothiazine ingestions and can be used to rapidly screen for these agents.

ED MANAGEMENT

Advanced life-support measures should be instituted as necessary. All patients require cardiac and respiratory monitoring along with intravenous access. Core temperature should be monitored for evidence of hypo- or hyperthermia. Endotracheal intubation may be required for respiratory or CNS depression. When paralysis is needed, nondepolarizing paralytic agents such as rocuronium (0.6–1 mg/kg IV) or vecuronium (0.08–0.1 mg/kg IV) are recommended, because succinylcholine (and other depolarizing neuromuscular blockers) can cause MH and potentiate rhabdomyolysis and hyperkalemia in neuroleptic-poisoned patients.

Hypotension should initially be treated with intravenous crystalloids. Norepinephrine and/or phenylephrine are the drugs of choice for refractory hypotension. Dopamine may be ineffective or even exacerbate the hypotension associated with antipsychotics agents. At modest doses, dopamine's activity may be impaired because it is unable to enter presynaptic terminals through the blocked catecholamine reuptake pump caused by the neuroleptic, whereas at higher doses, dopamine may encounter α-blocking effects of these drugs, leading potentially to unopposed β-receptor stimulation of blood vessels and vasodilation.

Unstable tachydysrhythmias should be treated with electrical cardioversion (8) or defibrillation for ventricular fibrillation and nonperfusing monomorphic or polymorphic ventricular tachycardia (VT). If the QRS complex is wide prior to or after termination of unstable tachydysrhythmias, sodium bicarbonate (1 mEq/kg IV) may be effective (see Chapter 26, "Antidysrhythmic Drugs and

Local Anesthetics," and Chapter 44, "Cyclic Antidepressants"). Amiodarone or lidocaine can also be used to treat refractory stable VT (11). Type Ia (disopyramide, quinidine, procainamide), Ic (encainide, flecainide, propafenone), II (β blockers), and IV (calcium channel blockers) antidysrhythmic drugs should be avoided in wide complex tachydysrhythmias. If the QTc interval is prolonged or torsades de pointes is observed, magnesium (50–100 mg/kg IV over 1 hour), isoproterenol, or overdrive pacing are preferred. Increasing the heart rate shortens the Q-T interval and is recommended for preventing the recurrence of torsades de pointes. Bradydysrhythmias should be treated according to current Advanced Cardiac Life Support protocols. Complete heart block may require temporary cardiac pacing after underlying metabolic abnormalities are corrected.

Seizures should be treated with benzodiazepines (e.g., lorazepam, 0.05 mg/kg IV, or diazepam, 0.1 mg/kg IV). Barbiturates (e.g., phenobarbital, 18–20 mg/kg IV, or pentobarbital, 5 mg/kg IV) and propofol may be added if necessary. Patients with refractory convulsions may require pharmacologic paralysis to prevent complications such as hyperthermia and rhabdomyolysis. Continuous or serial electroencephalographic monitoring should be instituted during paralysis. Diuresis with or without alkalinization of the urine may prevent myoglobinuric renal failure in patients with rhabdomyolysis. Physostigmine can reverse the delirium resulting from muscarinic receptor blockade if cardiac conduction intervals are normal and if there is no seizure activity (see Chapter 49, "Anticholinergic Agents").

Early and aggressive treatment of muscular hyperactivity and hyperthermia in patients with NMS appears to improve outcome. Initial management includes benzodiazepines, but therapeutic paralysis may be required for patients with refractory seizures or severe hyperthermia. Active cooling measures (e.g. cooling blankets, ice packs, and evaporative cooling methods) are necessary for most severely hyperthermic patients. Antipyretics are unlikely to be effective, and neuroleptic therapy must be discontinued. Although dantrolene (2.5–10 mg/kg/d IV) has been proposed to treat NMS, there are no convincing clinical data or theoretical reasons to suggest that it would be efficacious. The release of calcium from muscle sarcoplasmic reticulum is reduced by dantrolene through inhibition of ryanodine receptors. This mechanism is involved in the pathogenesis of MH but does not seem to cause or contribute to NMS.

Activated charcoal may be considered in patients with a secure airway and ingestion within 1 hour. Repeated oral doses of activated charcoal are not beneficial for these poisonings and are contraindicated when an ileus is present. Diuresis, dialysis, and hemoperfusion are not effective.

Patients with extrapyramidal syndromes who require continued neuroleptic therapy can be managed by reducing the dose, switching to an agent of lower potency, or giving an antimuscarinic agent (e.g., benztropine or diphenhydramine). Benzodiazepines, clonidine, propranolol, and short-acting barbiturates have also been used with moderate success. Patients who develop akathisia after a single therapeutic dose of neuroleptic (e.g., for migraine or vomiting) should be reassured that symptoms will resolve within 24 hours.

CRITICAL INTERVENTIONS

- Establish intravenous access, institute cardiac monitoring, obtain an ECG, and frequently re-evaluate the vital signs and clinical status of patients with actual or potential neuroleptic poisoning.
- Obtain a core temperature and CPK in patients with suspected NMS (altered mental status, autonomic dysfunction and muscle hyperactivity).
- Treat hyperthermia, muscle hyperactivity, and seizures aggressively with benzodiazepines or barbiturates, therapeutic paralysis for refractory cases, physical cooling measures for hyperthermia, and alkaline diuresis for rhabdomyolysis.
- Administer sodium bicarbonate to patients with monomorphic VT. Lidocaine or amiodarone may be used in refractory VT.
- Administer magnesium, isoproterenol, or overdrive pacing to patients with torsades de pointes.

DISPOSITION

Asymptomatic patients with an acute overdose should be observed for 6 hours.

Symptomatic patients with significant CNS depression, hypotension, seizures, or dysrhythmias should be admitted to an intensive care unit (ICU) or a similarly equipped observation area. Alert patients with a history of overdose and abnormal ECG should be monitored as ECG abnormalities can be seen with therapeutic doses and have been implicated as a cause of sudden death.

Except for NMS, extrapyramidal syndromes are not life-threatening and do not require admission, although the symptoms may be quite stressful to patients. Medication adjustment may be appropriate, but this should be done in consultation with the patient's psychiatrist. Patients with NMS will require ICU admission. Patients requiring transfer to a facility capable of providing intensive care should be accompanied by advanced life-support personnel and should have cardiac monitoring en route.

COMMON PITFALLS

- Failure to appreciate that neuroleptics can prolong QRS and QTc intervals causing cardiac dysrhythmias
- Failure to appreciate that atypical antipsychotics, although less likely to cause EPS than traditional agents, are more sedating and cause similar CV toxicity
- Failure to appreciate that antipsychotics can lower seizure threshold
- Failure to appreciate that attenuated forms of NMS can occur and to discontinue neuroleptic therapy in patients with any manifestation of NMS
- Use of type Ia, Ic, II (β blockers), and IV (calcium channel blockers) antidysrhythmic agents in wide complex tachydysrhythmias
- Failure to appreciate that dopamine agonists are not as effective as norepinephrine or phenylephrine in treating antipsychotic-induced hypotension

ICD9

969.3 Poisoning by other antipsychotics, neuroleptics, and major tranquilizers

REFERENCES

1. Acri AA, Henretig FM. Effects of risperidone in overdose. *Am J Emerg Med* 1998;16:498.
2. Baldessarini RJ, Tarazi FI. Drugs and the treatment of psychiatric disorders: psychosis and mania. In: Hardman JG, Limbird LE, Gilman AG, eds. *Goodman & Gilman's the Pharmacological Basis Of Therapeutics,* 10th ed. New York: McGraw-Hill, 2001:485.
3. Biswas AK, Zabrocki LA, Mayes KL, et al. Cardiotoxicity associated with intentional ziprasidone and bupropion overdose. *J Toxicol Clin Toxicol* 2003;4:101–104.
4. Buckley NA, White IM, Dawson AH. Cardiotoxicity more common in thioridazine overdose than with other neuroleptics. *J Toxicol Clin Toxicol* 1995;33:199.
5. Caravati EM, Juenke JM, Crouch BI, et al. Quetiapine cross-reactivity with plasma tricyclic antidepressant immunoassays. *Ann Pharmacother* 2005;39(9):1446–1449.
6. Haddad PM, Sharma SG. Adverse effects of atypical antipsychotics: differential risk and clinical implications. *CNS Drugs* 2007;21:911–936.
7. Li C, Gefter WB. Acute pulmonary edema induced by overdose of phenothiazines. *Chest* 1992; 101:102.
8. Nelson LS. Toxicological myocardial sensitization. *J Toxicol Clin Toxicol* 2002;40:867.
9. Palenzona S, Meier PJ, Kupferschmidt H, et al. The clinical picture of olanzapine poisoning with special reference to fluctuating mental status. *J Toxicol Clin Toxicol* 2004;42:27.
10. Richards JR, Schnier AB. Droperidol in the emergency department: is it safe? *J Emerg Med* 2003; 24:441.
11. Somberg JC, Bailin SJ, Molnar J et al. Intravenous lidocaine versus amiodarone for incessant ventricular tachycardia. *Am J Cardiol* 2002; 22(13):1209–1212.
12. Strawn JR, Keck PE, Caroff SN. Neuroleptic malignant syndrome. *Am J Psychiatry* 2007;164:6.

Cyclic Antidepressants

PRE-HOSPITAL CONSIDERATIONS

- Do not be lulled into a false sense of security by a well-appearing patient. The onset of altered mental status, seizures, and dysrhythmias may be rapid.
- Perform endotracheal intubation if there is any evidence of compromise.
- Secure intravenous access.
- Administer sodium bicarbonate if there is any evidence of QRS widening (>100–120 ms): one ampule in adults and 1–2 mEq/kg in children.
- Do *not* give ipecac (risk of aspiration with development of depressed mental status or seizures).

CLINICAL PRESENTATION

The presentation of cyclic antidepressant (CA) poisoning may rapidly change from asymptomatic to cardiopulmonary arrest within minutes as an alert patient may become comatose, have seizures, or develop hemodynamic and cardiac instability. CA-induced seizures typically occur early and are unlikely to recur beyond 12 hours after ingestion but may deteriorate into status epilepticus (6). Status myoclonic activity is seen with severe poisoning. Patients may initially be tachycardic and mildly hypertensive (as a result of the blockade of norepinephrine reuptake and anticholinergic effects), or they may be hypotensive (from α_1 blockade). Later, the metabolism of norepinephrine often leads to a catecholamine depletion state resulting in hypotension, bradycardia, and finally cardiogenic shock with refractory hypotension seen in most fatalities. Most patients recover in <24 to 48 hours with supportive care.

Cardiac dysrhythmias include both supraventricular tachydysrhythmias and ventricular dysrhythmias. Intraventricular conduction delay often makes it difficult to distinguish a ventricular tachycardia (VT) from a supraventricular tachycardia with aberrant conduction. Polymorphous VT (torsades de pointes) has also been reported. Aspiration pneumonia is relatively common in comatose patients, and adult respiratory distress syndrome may occur. Rhabdomyolysis and compartment syndrome are additional complications.

Patients with ingestions of <15 mg/kg display a predominant anticholinergic syndrome without cardiac conduction effects. Anticholinergic effects can also occur during recovery from severe poisoning and may last for days. Typical signs and symptoms include tachycardia, hypertension, absent bowel sounds, ileus, and urinary retention. Other anticholinergic effects, such as dilated pupils, flushed hot skin, and dry mucous membranes, however, are more variable. Central anticholinergic findings may vary from agitation to psychosis to coma. Additional neurologic manifestations include choreoathetosis, ataxia, myoclonus, status epilepticus, and coma.

DIFFERENTIAL DIAGNOSIS

The differential diagnosis of coma, seizures, and cardiac dysrhythmias includes hypoxia, metabolic abnormalities, and intrinsic neurologic and cardiac disease. Other drugs with toxicities that can appear similar to CAs include the antidysrhythmics, antihistamines, antimalarials, atypical antipsychotics, β-blockers, calcium channel blockers, carbamazepine, phenothiazines, and propoxyphene. Anticholinergic agents, camphor, cocaine, chloral hydrate, isoniazid, lithium, sympathomimetic poisoning, and drug withdrawal should also be considered.

ED EVALUATION

The history should be obtained from the patient, family, friends, or prehospital personnel. If possible, the time, amount, and identity of all agents ingested should be determined. When known, the amount of CA ingested often helps anticipate the potential for deterioration. The therapeutic dose of 5 mg/kg should be tolerated by all, including children. Observation without intervention would be the best approach for these patients. Conversely, patients who ingest 15 mg/kg (roughly 1 gram for a 70-kg adult) have the potential for serious poisoning.

The physical examination should focus on the vital signs and cardiovascular (CV), pulmonary, and neurologic function. The potential for rapid deterioration requires that intravenous access and continuous cardiac and oxygenation monitoring be initiated immediately. Vital signs and neurologic status should be evaluated continuously, and a limb lead QRS duration (discussion follows) should be checked every 30 minutes or if the monitor looks suspicious.

An electrocardiogram (ECG) should be performed early in the evaluation. A QRS duration >100 milliseconds is associated with seizures, and a QRS duration >160 milliseconds is associated with ventricular dysrhythmias. Patients with a QRS duration >120 milliseconds who have a seizure are at great risk for sudden CV toxicity including CV collapse (6). More subtle, early ECG changes include a rightward axis of the terminal 40 milliseconds of the QRS in the frontal plane. This manifestation can be quickly assessed by looking for the presence of a widened S wave in leads 1 and aVL, and an R wave in lead aVR (Fig. 44.1). These terminal 40-millisecond changes are good indicators for sodium channel blockade, as seen with CA poisoning, but they do not absolutely confirm or exclude the diagnosis.

Other than a lactic acidosis secondary to seizures or shock, CAs are not known to produce biochemical disturbances. However, evaluation of patients with altered mental status or cardiotoxicity includes assessment of serum electrolytes, blood urea nitrogen, creatinine, and glucose; a serum osmolality should also be obtained

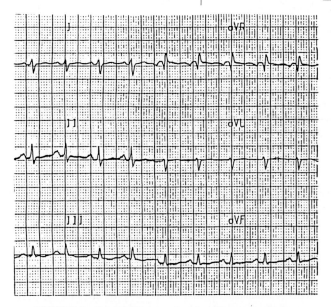

FIGURE 44.1. Terminal QRS changes in cyclic antidepressant poisoning.

in patients with metabolic acidosis. An arterial blood gas, creatine phosphokinase, calcium, magnesium, phosphorus, liver chemistries, and a chest radiograph should be considered for patients with abnormal vital signs, significant central nervous system depression, seizures, or an abnormal ECG.

Drug screening for CAs has very little impact on the management of the CA-poisoned patient. Qualitative screens may identify the presence of CAs in urine, although quantitative screens provide drug levels. Although serum levels >1,000 ng/mL generally correlate with significant toxicity, levels do not assist in emergency management. Monitoring the changes on the ECG and the patient's mental status are more clinically useful indicators of ongoing CA toxicity.

ED MANAGEMENT

Prehospital care for patients with coma, seizures, hypotension, and dysrhythmias includes endotracheal intubation, administration of anticonvulsants, intravenous crystalloids, and serum alkalinization with parenteral sodium bicarbonate boluses.

Parenteral benzodiazepines such as diazepam or midazolam (5–10 mg), or lorazepam (2–4 mg) are the agents of choice for the prevention and treatment of seizures. They should be administered to any patient with severe poisoning. Repeat doses may be required. When intubation is required, parenteral benzodiazepines may be useful for sedative and anticonvulsant effects. If benzodiazepines do not completely control seizures, phenobarbital or propofol should be considered. Phenobarbital or propofol may be necessary for the treatment of myoclonus. In the intubated patient, a phenobarbital loading dose of 18 mg/kg is usually sufficient. The dose for propofol sedation of the intubated patient begins with a bolus infusion of 0.3 mg/kg. The dose is titrated to the desired sedation level in increments of 0.3 to 0.6 mg/kg/hr every 5 to 10 minutes. Propofol's rapid onset and offset make it ideal for the management of these ventilated CA-poisoned patients. Seizures will rapidly produce a lactic acidosis that may further compromise the cardiac and hemodynamic status. Hence, an intravenous bolus of 1 to 2 ampules (44–100 mEq) of hypertonic sodium bicarbonate is recommended as adjunctive treatment for seizures. Neuromuscular paralysis with a short-acting agent should be considered for neuromuscular toxicity that does not respond to the foregoing treatment.

Hypotension should be treated with intravenous crystalloid boluses of 20 mL/kg. This treatment should overcome hypotension from α-adrenergic blockade and mild dehydration. For more seriously poisoned patients, vasopressors may be needed. Dopamine and norepinephrine have been used successfully; however, many cases have been refractory to dopamine. Because dopamine partially acts as an indirect sympathomimetic agent, causing catecholamine release from sympathetic nerve terminals, it may lose some of its effectiveness when norepinephrine stores are depleted as a result of CA poisoning. High infusion rates of dopamine should be tried initially. The dose should be at least 10 μg/kg/min to provide direct α-adrenergic agonism. Lower doses of dopamine have relatively more β-adrenergic effects that could cause vasodilation and actually worsen hypotension. If there is an inadequate response, norepinephrine should be given (substituted for or added to dopamine). Norepinephrine has been demonstrated to have greater efficacy than dopamine in successfully treating refractory hypotension (7). Patients usually respond to low infusion rates of 1 μg/kg/min. Glucagon has been used for refractory hypotension and warrants consideration (4). It increases intracellular cAMP producing both inotropic and chronotropic effects. It should be administered in a bolus of 5 to 10 mg IV and infusion of 3 to 7 mg/hr. In patients unresponsive to these measures, the insertion of a pulmonary artery catheter may be useful to guide additional fluid and vasopressor management.

Cardiac dysrhythmias can be terminated with the administration of sodium bicarbonate. Sodium and bicarbonate have proven to be beneficial treatments for toxins that have quinidine-like, sodium-channel blocking actions. In experimental models of amitriptyline toxicity, sodium loading and increasing pH each separately improve cardiac conduction, but both treatments together produced the greatest improvement (3). Hypertonic saline, 7.5% in dextran, without bicarbonate in a swine model also dramatically increases blood pressure and narrows the QRS interval after nortriptyline poisoning (2). The use of hypertonic saline has not gained widespread popularity as a clinical practice standard, however. The use of sodium bicarbonate boluses and normal saline infusions are usually sufficient but require careful monitoring as they have resulted in patients developing severe hypernatremia, fluid overload, and alkalemia.

Dysrhythmias should be treated with at least one or two ampules (44–100 mEq) of sodium bicarbonate (1 mEq/kg for pediatric patients). Sodium bicarbonate has acutely terminated VT and wide-complex tachycardia. The QRS duration shortens, and the terminal 40-millisecond changes become less evident. Respiratory alkalosis is advocated by many clinicians, but the pH increase is not as instantaneous as with bolus bicarbonate administration, and sustained respiratory alkalosis will lead to compensatory renal bicarbonate excretion, resulting in a relative deficiency state. The target pH for alkalinization is 7.45 to 7.55, but caution is needed to avoid overshooting the desired pH or causing hypernatremia or ionized hypocalcemia. Additionally, the administration of large amounts of bicarbonate for a number of hours may lead to respiratory acidosis and hypoventilation. Overdrive pacing including the use of β-agonist infusions, magnesium therapy and possibly glucagon warrant consideration for refractory ventricular dysrhythmias.

Ovine antibody (Fab fragment) has decreased free serum CA levels and reversed cardiovascular toxicity in overdose patients, but these antibody fragments are not readily available (1). Extracorporeal removal techniques are not helpful in the management of the CA-poisoned patient.

Because benzodiazepines can be therapeutic, flumazenil is contraindicated for patients with coma and a history or ECG suggestive for moderate or severe CA poisoning. Though physostigmine may be effective in reversing anticholinergic toxicity, it can cause asystole when used in severe CA poisoning, especially if there has been concomitant treatment with atropine. It is contraindicated for patients with a prolonged QRS interval or dysrhythmias suggestive of CA cardiotoxicity. Physostigmine may be beneficial in patients with the anticholinergic syndrome after mild overdose or in the recovery phase of severe poisoning (5). The dose is 2 mg IV (pediatric, 0.5–1 mg) over at least 3 minutes, which can be repeated as needed. Concomitant use of benzodiazepines is always recommended. Benzodiazepines alone do not effectively control anticholinergic delirium unless heavily sedating doses are used, which may extend the lengths of stay for many patients.

Gastrointestinal decontamination should be accomplished after the institution of any necessary life-support measures. Activated charcoal (AC) in a dose of 1 g/kg is the method of choice, when safe to administer. Multiple doses of AC have not been of clinical benefit and are not recommended. Care should be taken to avoid aspiration of charcoal into the lung, which can dramatically prolong hospital stays. Gastric lavage, though no longer routinely recommended for most poisonings, may benefit some CA-poisoned patients who present early (within 1–2 hours) after the ingestion because the toxicity of this overdose is high.

CRITICAL INTERVENTIONS

- Establish IV access and initiate continuous cardiac and oxygen saturation monitoring.
- Administer benzodiazepines for seizures and sodium bicarbonate for dysrhythmias and cardiac conduction disturbances >100 msec.
- Administer intravenous fluids and high-dose dopamine or norepinephrine for hypotension.
- Administer propofol or phenobarbital for refractory seizures or myoclonus.

DISPOSITION

The maximal severity of CA poisoning is usually apparent within 2 to 6 hours of an overdose. Patients who develop coma, hypotension, seizures, or dysrhythmias require intensive care unit admission. Those who remain or become asymptomatic after 6 hours of observation can be medically cleared for discharge or psychiatric evaluation (a requirement for all intentional ingestions). Patients with persistent but mild symptoms, such as lethargy or tachycardia, require additional monitoring and observation. Emergency department observation units or intermediate care units are appropriate.

If critically ill and complicated poisoned patients are transferred, either an air ambulance or an advanced cardiac life support–equipped crew, accompanied by a nurse or physician, is required.

COMMON PITFALLS

- Failure to appreciate that awake and stable-appearing patients with recent CA overdose may rapidly deteriorate
- Failure to recognize the subtle electrocardiographic changes consistent with cyclic antidepressant poisoning
- Failure to aggressively prevent and treat seizures and correct the resultant metabolic acidosis

ICD9

969.04 Poisoning by tetracyclic antidepressants
969.05 Poisoning by tricyclic antidepressants

REFERENCES

1. Heard K, Dart RC, Bogdan G, et al. A preliminary study of tricyclic antidepressant (TCA) ovine FAB for TCA toxicity. *Clin Toxicol* 2006;44:275–281.
2. McCabe JL, Menegazzi JJ, Cobaugh DJ, et al. Recovery from severe cyclic antidepressant overdose with hypertonic saline/dextran in a swine model. *Acad Emerg Med* 1994;1:111–115.
3. Nattel S, Mittleman M. Treatment of ventricular tachyarrhythmias resulting from amitriptyline toxicity in dogs. *J Pharmacol Exp Ther* 1984;231:430–435.
4. Sensky PR, Olczk SA. High-dose intravenous glucagon in severe tricyclic poisoning. *Postgrad Med J* 1999;75:611–612.
5. Suchard JR. Assessing physostigmine's contraindication in cyclic antidepressant ingestions. *J Emerg Med* 2003;25:185–191.
6. Taboulet P, Michard F, Muszynski J, et al. Cardiovascular repercussions of seizures during cyclic antidepressant poisoning. *J Toxicol Clin Toxicol* 1995;33:205–211.
7. Tran TP, Panacek EA, Rhee KJ, et al. Response to dopamine vs norepinephrine in tricyclic antidepressant-induced hypotension. *Acad Emerg Med* 1997;4:864–868.

45

Dystonic Reactions

PRE-HOSPITAL CONSIDERATIONS

- Pay direct attention to spasm of the larynx and the tongue to make sure that the dystonic reaction is not causing respiratory compromise. (However, a dystonic reaction is rarely life threatening.)
- Ask family and friends about ingestions of antipsychotic medications, antiemetics, and recreational drugs.
- Transport pills and pill bottles.

CLINICAL PRESENTATION

Any striated muscle group may be involved in a dystonic movement. Blepharospasm, progressing to oculogyric crisis, is the most common form of dystonia in the upper face. It usually begins with increased blinking of the eyelids. The muscles of the lower jaw most commonly involved are those of the pharynx and tongue. Oromandibular dystonia describes the involvement of any combination of these muscles. Specifically, mandibular dystonia is manifested as a pulling down or up of the jaw, and lingual dystonia is either a sustained protrusion of the tongue or an upward deflection so that the tongue curves and touches the hard palate. In the neck, torticollis is most common, although retrocollis and anterocollis may also occur. In most cases, the shoulder is elevated on the side toward which the chin is pointing. Jerking, rhythmic movements of the head may also occur. When the trunk is involved, twisting movements and postures such as lordosis, scoliosis, kyphosis, tortipelvis, and opisthotonos develop. Dystonic movements may begin focally but become segmental as they spread in a contiguous manner. Generalized dystonia refers to involvement of the leg plus other body parts, with or without the trunk. Dystonic movements are usually continual, repetitive, and twisting, varying in speed from rapid to slow and being sustained from seconds to minutes at the height of the involuntary contraction.

The prognosis is excellent for patients with drug-induced dystonias when correctly treated. However, cardiorespiratory arrest and death have been linked to metoclopramide when diagnosis and treatment were delayed (4).

DIFFERENTIAL DIAGNOSIS

Dystonic reactions have been misdiagnosed as tetanus, hysterical conversion, and even seizure disorders. Children with such abnormal movements have been thought to have encephalitis or meningitis. Strychnine poisoning and the choreiform movements sometimes seen with sympathomimetic abuse ("crack dancing") or with rheumatic fever may appear similar to dystonic reactions as well. Some rigid patients with serotonin syndrome may also appear dystonic.

ED EVALUATION

The patient, family, or friends should be asked about the recent use of medications. Physical examination is remarkable for typical abnormal posturing or movements. Response to antimuscarinic treatment supports the diagnosis.

ED MANAGEMENT

As dystonic reactions are not usually associated with an acute drug overdosage, gastrointestinal decontamination is not necessary. Administration of an antimuscarinic medication rapidly reverses the symptoms of dystonia in most cases, presumably because of restoration of the cholinergic-dopaminergic balance in nigrostriatal neurons. Diphenhydramine (Benadryl) and benztropine mesylate (Cogentin) are the two medications most frequently used. Intravenous administration is preferable to intramuscular or oral administration. Symptoms typically abate within 2 minutes and completely resolve within 15 minutes when the intravenous route is used. Muscle relaxation begins within 30 minutes but may not be complete for 90 minutes when the antidote is given intramuscularly or orally. Benztropine has been advocated over diphenhydramine because of fewer side effects and more rapid improvement of both objective and subjective findings, regardless of route of administration (3). One report describes a patient who responded minimally to multiple doses of diphenhydramine but completely to a subsequent dose of benztropine (1). Diphenhydramine should be used in children younger than age 3, as the greater antimuscarinic effects of benztropine are considered contraindicated in children this age, who may be more sensitive. Drowsiness should be anticipated as a side effect of antimuscarinic drug administration, especially with diphenhydramine.

After reversal of the reaction, an oral agent should be continued for 72 hours to prevent a relapse (2).

The usual dose of benztropine is 1 to 2 mg for adults and 0.02 to 0.05 mg/kg for children age 3 years or older, given intravenously over 2 minutes, followed by the same dose orally twice a day for 3 days. The dose of diphenhydramine is 50 to 100 mg for adults and 1 to 2 mg/kg for children, given intravenously over 2 minutes, followed by 12.5 to 50.0 mg orally three or four times a day for 3 days. Some patients may require more than one dose of intravenous medication to control the reaction.

Rare cases of dystonia may not respond to antimuscarinic therapy, and benzodiazepines should be used as a second agent. Unlike diphenhydramine and benztropine, side effects from the benzodiazepines are limited to drowsiness. Antimuscarinic sequelae such as dry mouth, blurred vision, and urinary retention are not expected. Although any benzodiazepine should be effective, diazepam and lorazepam are favored because of their longer duration of action. Diazepam can be administered intravenously in 5-mg increments every 5 minutes as needed for reversal, whereas intravenous lorazepam doses of 2 mg every 5 minutes as needed can be used. Lorazepam can also be administered intramuscularly.

Prophylactic use of benztropine and diphenhydramine has reduced the incidence of dystonic reactions in patients receiving either antiemetic or antipsychotic medications (5). Sedation may be increased, however, and should be considered.

CRITICAL INTERVENTIONS

- Recognize acute dystonia as an adverse drug reaction rather than due to other medical or psychiatric causes.
- Treat dystonic reactions with anticholinergic medications, such as benztropine or diphenhydramine, can be diagnostic and therapeutic.
- Prescribe oral antimuscarinic medication for 3 days after acute treatment to prevent relapse.

DISPOSITION

The patient may be discharged after the acute dystonia resolves. Consultation with the prescribing psychiatrist is advisable if the patient is to remain on neuroleptic medication. When antimuscarinics are prescribed, patients should be advised not to drive or perform potentially dangerous activities for 72 hours. They should be instructed to return if symptoms recur.

COMMON PITFALLS

- Failure to recognize that dystonic reactions may be delayed for 12 to 24 hours from the time of drug ingestion.
- Failure to realize that dystonic reactions are not usually the result of an overdose; because of their delayed onset, gastrointestinal decontamination is seldom indicated and may be dangerous in patients with head or neck involvement.

ICD9

333.72 Acute dystonia due to drugs

REFERENCES

1. Bailie GR, Nelson MV, Krenzelok EP, et al. Unusual treatment response of a severe dystonia to diphenhydramine. *Ann Emerg Med* 1987;16:705–708.
2. Corre K, Niemann J, Bessen H. Extended therapy for acute dystonic reactions. *Ann Emerg Med* 1984;13:194–197.
3. Lee AS. Treatment of drug-induced dystonic reactions. *JACEP* 1979;8:453–457.
4. Pollera CF, et al. Sudden death after acute dystonic reaction to high-dose metoclopramide. *Lancet* 1984;2(8400):460–461.
5. Vinson DR, Drotts DL. Diphenhydramine for the prevention of akathisia induced by prochlorperazine: a randomized, controlled trial. *Ann Emerg Med* 2001;37:125–131.

CHAPTER 46

Lithium

PRE-HOSPITAL CONSIDERATIONS
- Transport all appropriate pill bottles to the hospital.
- Provide intravenous access, oxygen, and cardiac monitoring.

CLINICAL PRESENTATION

Toxic effects depend on the dose of lithium, the time since ingestion, underlying medical conditions such as renal disease or dehydration, concomitant ingestions, and the patient's age (1,7). It is useful to classify the overdose as acute (single ingestion), acute overdose in association with chronic therapy, or chronic (10). Chronic toxicity can occur in dehydrated patients or those with renal insufficiency even without a change in dosage. Because it is likely to result in the greatest lithium distribution into tissues, it may be the most dangerous of the three types. Acute-on-chronic is probably the most common presentation. The clinical classification given in Table 46.1 can be used in the initial assessment.

DIFFERENTIAL DIAGNOSIS

The classic painless rigidity, tremor, and hyperreflexia may not be present early in the clinical course. Neurologic manifestations might mimic a cerebrovascular accident, a postictal state, metabolic disorders such as hypercalcemia or hyperthyroidism, or infection including sepsis or meningitis. The common nausea and vomiting seen after an acute overdose may be easily confused with gastroenteritis or food poisoning. Particularly in the elderly, parkinsonism or tardive dyskinesia should be considered. Co-ingestants should be considered, especially other psychiatric medications such as antipsychotics, antidepressants, and carbamazepine and sodium valproate, which are also used to treat bipolar illness. The serotonin syndrome from selective serotonin reuptake inhibitors or neuroleptic malignant syndrome from antipsychotics can closely mimic lithium toxicity.

ED EVALUATION

Attention should focus on the patient's mental status and neurologic examination, searching particularly for tremor, myoclonus, hyperreflexia, and stiffness.

TABLE 46.1	Severity of Lithium Poisoning

Grade 1 (mild): Nausea, vomiting, tremor, hyperreflexia, agitation, muscle weakness, ataxia
Grade 2 (moderate): Confusion, dysarthria, rigidity, hypertonia, hypotension, stupor
Grade 3 (severe): Convulsions, myoclonic jerking, coma, cardiovascular collapse

Hydration and serum sodium status and renal function must be addressed. A serum lithium level should be performed; lithium levels are not included in broad toxicology screens and must be ordered separately. Green-top tubes may contain lithium heparin and should not be used. A toxicology screen and blood alcohol level are indicated if the patient is ill enough to require admission to the hospital or will assist in the psychiatric assessment of the patient. More than one lithium level separated by several hours should be drawn if the patient has taken an acute overdose, particularly if the preparation is of the sustained-release type (3,5). Lithium can be nephrotoxic, targeting distal and collecting tubules, resulting in proteinuria (11). Lithium overdose can also result in electrocardiographic (ECG) changes which appear ischemic but are not (12).

Electrolytes and creatinine should be checked. ECG changes are nondiagnostic and may occur in patients with therapeutic levels who are not clinically toxic. Common changes include nonspecific ST-T wave changes, T wave inversion (which may mimic cardiac ischemia), and first-degree atrioventricular block; much more unusual findings are intraventricular conduction delay or prolonged Q-T interval (6). Cardiovascular collapse may occur as a result of severe central nervous system toxicity. Permanent neurologic sequelae can result from lithium intoxication in the absence of cardiovascular collapse (2).

ED MANAGEMENT

Advanced life-support measures are instituted as necessary. An intravenous line of normal saline should be started, and the patient should be rehydrated aggressively. However, once euvolemia and normal urine output have been established, there is little added advantage to aggressive saline diuresis, and fluid overload may occur from overly aggressive saline administration.

Lavage should be avoided, as it is unlikely to remove significant quantities of drug. Activated charcoal does not bind lithium and should only be given if co-ingestants are suspected. There is experimental evidence that sodium polystyrene sulfonate (Kayexalate), an ion-exchange resin usually used to treat hyperkalemia, can both prevent absorption of lithium and enhance its removal once absorbed (9). The clinical efficacy of this therapy is unproved, and it is probably best reserved for patients who have taken a massive overdose, have high or rising levels, or are otherwise severely ill. The optimum dose and dosing intervals have not been defined; 15 to 50 g orally or by nasogastric tube every 4 to 6 hours might be a reasonable starting point. Kayexalate can cause nausea, vomiting, and constipation. The serum potassium level should be carefully monitored and replaced as needed to prevent hypokalemia.

Whole-bowel irrigation has also been recommended as a gastrointestinal decontamination measure for lithium overdose, especially for slow-release formulations. It is uncertain whether this technique is as effective as using Kayexalate or whether, in fact, either approach alters clinical outcome.

Hemodialysis is the most efficient method of removing lithium from the intravascular compartment, allowing lithium to redistribute into it from the brain. Because this redistribution is relatively slow, however, clinical improvement lags behind the fall in serum lithium levels (4,8). A significant rebound of the serum lithium level usually occurs, which may necessitate a second or third round of dialysis in the sickest patients. It may take days or longer for toxicity to resolve, despite hemodialysis.

Hemodialysis is recommended for patients with severe or progressive lithium toxicity and those with renal failure. There is no serum lithium level above which all patients need to be hemodialyzed. Patients on chronic therapy may manifest some toxicity even though their levels may be within the therapeutic range. Other patients may be relatively asymptomatic with levels >5 mEq/L after acute overdose. Clinical judgment, preferably by a physician experienced in the treatment of lithium-poisoned patients, is necessary in making these important decisions. In general, serum lithium levels above 3 meq/L (mmol/L) in any patient are an indication that the patient could deteriorate. Levels less than that may still result in serious illness in some patients, particularly those who are dehydrated, hyponatremic, or have renal insufficiency or other serious chronic disease (10).

CRITICAL INTERVENTIONS

- Administer normal saline intravenously for rehydration and treatment of hyponatremia; establish and maintain a normal urine output.
- Obtain a serum lithium level and repeat to determine if levels are rising significantly.
- Consider hemodialysis in patients with significant clinical toxicity and high lithium levels, especially those with renal insufficiency.
- Consider Kayexalate or early whole-bowel irrigation for large acute ingestions.

DISPOSITION

Patients should be admitted if they have significant neurologic findings from lithium such as altered mental status, tremor, hyperreflexia, or stiffness. If patients are dehydrated, are in renal failure, or have a high or rising lithium level, they should be admitted to an intensive care unit. Consultation with a poison center or toxicologist is also recommended. Although hemodialysis may not be necessary and is not usually performed in the emergency department, nephrology consultation can result in the dialysis team's being mobilized more quickly when needed. In all cases of overdose with suicidal intent, psychiatric consultation should be obtained before discharge.

COMMON PITFALLS

- Failure to consider the possibility of chronic lithium toxicity in patients taking lithium who develop hyponatremia, dehydration, or renal compromise
- Failure to obtain serial lithium levels in patients with acute overdose, especially with a sustained-release lithium preparation
- Failure to appreciate that severe lithium poisoning can lead to permanent neurologic impairment and that aggressive treatment is warranted

ICD9

985.8 Toxic effect of other specified metals

REFERENCES

1. Amdisen A. Clinical features and management of lithium poisoning. *Med Toxicol Adverse Drug Exp* 1988;3:18.
2. Apte SN, Langston JW. Permanent neurological deficits due to lithium toxicity. *Ann Neurol* 1983;13:453.
3. Astruc B, Petit P, Abbar M. Overdose with sustained-release lithium preparations. *Eur Psychiatry* 1999;14:172–174.
4. Bailey B, McGuigan M. Comparison of patients hemodialyzed for lithium poisoning and those for whom dialysis was recommended by PCC but not done: what lesson can we learn? *Clin Nephrol* 2000;54:388–392.
5. Bosse GM, Arnold TC. Overdose with sustained-release lithium preparations. *J Emerg Med* 1992; 10:719.
6. Brady HR, Horgan JH. Lithium and the heart: unanswered questions. *Chest* 1988;93:166–169.
7. Hansen HE, Amdisen A. Lithium intoxication: report of 23 cases and review of 100 cases from the literature. *Q J Med* 1978;47:123.
8. Jaeger A, Sauder P, Kopferschmitt J, et al. When should dialysis be performed in lithium poisoning? A kinetic study in 14 cases of lithium poisoning. *J Toxicol Clin Toxicol* 1993;31:429.
9. Tomaszewski C, Musso C, Pearson JR, et al. Lithium absorption prevented by sodium polystyrene sulfonate in volunteers. *Ann Emerg Med* 1992;21:1308.
10. Waring WS, Laing WJ, Good AM, et al. Pattern of lithium exposure predicts poisoning severity: evaluation of referrals to a regional poisons unit. *Q J Med* 2007;100:271–276.
11. Markowitz GS, Radhakrishnan J, Kambham N, et al. Lithium nephrotoxicity: A progressive combined glomerular and tubulointerstitial nephropathy. *J Am Soc Nephrol* 2000;11:1439–1448.
12. Puhr J, Hack J, Early J, et al. Lithium overdose with electrocardiogram changes suggesting ischemia. *J Med Toxicol* 2008;4:170–172.

CHAPTER 47

Monoamine Oxidase Inhibitors

PRE-HOSPITAL CONSIDERATIONS

- Keep in mind that the patient may be uncooperative or violent.
- Secure intravenous access.
- Protect from self-induced trauma.

CLINICAL PRESENTATION

Drug or food interactions with monoamine oxidase (MAO) inhibitors are common, with hypertensive crisis occurring in 1% to 8% of those taking MAO inhibitors therapeutically (2,6). The clinical presentation may include headache, hypertension, tachycardia (or reflex bradycardia), diaphoresis, agitation, hypertonicity, hyperreflexia with myoclonus, rigidity, seizures, and coma (6). Hyperpyrexia, intracranial hemorrhage, and death may occur. Toxicity begins within 30 to 90 minutes of the ingestion or administration of sympathomimetic amines (2). The duration of effect is variable but often resolves within a few hours.

MAO inhibitor overdose follows a distinctly different time course (3–5). The absence of early symptomatology is typical with nonselective irreversible agents. Onset of toxicity is usually delayed from 6 to 12 hours after the overdose, peaks from 24 to 48 hours for severe cases, and may last for 72 to 96 hours (5). A latent period as long as 29 hours has been described after tranylcypromine overdose (2). During the latent phase, the patient usually appears well or mildly sedated (2,3,5). Poisoning is characterized by alterations in behavior, cognition, autonomic nervous system function, and neuromuscular activity and may be classified as mild, moderate, or severe (Table 47.1) (5). Signs and symptoms vary greatly in their onset, severity, and duration. Patients with early or mild toxicity may demonstrate mild lethargy or restlessness, dysarthria, nausea, headache, ataxia, palpitations, flushing, shivering, sweating, tremor, nystagmus, incoordination, or hyperreflexia. Moderate toxicity may include confusion, hallucinations, disorientation, agitated delirium, mutism, salivation, diarrhea, marked diaphoresis, myoclonus, fasciculations, trismus, writhing movements, and mild-to-moderate elevations of temperature, pulse, respiratory rate, and blood pressure. Severe toxicity may be characterized by unresponsive coma; fixed, dilated pupils; "ping-pong" gaze; pathologic reflexes; generalized rigidity; seizures; hyperpyrexia (temperature >104°F); marked tachypnea or respiratory depression; extreme sinus tachycardia or bradycardia; malignant cardiac dysrhythmias;

TABLE 47.1 Clinical Course of Monoamine Oxidase Inhibitor Poisoning

Phase-Severity*	Time after Ingestion*	Cognitive-Behavioral Dysfunction	Autonomic Dysfunction	Neuromuscular Dysfunction
0-Latent	0–24 h	Mild lethargy	Absent	Absent
I-Mild	6–12 h	Mild lethargy Dysarthria Ataxia Headache Anxiety Insomnia	Nausea Flushing Diaphoresis Shivering Irritability	Mild tremor Hyperreflexia Incoordination Nystagmus Mydriasis
II-Moderate	10–24 h	Confusion Disorientation Agitated delirium Mumbling/rambling speech Mutism Hyperactivity	Mild hyperthermia (temperature <104°F) Marked diaphoresis Salivation Piloerection Hypertension Sinus tachycardia (P <150 beats/min) Hyperventilation	Myoclonus Fasciculations Trismus Facial grimacing Writhing extremities
III-Severe	16–72 h	Incomprehensible speech Coma Seizures	Hyperventilation to respiratory arrest Extreme sinus tachycardia to sinus bradycardia Malignant dysrhythmias (VT, VF, bradyasystole) Hypotension Pale, clammy, mottled skin Severe hyperthermia (temperature <104°F)	Generalized rigidity Opisthotonus Fixed, dilated pupils "Ping-pong" gaze Pathologic reflexes (decorticate, decerebrate, Babinski)
IV-Complications	24–96 h	Aspiration pneumonitis Adult respiratory distress syndrome	Anion gap metabolic acidosis Hemolysis	Rhabdomyolysis Acute renal failure Disseminated intravascular coagulation Hepatic failure

*Signs and symptoms vary greatly in their onset, severity, and duration.

hypotension; and death (2–4,5). Death from cardiovascular (CV) collapse is most likely to occur in patients with severe hyperpyrexia (3,5).

Although seizures may occur after MAO overdose, they are uncommon and can be confused with neuromuscular hyperactivity produced by these agents (2,3). Secondary complications may occur in patients with moderate-to-severe toxicity and include aspiration pneumonitis, adult respiratory distress syndrome, rhabdomyolysis, acute renal failure, metabolic acidosis, and disseminated intravascular coagulation (DIC) (5). The likelihood of secondary complications (e.g., rhabdomyolysis, DIC) and death is related to the degree and duration of hyperthermia. Patients with severe toxicity can manifest fixed, dilated pupils, posturing, and extensor plantar response, yet make a complete neurologic recovery (2–4).

When taken alone, reversible inhibitors of MAO-A, a subtype of MAO, appear to have a benign course after acute overdose. Ingestion of doses as high as 20.5 g has resulted in only mild to moderate toxicity. Large overdoses are characterized by mild central nervous system (CNS) depression, agitation, tachycardia, hypertension, and mydriasis. Although death is rare after overdose with moclobemide alone, mixed-drug overdoses are more serious. Many fatalities have been reported from the serotonin syndrome when moclobemide has been combined with other serotonin-potentiating drugs (e.g., citalopram, clomipramine, methylenedioxymethamphetamine, paroxetine, and sertraline). Chronic use of irreversible nonselective inhibitors has been associated with hyperadrenergic adverse effects similar to the chronic use of amphetamines. These effects include agitation, confusion, hallucinations, hyperhidrosis, hypomania, insomnia, tremors, and seizures (2).

DIFFERENTIAL DIAGNOSIS

Amphetamine, cocaine, and sympathomimetic (including over-the-counter appetite suppressants) overdose produce a clinical picture similar to the hypertensive reactions associated with MAO inhibitors and dietary and drug monoamines. The clinical presentation of anticholinergic, hallucinogen (e.g., lysergic acid diethylamide, phencyclidine), lithium, salicylate, sympathomimetic (e.g., amphetamines, cocaine), and strychnine poisoning may be similar to that of MAO inhibitor overdose. MAO inhibitor toxicity may be confused with the neuroleptic malignant syndrome and withdrawal from alcohol or sedative hypnotic agents. Clinical features of the serotonin syndrome are nearly identical to those after overdose with MAO inhibitors. Medical emergencies such as hypoglycemia, malignant hyperthermia, intracranial hemorrhage, meningitis, encephalitis, pheochromocytoma, septicemia, tetanus, and thyrotoxicosis may present in a similar manner.

ED EVALUATION

The history should include the time, dose, and duration of exposure; the time of onset, nature, and severity of symptoms; the type of first aid undertaken; and the medical and psychiatric history. Accurate and complete historical data are essential in differentiating the toxic syndromes related to MAO inhibitors. The physical examination should focus on the vital signs and CV and neurologic function. Except for "ping-pong" gaze, there are no pathognomonic physical findings or laboratory abnormalities. Initial testing for patients with suspected intentional overdose should include an electrocardiogram and routine serum chemistries. Patients with toxicity should also have a complete blood count; prothrombin and partial thromboplastin times; creatine phosphokinase, calcium, magnesium, and liver function tests; and a urinalysis. Patients with altered mental status should have a bedside fingerstick glucose determination and appropriate intervention, as necessary. A lumbar puncture and computed tomography scanning may be necessary to differentiate drug intoxication from intracranial hemorrhage, meningitis, and encephalitis.

Toxicology screening may be useful to exclude other intoxications (e.g., acetaminophen and salicylate), but it rarely detects MAO inhibitors because of their low concentrations in blood and urine samples (5). Overdose of selegiline or tranylcypromine, however, may produce a false-positive qualitative screen for amphetamines (5). Quantitative MAO inhibitor levels are not generally available and do not correlate with the severity of poisoning (5,6). Similarly, the degree of MAO enzyme activity inhibition does not correlate with clinical toxicity.

ED MANAGEMENT

Supportive care is the primary treatment for MAO inhibitor overdose. Advanced life-support measures should be instituted, as necessary. The administration of glucose, oxygen, naloxone, and thiamine should be considered for patients with altered mental status. Activated charcoal is the preferred method of gastrointestinal decontamination for recent acute MAO inhibitor overdose. Before any drug or food is given, the potential for an adverse interaction with MAO inhibitors must be considered.

Agitation, neuromuscular hyperactivity, and seizures should be treated promptly with liberal doses of benzodiazepines (e.g., diazepam, lorazepam) or barbiturates (e.g., phenobarbital) (5). Phenytoin is unlikely to be as effective for seizures associated with MAO inhibitors. Pyridoxine administration (see Chapter 22, "Isoniazid") is recommended for seizures that occur after overdose with a hydrazine MAO inhibitor.

Rapid cooling is essential to minimize patient morbidity and mortality from hyperthermia. Because hyperthermia is almost invariably associated with CNS agitation and neuromuscular hyperactivity, initial treatment with benzodiazepines or barbiturates is recommended. In conjunction with these initial pharmacologic measures, evaporative and convective cooling methods, using wet sheets or cool mist sprays and fans, are recommended (5). Antipyretics and cooling blankets are generally ineffective. If these initial maneuvers do not provide rapid patient cooling, neuromuscular paralysis is strongly recommended (3–5).

Animal studies and human case reports suggests that neuromuscular paralysis is effective for the treatment of severe hyperthermia (3,4). Cooling times of <1 hour have been achieved with this method of treatment. Although dantrolene

(2.5 mg/kg orally or intravenously every 6 hours) has also been reported to be effective, it is itself toxic and does not terminate muscular rigidity and hyperthermia as rapidly as paralyzing agents. Because the pathophysiology of serotonin syndrome overlaps considerably with MAO inhibitor overdose, nonspecific serotonin receptor antagonists (e.g., cyproheptadine, methysergide) could be of benefit. Because there are no clinical data in this regard, such therapy cannot currently be recommended.

Severe hypertension may be treated with rapid-onset, short-acting intravenous agents such as sodium nitroprusside or phentolamine (5,6). Phentolamine (2–10 mg intravenously) is attractive because it blocks α-adrenergic receptors and antagonize the effects of norepinephrine (NE). It is effective for the treatment of hypertension associated with the cheese reaction. Dexmedetomidine is a parenteral, selective, α_2-adrenergic agonist that might be used for rapid, titratable control of hypertension, but its use for this purpose cannot yet be recommended owing to lack of published data. Long-acting agents (tolazoline, clonidine) also have been used but are not recommended, as hypertension is often followed by severe hypotension (5). β-adrenergic antagonists are not recommended for hypertension because of potential unopposed α-adrenergic vasoconstriction and worsened hypertension.

Hypotension should initially be treated with fluid resuscitation. When pressors are required, direct-acting agents (e.g., epinephrine, NE) are recommended (5,6). The use of indirectly acting agents (e.g., dopamine), which require the release of intracellular amines for their pressor effect, may either precipitate a hypertensive crisis or be ineffective on account of depleted stores of catecholamines (2). Additionally, MAO inhibition is less likely to potentiate the effects of exogenously administered, direct-acting pressors, which circulate extracellularly and are primarily metabolized by catechol-o-methyltransferase. Regardless, low doses of direct-acting pressors should be used initially to minimize the risk of an exaggerated pressor response. Phenylephrine, a direct-acting agent, has been associated with an exaggerated pressor response and is not recommended for the treatment of hypotension in MAO inhibitor poisoning.

Ventricular dysrhythmias and severe bradycardias, usually premorbid signs, should be treated according to current advanced cardiac life-support protocols.

Diuresis, urinary acidification, hemodialysis, and hemo perfusion play no role in the management of MAO inhibitor poisoning (1,5,7).

CRITICAL INTERVENTIONS

- Admit all patients with known or suspected MAO inhibitor overdose to an intensive care unit for 24-hour monitoring.
- Treat neuromuscular hyperactivity with benzodiazepines or barbiturates; if severe or accompanied by hyperthermia or rhabdomyolysis, institute neuromuscular paralysis.
- Rapidly and aggressively cool patients with hyperthermia.
- Administer a direct-acting pressor (e.g., NE) for hypotension unresponsive to fluid administration.

DISPOSITION

All patients with suspected MAO inhibitor overdose should be admitted for extended observation (24 hours) in a monitored setting. Symptomatic patients and those with abnormal vital signs should be admitted to an intensive care unit. If intensive care is unavailable, patients should be transferred to an institution with this capacity.

Patients who present with drug or dietary interactions may not require hospital admission if the clinical response has been mild. Patients with severe reactions, those with persistent symptoms after a 4- to 6-hour observation period, and those with symptoms that necessitate active intervention should be admitted. The level of in-hospital care required (intensive care or floor) depends on the severity of symptoms. For patients well enough to eat, an MAO inhibitor diet (e.g., low tyramine) should be ordered.

COMMON PITFALLS

- Failure to check for or recognize MAO inhibitor use before prescribing sympathomimetics or giving pain medications, particularly meperidine
- Failure to appreciate that the history is key to differentiating acute overdose from drug and food interactions, including the serotonin syndrome
- Failure to appreciate that the onset of toxicity may be delayed and gradual in onset after MAO inhibitor overdose
- Failure to appreciate that early sympathetic stimulation may be followed by catecholamine depletion and CV collapse in patients with acute MAO inhibitor overdose

ICD9

969.01 Poisoning by monoamine oxidase inhibitors

REFERENCES

1. Baker GB, Urichuk LJ, McKenna KF, et al. Metabolism of monoamine oxidase inhibitors. *Cell Mol Neurobiol* 1999;19:411–426.
2. Baldessarini RJ. Drug therapy of depression and anxiety disorders. In: Brunton LL, Lazo JS, Parker KL, eds. *Goodman & Gilman's: The Pharmacological Basis of Therapeutics,* 11th ed. New York, McGraw-Hill, 2006:429–459.
3. Ciocatto E, Gagiano G, Bava GL. Clinical features and treatment of overdosage of monoamine oxidase inhibitors and their interaction with other psychotropic drugs. *Resuscitation* 1972;1:69.
4. Erich JL, Shih RD, O'Connor RE. "Ping-pong" gaze in severe monoamine oxidase inhibitor toxicity. *J Emerg Med* 1995;13:653.
5. Linden CH, Rumack BH. MAO inhibitor overdose. *Ann Emerg Med* 1984;13:1137.
6. Lipson RE, Stern TA. Management of monoamine oxidase inhibitor-treated patients in the emergency and critical care setting. *J Intensive Care Med* 1991;6:117.

CHAPTER

48

Serotonin Reuptake Inhibitors and the Serotonin Syndrome

PRE-HOSPITAL CONSIDERATIONS

- In cases of suspected overdose, bring all medication bottles to the hospital.
- Check airway, breathing, and circulation.
- Give 0.9% normal saline intravenously for blood pressure stabilization.
- Give benzodiazepine for seizures.
- In cases of wide-complex tachycardia, administer sodium bicarbonate by intravenous fluid bolus to standard advanced cardiac life support measures.

CLINICAL PRESENTATION

Though serotonin reuptake inhibitors (SRIs) are well tolerated in moderate overdoses presenting with little more than nausea or tremor, more significant symptoms such as sedation, QTc prolongation, and seizures do occur (1). Patients can present with serotonin syndrome after overdose of an SRI. Seizures appear to be most common with citalopram and venlafaxine (8), particularly in doses >3 g, and a case report of seizures due to drug-induced syndrome of inappropriate antidiuretic hormone has been attributed to duloxetine (9).

Cardiac conduction effects are seen primarily as QTc prolongation, especially with citalopram (7). A prolonged QTc places the patient at risk for torsades de pointes. Venlafaxine can cause blockade of fast inward sodium channels in cardiac myocytes (11,14). This contributes to widening of the QRS, similar to toxicity seen with tricyclic antidepressants (TCAs). Cardiac dysrhythmias, including ventricular tachycardia, have been reported in large venlafaxine overdoses (>5–8 g) (11,14). Seizures and electrocardiographic QRS prolongation have been reported after overdose with fluoxetine.

In overdose, antimuscarinic (anticholinergic) effects can be seen, depending on the agent ingested. These may manifest as sedation, delirium, coma, hyperthermia, tachycardia, hypertension, dry mucus membranes, decreased bowel sounds, or urinary retention.

DIFFERENTIAL DIAGNOSIS

It is important to remember that poly-drug ingestions are the norm rather than the exception, especially in intentional adult overdoses. Other agents with sedating or antimuscarinic properties must be considered as co-ingestants. Sympathomimetic agents (such as cocaine or amphetamines); dextromethorphan; anticholinergic agents such as diphenhydramine; hallucinogens such as lysergic acid diethylamide or phencyclidine (PCP); alcohol; or withdrawal from benzodiazepines or alcohol can present with altered mental status, hallucinations, agitation, seizures, or autonomic instability. Access to other psychotropic medications should also be considered, as many patients may have multiple agents at home that are "left over." When evaluating a patient with hyperthermia and altered mental status, one should always consider a possible infectious etiology such as meningitis, encephalitis, or septicemia. Neurotrauma, hypoxia, hyponatremia, and hypoglycemia should also be considered when there is altered mental status. Though cardiac conduction delays can be common in SRI intoxications, they can also be a sign of ischemic injury, so the patient's underlying cardiac status should be taken into account.

ED EVALUATION

As potentially profound sedation can be seen in SRI intoxications, evaluation of a patient's ability to protect the airway is vital. Breathing and circulation should be immediately assessed. The patient should have cardiac monitoring with telemetry and serial electrocardiograph (ECG) evaluations. Blood chemistries should be obtained to look for acid-base and electrolyte abnormalities. Serum acetaminophen levels should be obtained on intentional overdose patients to detect this possible co-ingestant.

ED MANAGEMENT

Excellent symptomatic and supportive care is essential. The emergency physician should protect the airway and assist breathing, with endotracheal intubation if indicated. Blood pressure should be supported with pressor agents as necessary to maintain perfusion. Glucose (with thiamine) and naloxone can be considered for patients with altered mental status. Flumazenil is contraindicated in suspected SRI overdoses or any suspected poly-drug overdose. It will not reverse the sedation from the SRIs. Additionally, it may induce withdrawal seizures in a benzodiazepine-dependent patient and decrease the ability to control seizures should they occur from the overdose. Physostigmine may produce brief reversal of significant antimuscarinic side effects, but its primary utility is as a diagnostic agent in patients with a normal ECG. Physostigmine has caused asystole with cyclic antidepressants and, because some SRIs have similar sodium channel–blocking effects, it may be best avoided (5).

Seizures should be treated with benzodiazepines as first-line agents. If seizures persist and are not controlled by benzodiazepines, consider barbiturates, propofol, and finally general anesthesia with electroencephalographic monitoring. Status epilepticus is not a typical feature of SRI-induced seizure activity, and its presence should prompt evaluation of other causes such as trauma, infection, or a secondary toxic exposure or an unknown co-ingestant such as isoniazid.

If there is QRS prolongation (>100 msec or increasing on serial ECGs), serum alkalinization with sodium bicarbonate ($NaHCO_3$) should be considered. Initial dosing of one to three ampoules (50 mEq each) IV, usually followed by continuous infusion of three ampoules $NaHCO_3$ in one liter of D5W at a high maintenance infusion rate. The goal is normalization of the QRS or a maximum serum pH of 7.5 to 7.55. Serum alkalinization with $NaHCO_3$ is the mainstay of treatment for TCA-induced QRS prolongation. The efficacy of this modality in QRS prolongation from other psychotropic agents is variable, but it should be attempted if the patient has no contraindication to the sodium and volume load.

Drug-induced QTc prolongation from SRIs should be followed closely with serial ECGs, as the patient is at increased risk for torsades de pointes. QTc >470 msec on serial ECGs should be considered abnormal. Potassium, magnesium, and calcium levels should be normalized if possible, to mitigate their potential contribution to QTc prolongation.

Hyperthermia should be treated with active cooling and intravenous benzodiazepines if muscle hyperactivity and rigidity are contributing components. Oral activated charcoal (1 gm/kg) should be considered in any patient within 1 to 2 hours of acute overdose who is alert enough to protect the airway. Orogastric lavage should rarely be performed, as these agents have relatively low toxicity. Whole bowel irrigation (WBI) with polyethylene glycol solution should be considered for acute ingestions of extended release preparations. The WBI solution should be given at 1 to 2 liters per hour per nasogastric tube until the rectal effluent is clear. There is no role for hemodialysis, given the high level of protein binding and large volumes of distribution.

Beta blockers or calcium channel blockers should generally be avoided in attempts to control drug-induced tachycardia or hypertension, unless there are signs of end-organ injury from these. It is best to use agents with a short duration of actions (e.g., nitroglycerin, nitroprusside, or esmolol), as they can be titrated down rapidly if necessary.

CRITICAL INTERVENTIONS

- Evaluate airway, breathing, and circulation.
- Establish intravenous access and cardiac monitoring with serial ECGs for QRS and QT prolongation.
- Benzodiazepines for agitation, muscle hypertonicity, hyperthermia, and seizures.
- Bicarbonate for QRS prolongation.

DISPOSITION

Admission to the hospital is indicated for the rare patient with persistent sedation, antimuscarinic effects, QRS or QT prolongation, seizures or any clinical manifestations of serotonin syndrome. Persistently asymptomatic patients with no evidence of drug-induced conduction delays on their ECGs who have had an ingestion of a nonsustained-release preparation can be observed and discharged after 6 hours. Psychiatric services should be considered for all intentional overdoses. Patients who have ingested sustained release preparations should be considered for observation up to 24 hours for possibly delayed toxic effects or serotonin syndrome.

SEROTONIN SYNDROME

Serotonin syndrome is the result of excess serotonergic stimulation in the central nervous system and remains the most common significant complication of selective serotonin reuptake inhibitor (SSRI) overdose. Serotonin syndrome can occur when a second agent with serotonergic properties is added during therapeutic dosage of an SRI and rarely after initiation of a single SRI medication. The 5HT-2A receptor has been implicated in most of the manifestations of serotonin syndrome, but it is likely that there is a significant contribution from other serotonergic receptors and possibly interactions with other neurotransmitters (3). As some of the SSRIs have prolonged elimination half-lives and pharmacologically active metabolites, serotonin syndrome can occur when a patient is switched from one SRI to another SRI or to another agent with similar serotonergic activity. The emergency physician should be aware of this possibility and record a careful medication history that includes discontinued medications (Table 48.1). The syndrome is evident in up to 16% of patients who overdose on SSRIs (3). Clinical effects occur on a spectrum of mild to severe, and the history is vital in making the diagnosis and differentiating it from other etiologies, in particular neuroleptic malignant syndrome (NMS), which shares many clinical characteristics (see Table 48.3).

TABLE 48.1	Drugs with the Potential to Produce Serotonin Syndrome

Increased serotonin production
    L-tryptophan

Increased presynaptic serotonin release
    Amphetamines
    MDMA (Ecstasy)
    Cocaine

Decrease serotonin breakdown by MAO
    Phenelzine, tranylcypromine, isocarboxazid
    Moclobemide
    Selegiline

Inhibition of serotonin reuptake
    Fluoxetine, citalopram, escitalopram, paroxetine, sertraline, fluvoxamine, cyclic antidepressants, clomipramine
    Meperidine, dextromethorphan, tramadol

TABLE 48.2 Comparison of Serotonin Syndrome and Neuroleptic Malignant Syndrome (NMS)

	Serotonin Syndrome	NMS
Cause	Serotonin excess	Dopamine blockade/depletion
Onset of symptoms	$\leq$ 24h	Days to weeks
Neuromuscular effects	Hyperreflexia, clonus, hypertonicity (greater in lower extremities)	"Lead pipe" muscle rigidity in all muscle groups Bradyreflexia (tremor, hyperreflexia and clonus not as common)
Length of symptoms	Days	Days to weeks

Note: Varying degrees of altered mental status and autonomic instability are seen with both syndromes.

The signs and symptoms of serotonin syndrome can be divided into three major categories: neuromuscular hyperactivity, altered mental status, and autonomic nervous system instability (Table 48.2). There may be abnormalities in only one or two of these categories. The most common clinical findings are myoclonus, hyperreflexia, confusion, hyperthermia, diaphoresis, and sinus tachycardia (13), but there is no single abnormality that is required for the diagnosis (12). Patients often have a combination of signs and symptoms, and these may not match one another in severity (e.g., a patient may have significant muscle hypertonicity with only mildly altered mental status and autonomic abnormalities). The diagnosis should thus be considered in patients with a history of recent exposure to serotonergic agents and findings in any of the major categories with some of the typical findings (Table 48.3).

TABLE 48.3 Summary of Potential Clinical Findings Associated with Serotonin Syndrome

Autonomic Instability	Altered Mental Status	Hyperactivity Neuromuscular
Tachycardia	Anxiety	Myoclonus
Fluctuating blood pressure	Confusion	Hyperreflexia
Diaphoresis	Drowsiness	Muscle rigidity
Flushed skin	Hallucinations	Tremor
Hyperthermia	Coma	Agitation
Tachypnea	Insomnia	Restlessness
Mydriasis	Dizziness	Ataxia
Unreactive pupils	—	Nystagmus
Diarrhea	—	Trismus
Abdominal pain	—	Opisthotonus
Excessive salivation	—	

The time of onset of symptoms after exposure to serotonergic agents is variable. Symptoms are often reported to develop within 1 to 2 hours of ingestion (10). The syndrome has also been reported to occur several days after gradual increases in dosing of antidepressant medications (3). There appears to be no relationship between the amount of drug ingested and the risk of serotonin syndrome, as it can occur with both therapeutic dosing and in overdose. Serum drug levels measured in patients with the serotonin syndrome have been either at therapeutic or below therapeutic levels in up to 90% of cases (13).

Mild neuromuscular effects can include tremor and akathisia that progress to increased reflexes and clonus and then to frank hypertonicity of muscles, which contributes to hyperthermia. Hypertonicity often occurs to a greater extent in the lower extremities. Mild confusion, agitation, and sedation can worsen to profoundly altered mental status, coma, and seizures. Autonomic instability ranges from minimally elevated heart rate, blood pressure, and temperature to frankly unstable vital signs with significant hypertension, tachycardia and life-threatening hyperthermia ($>41°C$).

Laboratory abnormalities may include evidence of rhabdomyolysis, with elevation of creatine phosphokinase, serum creatinine, and lactic acidosis from muscle tissue breakdown, seizures, or hyperthermia. Coagulation abnormalities (including disseminated intravascular coagulopathy), hypotension, and death have also been reported (12).

The differential diagnosis of serotonin syndrome includes sympathomimetic toxicity from agents such as cocaine, amphetamines, phencyclidine (muscle hyperactivity, autonomic instability, potentially altered mental status), tetanus (opisthotonus, muscle spasms), strychnine poisoning (muscle spasms and rigidity), lithium toxicity (altered mental status, tremor, and clonus), and severe dystonic reactions. Infectious etiologies and metabolic derangements should also be ruled out. The most similar condition, however, is the NMS (see Chapter 43, "Antipsychotic Drugs"). In contrast to patients with the serotonin syndrome, those with NMS have a history of recent commencement of, or increase in, dosage of neuroleptic medications. Symptoms tend to develop (and later resolve) over days rather than hours; muscular hyperactivity is characterized by sustained "lead pipe" rigidity rather than by myoclonus; and hyperreflexia is rarely, if ever, seen.

Both the history and physical examination should focus on excluding other causes of the clinical picture. Vital signs should include an accurate temperature. A thorough search for trauma should be made. Patients should be questioned about the presence of visual or auditory hallucinations and examined for neuromuscular features of serotonin syndrome. In patients presenting with a clinical picture suggestive of serotonin syndrome the history should focus on drug use. Specifically, any evidence of drug overdose and use of multiple serotonergic medications, drugs of abuse, and over-the-counter medications containing dextromethorphan should be sought. The vital signs should be repeated frequently, as autonomic instability can result in fluctuating blood pressure and pulse. Laboratory investigation should focus on excluding other causes of the clinical picture and evaluating for potential complications of the serotonin syndrome.

The treatment of serotonin syndrome consists primarily of aggressive symptomatic and supportive care. This includes active external cooling, airway management, and control of muscle tone with benzodiazepines. Agitation, myoclonus, hypertonia, or hyperpyrexia should be treated with intravenous benzodiazepines, crystalloids, and rapid external cooling measures. Untreated hyperthermia from serotonin syndrome increases a patient's morbidity and mortality (4). If no response is observed, chemical paralysis and sedation should be used to reduce muscle tone and decrease hyperthermia. All medications with serotonergic activity should be discontinued, and care should be used in choosing medications for treatment. Consultation with a clinical pharmacist may be helpful to tailor therapy, as certain commonly used medications have potentially unrecognized serotonergic activity (e.g., ondansetron, fentanyl, valproate, metoclopramide) (3).

Various serotonin receptor antagonists have been utilized to treat serotonin syndrome, with inconsistent efficacy. Cyproheptadine is an oral antihistamine with antagonist effects at 5HT-1A and 2 receptors that has shown some efficacy in case reports in mitigating symptoms, though its impacts on outcome is still unclear (6). Initial control of symptoms can be attempted using 4 to 12 mg of cyproheptadine orally (or per nasogastric tube), followed by dosing of 2 mg every 2 hours until symptoms improve, followed by maintenance dosing of 8 mg every 6 hours (3,6). The maximum dose in a 24-hour period is 32 mg. It is most effective with mild-to-moderate toxicity typically within 1 to 2 hours of initial administration (6). Patients with more severe or progressive serotonin syndrome do not respond as well, if at all (6).

The antipsychotic chlorpromazine is another serotonin receptor antagonist and has the advantage of being available for parenteral administration. It has been used successfully in doses of 50 to 100 mg intravenously and intramuscularly. Dosing should be preceded by adequate intravenous fluid hydration to prevent hypotension. Other side effects include sedation and dystonic reactions. The use of chlorpromazine in patients with NMS misdiagnosed as serotonin syndrome has the potential to worsen the former condition. Preliminary observations also suggest that olanzapine, a newer atypical antipsychotic agent, may also be effective in reversing serotonergic toxicity. Olanzapine also antagonizes 5-HT$_2$ receptors and has a higher affinity for these than either cyproheptadine or chlorpromazine. Further study is required to delineate its role in the treatment of serotonin syndrome.

Serotonin syndrome is usually self-limited and resolves in days as long as there is cessation of any serotonergic agent and aggressive symptomatic and supportive care.

CRITICAL INTERVENTIONS

- Initiate aggressive active cooling for hyperthermia.
- Initiate aggressive benzodiazepine therapy and paralysis for neuromuscular stimulation.

Any patient manifesting even mild signs and symptoms of serotonin syndrome should be admitted to the hospital for further care until symptoms resolve. Patients with significant autonomic instability are best managed in an intensive care setting.

SELECTIVE SEROTONIN REUPTAKE INHIBITOR DISCONTINUATION SYNDROME

After abrupt discontinuation of an SSRI, a mild and transient syndrome can occur. Typically starting in the first few days after discontinuation of an SSRI and lasting 1 to 2 weeks, symptoms can include headache, dizziness, nausea, irritability, insomnia, and paresthesias (2). Symptoms resolve spontaneously, but resolution is more rapid when the medication is restarted (2). Though abrupt cessation of SSRIs is to be avoided in the outpatient setting because of these symptoms, this should not be a concern for the emergency physician in patients with an overdose. Resumption of treatment with an SSRI should be delayed until after any acute toxicity has resolved.

COMMON PITFALLS

- Prescribing medication with serotonergic effects (e.g., meperidine, tramadol, or dextromethorphan) in patients who are taking serotonergic medications, especially monoamine oxidase inhibitors
- Failing to admit patients with cardiac conduction delays (e.g., prolonged QTc) to telemetry
- Failure to measure the temperature and begin cooling measures as indicated
- Failure to recognize that a diagnosis of serotonin syndrome does not require all three elements of altered mental status, autonomic instability, and neuromuscular hyperactivity

ICD9

969.02 Poisoning by selective serotonin and norepinephrine reuptake inhibitors
969.03 Poisoning by selective serotonin reuptake inhibitors

REFERENCES

1. Barbey JT, Roose SP. SSRI safety in overdose. *J Clin Psychiatry* 1998;59(Suppl 15):42–48.
2. Black K, Shea C, Dursun S, Kutcher S. Selective serotonin reuptake inhibitor discontinuation syndrome: proposed diagnostic criteria. *J Psychiatry Neurosci* 2000;25(3):255–261.
3. Boyer EW, Shannon M. The serotonin syndrome. *N Engl J Med* 2005;352:1112–1120.
4. Callaway CW, Clark RF. Hyperthermia in psychostimulant overdose. *Ann Emerg Med* 1994; 24(1):68–76.
5. Frascogna N. Physostigmine: Is there a role for this antidote in pediatric poisonings? *Curr Opin Pediatr* 2007;19:201–205.
6. Graudins A, Stearman A, Chan B. Treatment of the serotonin syndrome with cyproheptadine. *J Emerg Med* 1998;16(4):615–619.

7. Isbister GK, Bowe SJ, Dawson A, Whyte IM. Relative toxicity of selective serotonin reuptake inhibitors (SSRIs) in overdose. *J Toxicol Clin Toxicol* 2004;42(3):277–285.

8. Kelly CA, Dhaun N, Laing WJ, et al. Comparative toxicity of citalopram and the newer antidepressants after overdose. *J Toxicol Clin Toxicol* 2004;42(1):67–71.

9. Maramattom BV. Duloxetine-induced syndrome of inappropriate antidiuretic hormone secretion and seizures. *Neurology* 2006;66(5):773–774.

10. McKenzie MS, McFarland BH. Trends in antidepressant overdoses. *Pharmacoepidemiol Drug Saf* 2007;16:513–523.

11. Peano C, Leikin JB, Hanashiro PK. Seizures, ventricular tachycardia and rhabdomyolysis as a result of ingestion of venlafaxine and lamotrigine. *Ann Emerg Med* 1997;30:704–708.

12. Sternbach H. The serotonin syndrome. *Am J Psychiatry* 1991;148(6):705–713.

13. Taylor, MJ, Freemantle N, Geddes JR, et al. Early onset of selective serotonin reuptake inhibitor antidepressant action: systematic review and meta-analysis. *Arch Gen Psychiatry* 2006;63:1217–1223.

14. Whyte IM, Dawson AH, Buckley NA. Relative toxicity of venlafaxine and selective serotonin reuptake inhibitors in overdose compared to tricyclic antidepressants. *QJM* 2003;96:369–374.

Stimulants and Hallucinogens

Anticholinergic Agents

PRE-HOSPITAL CONSIDERATIONS

- Transport all pills and pill bottles in overdose for identification in the emergency department.

CLINICAL PRESENTATION

The patient presenting with anticholinergic syndrome (ACS) may exhibit peripheral or central manifestations or both (Table 49.1). Usually, peripheral stigmata of ACS predominate, with some central features. Mydriasis, tachycardia, dry skin and mucous membranes, fever, and altered mentation are common. These features provide the basis for the mnemonic "hot as a hare, mad as a hatter, red as a beet, dry as a bone." Although this mnemonic describes many of the features of the ACS, it ignores tachycardia, one of the most consistent and reliable clinical findings. However, in patients taking β-blockers or calcium channel blockers, infants, the elderly, and alcoholics with autonomic neuropathy, tachycardia may be absent. Hence, the absence of tachycardia does not rule out ACS. Central effects vary with lipid solubility, which affects the ability of an agent to penetrate the central nervous system (CNS), and have been described in patients who were found confused for a prolonged time after ingesting alcoholic beverages adulterated with scopolamine eye drops. Some medications such as benztropine can also cause relatively isolated CNS effects. Impaired perception of the environment may result in dangerous behavior. At the extremes of age, delirium may persist for several days (9).

Patients with severe ACS can present with seizures, hypotension, rhabdomyolysis, and respiratory or cardiac arrest (10). It is unclear whether these complications are direct anticholinergic effects, the end result of severe physiologic stimulation, or the result of other pharmacologic properties of the agents involved. Most patients have a self-limited course, with the extent and duration determined by the amount and nature of the agent. Finally, in patients who present to the hospital several hours following poisoning with an anticholinergic agent, the peripheral features of the toxidrome may be absent (5).

Although tricyclic antidepressants can cause ACS when taken in small overdoses (<10 mg/kg), large overdoses (>15 mg/kg) are dominated by hypotension, seizures, and cardiac-conduction delay resulting from nonanticholinergic effects.

TABLE 49.1	Anticholinergic Symptoms and Signs

Peripheral Muscarinic Effects	Central Nervous Effects
Tachycardia	Fever
Mydriasis	Delirium
Loss of accommodation	Seizures
Dry skin and mucous membranes	Coma
Constipation	Agitation
Flushed skin	Psychotic behavior
Decreased bowel motility	Extrapyramidal signs
Ileus	Respiratory depression
Urinary retention	Cardiovascular collapse

Toxicity resulting from H_1-receptor blockers can be divided into CNS, cardiovascular (CV), and anticholinergic effects. CNS depression (drowsiness, ataxia, coma) is common in adults following overdose of first-generation agents (7). In children, CNS excitation is more common as a result of their sensitivity to the anticholinergic effects. Tremors, confusion, hyperpyrexia, agitation, and seizures are often seen with significant overdose. Children and the elderly may develop anticholinergic toxicity or encephalopathy, following exposure to topical antihistamines, especially if used on broken skin.

The most common CV effect is sinus tachycardia, the result of cholinergic blockade. Conduction disturbances can occur with large overdoses. Diphenhydramine can cause QRS-interval prolongation and ventricular dysrhythmias (3). Astemizole overdose can cause QT prolongation, atrioventricular block, ventricular tachycardia, and ventricular fibrillation (6).

After large H_1-receptor blocker exposures, coma and seizures may occur within 30 minutes of ingestion and increase the patient's risk of death. In children <2 years old, seizures have occurred with doses as little as 150 mg diphenhydramine. Fatal doses in adults may range from 20 to 40 mg/kg; in children, as little as 500 mg may result in death.

Significant toxicity with isolated H_2-antagonist overdose is rare. Sinus bradycardia, atrioventricular block, and QT segment prolongation have been reported in patients on oral or parenteral cimetidine and ranitidine (4).

DIFFERENTIAL DIAGNOSIS

ACS should be considered in any patient who presents with altered mental status, fever, urinary retention, tachycardia, or seizures. Given the clinical features of the ACS, it may easily be misdiagnosed as a CNS infection, dehydration, psychiatric disorder, or sepsis. Intoxications with sympathetic stimulants, hallucinogens, and drug withdrawal should also be considered in the differential diagnosis.

The history and physical examination are crucial in this regard. The history should focus not only on prescribed medications but also on over-the-counter agents, plant or mushroom ingestions, anticholinergic eye drops (2), antihistamine-containing skin lotions, or circumstances in which illegitimate use of these agents may be a possibility. Often overlooked exposures include anticholinergic drops used to treat infantile colic and as mydriatics for funduscopic examination (2,7,8). ACS should be considered in patients with characteristic signs and symptoms such as delirium, hallucinations, tachycardia, mydriasis, dry skin, decreased bowel sounds, and a distended bladder, even without a supporting history. ACS can also present with isolated CNS symptoms.

Antihistamines are widely available as over-the-counter preparations, are often abused or used in suicide gestures, and should be considered in any patient presenting with ACS, CNS depression, psychosis, encephalopathy, and cardiac dysrhythmias and conduction disturbances. Other agents capable of producing similar toxicity include antidysrhythmics, cyclic antidepressants, neuroleptics, anticholinergic medications, and ingestions of plants such as jimsonweed, henbane, and deadly nightshade. Antihistamine poisoning must be differentiated from varicella encephalitis in children with altered mental status who have chickenpox and have been treated with topical or oral antihistamines. The effects of sympathomimetics can be confused with ACS, but patients typically have diaphoresis rather than dry skin. Patients with isolated CNS symptoms may be thought to be suffering from schizophrenia, heat illness, or the effects of illicit drug use.

ED EVALUATION

A detailed history and complete physical examination are essential in the evaluation of ACS or antihistamine poisoning. The physical examination should specifically search for the features of an ACS. Flushing of the skin may also be present as a result of excessive ingestion of anticholinergic agents, but this occurs infrequently. Cardiac monitoring and a 12-lead electrocardiogram (ECG) should be obtained, particularly in the presence of tachycardia. If seizures or altered mentation are present, a neurologic evaluation, including a cranial computed tomography scan and a lumbar puncture, is required, if it cannot be proven that these effects are secondary to anticholinergic poisoning. Administration of physostigmine may be able to obviate the need for the investigations mentioned previously (2). In patients with significant ACS or intentional overdoses, routine laboratory evaluation should include electrolytes, blood urea nitrogen, creatinine, glucose, and creatine kinase. Serum levels of acetaminophen and salicylate should be obtained to rule out coingestion of these agents, especially from over-the-counter products.

Toxicology screens are rarely helpful in defining the agents that may be implicated in producing ACS. Many of the medications and all of the plants that cause ACS are not detected by routine toxicology screens. Antihistamines are not detected by standard immunoassay tests for drugs of abuse. Antihistamines can be detected by thin-layer and gas chromatography, but these techniques are unavailable in most hospital laboratories. As a result, the diagnosis must be made predominantly by the history and physical examination.

ED MANAGEMENT

The mainstay of therapy for poisoning with anticholinergic agents is supportive care. Patients with ACS require a safe environment in which they cannot do themselves any harm. Comatose or hypoventilating patients should have appropriate airway intervention on arrival. Hypotension should be treated initially with intravenous crystalloid boluses. Hypotension refractory to fluids may necessitate the use of pressor agents such as norepinephrine. Agitation and seizures can commonly be controlled using parenteral benzodiazepines. Large doses may be required, resulting in impaired airway reflexes and necessitating endotracheal intubation.

Gastrointestinal decontamination with appropriate airway protection should be considered in patients presenting within 2 hours of ingestion. A single dose of oral activated charcoal is adequate in most instances. However, the benefit of activated charcoal in patients presenting with minimal or no signs of toxicity more than 2 hours following ingestion is questionable. Enhancing the elimination of antihistamines by extracorporeal methods or multiple-dose activated charcoal is ineffective in view of their large volumes of distribution and high protein binding.

The short-acting reversible acetylcholinesterase inhibitor physostigmine (1,2) rapidly reverses anticholinergic delirium and may prevent the need for escalating doses of benzodiazepines to control agitation. Physostigmine should never be used in patients with suspected acute cyclic antidepressant poisoning and ECG evidence of cardiac conduction delay (QRS prolongation or terminal r wave in lead AVr) because of the risk of precipitating sinus bradycardia, cardiac-conduction delays, and asystole. Other contraindications include bowel obstruction, significant cardiac or peripheral vascular disease, asthma, chronic obstructive pulmonary disease, and pre-existing urinary tract obstruction.

When using physostigmine, patients require continuous cardiac monitoring. An initial test dose, 0.5 mg, is followed by 1 to 2 mg in the next 2 to 3 minutes in an adult (0.02 mg/kg in a child to a maximum of 0.5 mg). A partial response may necessitate further 0.5 to 1.0 mg boluses. Clinical effects may last from 30 to 120 minutes, and dosing may be repeated as needed for recurrence of symptoms. In true anticholinergic poisoning, dramatic resolution of the syndrome is expected within minutes of physostigmine administration. The ideal response to physostigmine is complete or near-complete reversal of abnormal mental status, after which the patient can verbally confirm the history of poisoning with an anticholinergic agent and can deny symptoms consistent with alternative diagnoses (e.g., preceding fever, headache, and neck stiffness). A lack of a response should cause the diagnosis of ACS to be questioned. In the uncommon situation of excessive cholinergic effects following physostigmine administration, atropine can be used to reduce cholinergic signs (atropine dose in this case is half the dose of physostigmine that precipitated cholinergic effects).

When the diagnosis of ACS is questionable, agitation may be controlled with parenteral benzodiazepines. Neuroleptic agents such as phenothiazines or butyrophenones should be avoided because of their associated anticholinergic effects.

Wide-complex tachycardia associated with massive diphenhydramine overdose may respond to endotracheal intubation with hyperventilation and serum alkalinization with sodium-bicarbonate infusion given intravenously. Torsade de pointes associated with astemizole overdose may respond to intravenous magnesium sulfate and overdrive pacing. Class IA antidysrhythmics (e.g., procainamide) and class III agents (e.g., sotalol) should be avoided as they can promote dysrhythmias as a result of prolongation of cardiac muscle cell repolarization.

CRITICAL INTERVENTIONS

- Rapidly control agitation from ACS with intravenous physostigmine or intravenous benzodiazepines to prevent rhabdomyolysis, hyperthermia, and injury to the patient or staff.
- Obtain an ECG, and ensure that cardiac conduction delays are not present prior to the administration of physostigmine.
- Alkalinize the serum with intravenous sodium bicarbonate and hyperventilation in patients with evidence of sodium channel blockade-type cardiac conduction delays from first generation H1-receptor antagonist poisoning.

DISPOSITION

Patients with significant ACS should be observed until the clinical signs, including tachycardia, resolve, and the patient has a normal mental state examination. This observation often requires admission to a monitored bed. The duration of anticholinergic delirium may be from 12 hours to several days depending on the agent and dose ingested.

Patients with antihistamine poisoning who become or remain asymptomatic after a 4- to 6-hour observation period may be medically cleared. Patients with hallucinations, agitation, coma, seizures, or CV instability should be admitted to the intensive care unit. Patients with persistent but mildly depressed levels of consciousness and stable vital signs may be monitored in a telemetry unit. Patients with intentional overdoses should have a psychiatric evaluation.

COMMON PITFALLS

- Failure to consider the diagnosis of the ACS in patients with altered mental status (particularly agitated delirium), tachycardia, urinary retention, fever, or seizures
- Failure to appreciate that ACS may present with isolated central or peripheral manifestations
- Using physostigmine without adequate monitoring and resuscitation capability

- Using neuroleptics to treat ACS agitation and hallucinations
- *Giving a class IA, class IC (e.g., procainamide, flecainide), or class III (e.g., sotalol, amiodarone) antidysrhythmic agent to patients with ventricular tachydysrhythmias caused by antihistamines*

ICD9

971.1 Poisoning by parasympatholytics (anticholinergics and antimuscarinics) and spasmolytics

REFERENCES

1. Beaver KM, Gavin TJ. Treatment of acute anticholinergic poisoning with physostigmine. *Am J Emerg Med* 1998;16:505–507.
2. Burns MJ, Linden CH, Graudins A, et al. A comparison of physostigmine and benzodiazepines for the treatment of anticholinergic poisoning. *Ann Emerg Med* 2000;35:374–481.
3. Clark RF, Vance MV. Massive diphenhydramine poisoning resulting in a wide-complex tachycardia: successful treatment with sodium bicarbonate. *Ann Emerg Med* 1992;21:318–321.
4. Cohen ND, Modai A, Golik, et al. Cimetidine-related cardiac conduction disturbances and confusion. *J Clin Gastroenterol* 1989;11:68.
5. Feinberg M. The problems of anticholinergic adverse effects in older patients. *Drugs Aging* 1993; 3:335–348.
6. Heidemann SM, Sarnaik AP. Arrhythmias after astemizole overdose. *Pediatr Emerg Care* 1996; 12:102–104.
7. Koppel C, Ibe K, Tenczer J. Clinical symptomatology of diphenhydramine overdose: an evaluation of 136 cases in 1982 to 1985. *J Toxicol Clin Toxicol* 1987;25:53–70.
8. Myers JH, Moro-Sutherland D, Shook JE. Anticholinergic poisoning in colicky infants treated with hyoscyamine sulfate. *Am J Emerg Med* 1997;15:532–535.
9. Scott J, Pache D, Keane G, et al. Prolonged anticholinergic delirium following antihistamine overdose. *Australasian Psychiatry* 2007;15:242–244.
10. Winn RE, McDonnell KP. Fatality secondary to massive overdose of dimenhydrinate. *Ann Emerg Med* 1993;22:1481.

CHAPTER 50

Cocaine

PRE-HOSPITAL CONSIDERATIONS

- Establish intravenous access.
- Provide cardiac monitoring. Chest pain may be ischemic.
- Use benzodiazepine therapy to control agitation.
- When the drug is used as a "speedball" (combination of heroin and cocaine), administer naloxone in increments to reverse coma.

CLINICAL PRESENTATION

The most commonly seen manifestations of cocaine poisoning in the emergency department (ED) involve the cardiovascular (CV) and neurologic systems. Signs and symptoms of mild cocaine intoxication include normal or minimally increased blood pressure, pulse, respiratory rate, and temperature; agitation; anxiety; euphoria; headache; hyperreflexia; nausea; vomiting; mydriasis; pallor; diaphoresis; tremors; and twitching. Moderate intoxication may result in hypertension, tachycardia, dyspnea, tachypnea, hyperthermia, confusion, hallucinations, marked hyperactivity, increased muscle tone and deep tendon reflexes, abdominal cramps, formication, and generalized but brief tonic-clonic seizures. Severe intoxication results in hypotension, tachycardia (or preterminal bradycardia), ventricular dysrhythmias, Cheyne-Stokes respirations, apnea, cyanosis, severe hyperthermia, coma, flaccid paralysis, and status epilepticus.

Chest pain is a common chief complaint associated with cocaine use. Myocardial infarction (MI) as a result of cocaine is well established (4,5) and occurs in approximately 6% of patients presenting with this complaint. Cocaine causes coronary ischemia through coronary artery vasoconstriction, in situ thrombus formation, platelet activation, inhibition of endogenous fibrinolysis, and triggering an increase in the myocardial oxygen demand through generation of tachycardia and hypertension (4). Chronic users develop premature atherosclerosis and left ventricular hypertrophy, which can further exacerbate the oxygen supply-demand mismatch (4). Other less common but equally important CV complications of cocaine use include atrial and ventricular dysrhythmias, both systolic and diastolic congestive heart failure, coronary and aortic dissection, dilated cardiomyopathy, and ischemia in other vascular beds (e.g., intestinal, renal).

Euphoria, the impetus for the recreational use of cocaine, is typically short-lived and without serious sequelae. The stimulatory effects of cocaine can lead to seizures. Cocaine-induced seizures are typically single and generalized with rare status epilepticus (8). Focal neurologic events such as hemorrhagic cerebral infarction, and subarachnoid hemorrhage are uncommon. Severe, persistent lethargy with an altered mental status can occur after prolonged and intense cocaine usage and has been termed the *cocaine washout syndrome.* This diagnosis should be made only after exclusion of the aforementioned neurologic catastrophes (i.e., after a normal computed tomography (CT) of the head and lumbar puncture, if indicated). The syndrome is thought to follow such excessive cocaine usage that essential neurotransmitters are depleted and requires 12 to 24 hours to resolve.

Rhabdomyolysis is another common manifestation of cocaine toxicity. Cocaine's stimulatory effects lead to severe agitation and marked muscular agitation and rigidity. Ischemia of the skeletal muscle beds may also contribute. Profound elevations in creatinine kinase (CK) may be seen. Concurrent development of severe hyperthermia and acute renal failure can be life-threatening. Hyperthermia is most commonly a result of a combination of environmental exposure and heat production from excessive muscle activity. Renal failure is a result of muscle breakdown and renal tubular precipitation of the released muscle myoglobin.

Cocaine has a number of direct and indirect effects on the lungs. Many of these effects are a result of the inhalation rather than direct toxin effects. Asthma exacerbations are frequently reported with crack cocaine, most likely a result of particulate by-products of combustion. Further, crack usage is typically associated with deep Valsalva maneuvers to maximize drug delivery, which can cause pneumothorax, pneumomediastinum, and noncardiogenic pulmonary edema. Other less common effects on the lung include pulmonary infarction, bronchiolitis obliterans, pulmonary artery hypertrophy, and alveolar hemorrhage. Treatment of these conditions follows standard management protocols, whether they are related to cocaine or are not.

The intestinal vascular system is very sensitive to the effects of cocaine. Acute intestinal vascular infarction has been associated with all routes of administration. Although oral ingestion is not a common route of abuse, local intestinal and systemic effects can occur when containers of cocaine leak or rupture in body stuffers and packers. Body packers most often have been discovered by customs officers and present asymptomatically.

Habitual cocaine usage during pregnancy is associated with low birth weight, small head circumference, developmental problems, and a number of birth defects. Acute toxicity can also induce premature labor, eclampsia, and abruptio placentae. After delivery, neonates exposed to cocaine in utero are at risk for the development of neonatal withdrawal. This diagnosis of exclusion is manifested as irritability, jitteriness, and poor eye contact.

DIFFERENTIAL DIAGNOSIS

Cocaine toxicity is associated with sympathomimetic effects. These effects can also be seen with hypoglycemia, environmental and malignant hyperthermia, pheochromocytoma, manic psychiatric conditions, status epilepticus, and thyroid

TABLE 50.1	Differential Diagnosis of Cocaine-Associated Chest Pain

Aortic dissection	Pericarditis
Bacterial endocarditis	Pleurisy
Bronchospasm	Pneumonia
Esophageal illnesses	Pneumomediastinum
Gastrointestinal illnesses	Pneumothorax
Musculoskeletal injury	Pulmonary emboli
Myocardial infarction	Pulmonary infarction
Myocardial ischemia	
Myocarditis	

storm. Drugs with anticholinergic properties and other stimulants such as amphetamines can present with a similar picture. Patients with persistent altered mental status need to be evaluated for possible meningitis and central nervous system (CNS) lesions. Table 50.1 lists the differential diagnosis of chest pain related to cocaine use, which also includes reasons to be short of breath. New-onset seizures, epistaxis, hypertension, MI, intracranial hemorrhage, or psychiatric illness, especially in young patients, should suggest the possibility of cocaine use.

ED EVALUATION

The diagnostic evaluation of patients with cocaine toxicity relies on a history of cocaine use, recognition of signs and symptoms consistent with a sympathomimetic toxidrome, and evaluation of specific organ system complaints. The history should include the total amount and time of cocaine use in relation to symptom onset. Friends (or witnesses) of confused patients should be questioned about a history of seizures or syncope and antecedent activities. Many patients deny cocaine use unless approached with reassurance and compassion or confronted with a positive urine test.

The physical examination should include complete vital signs and a detailed examination of the cardiac, pulmonary, and neurologic systems. Patients should initially have continuous cardiac monitoring.

When the history is clear and symptoms are mild, laboratory evaluation is unnecessary. In contrast, if the history is absent or unreliable or the patient manifests moderate or severe toxicity, routine laboratory evaluation should include a complete blood count; determination of electrolyte, glucose, blood urea nitrogen, and creatinine levels; arterial blood gas analysis; urinalysis; and CK. Qualitative toxicologic screening of blood and urine can confirm the diagnosis and rule out other intoxicants, but toxicology testing is indicated only when confirmation of drug use would change management, counseling, or referral patterns.

A chest radiograph and electrocardiogram (ECG) should be obtained in patients with chest pain or moderate-to-severe toxicity. Those with prolonged, unexplained pain should have serial ECG and cardiac marker measurements to rule out MI. Many of the clinical parameters to assess ischemia or infarction are not as reliable as when they are used for patients with traditional coronary artery disease. The ECG is less sensitive and specific for identifying ischemia or infarction in this setting, the CK is often elevated as a result of associated rhabdomyolysis, and false elevations in the MB fraction can occur. Cardiac troponin I testing can help distinguish true-positive from false-positive CK-MB elevations (6). Observation for a 9- to 12-hour period can be used to evaluate patients with cocaine-associated chest pain. Patients without new ischemic changes on ECG, a normal troponin test, and no cardiovascular complications during this observation (dysrhythmias, acute myocardial infarction, or recurrent symptoms) can safely be sent home with follow-up and a planned outpatient workup (7).

Persistent headache despite normalization of blood pressure is an indication for evaluation by CT scan and lumbar puncture to rule out intracranial hemorrhage. Patients with severe abdominal or back pain should be evaluated for intestinal or renal infarction. The urine should be inspected and the serum CK level determined, to detect myoglobinuric renal failure.

Occult infections should be excluded in patients with fever, even though fever can be due solely to cocaine toxicity. A brief seizure clearly related temporally to cocaine use in an otherwise healthy person should be evaluated with CT to exclude serious underlying pathology, but it does not require further workup, provided the patient is alert and coherent, has no headache, and has a normal neurologic examination. Patients suspected of body packing or stuffing should be evaluated by abdominal radiographs (including contrast imaging) and cavity searches (digital or visual examination of the rectum or vagina). Toxicity lasting for more than 4 hours suggests continued drug absorption and should prompt a similar workup.

The route of administration may influence the patient's chief complaint or which organ system is affected. Intravenous users may present with fever and malaise secondary to infectious complications such as cellulitis, endocarditis, hepatitis, pneumonia, and the acquired immunodeficiency syndrome. Chronic nasal use may lead to rhinitis, septal perforation, and epistaxis. Inhalational use may produce dyspnea, cough, or hemoptysis from reactive airway disease, "crack lung" pneumonitis, or pulmonary edema or may result in pulmonary barotrauma (e.g., pneumothorax, pneumomediastinum, pneumopericardium) from a Valsalva maneuver or from blowing smoke into the mouth of a partner. Patients with barotrauma may also complain of neck and chest pain with tachypnea, subcutaneous emphysema, or Hamman's sign.

Behavioral disorders (e.g., agitation, combative behavior), headache, back pain (renal infarction or aortic dissection), abdominal pain (mesenteric ischemia), altered level of consciousness, or cardiopulmonary arrest are other common presentations that may follow the use of cocaine by any route. Patients with excited delirium with severe agitation, an elevated temperature, and metabolic acidosis deserve immediate attention. Patients may present as victims of trauma because of the violent, irrational, and risk-taking behavior associated with drug use. Delayed

CV complications can sometimes occur. MI has been reported in the first few days after cocaine use but has also been reported 1 to 2 weeks after last use.

Manifestations of chronic cocaine abuse include anorexia, insomnia, formication, depression, impotence, weight loss, paranoia, and psychosis. Halo vision (lights around objects) and "snow lights" (flashes in the peripheral fields) have also been described.

ED MANAGEMENT

Management depends on the specific complaint and presentation. Patients presenting with a sympathomimetic toxidrome are at risk for hyperthermia and rhabdomyolysis. After initial attention to the airway and CV status, management should focus on lowering core body temperature, halting further muscle agitation and heat production, and giving IV fluids to ensure a good urinary output. The agents of choice for muscle relaxation in this setting are benzodiazepines. Supranormal cumulative doses may be necessary in severely agitated individuals.

Patients with severe hypertension or tachycardia necessitating pharmacologic measures can usually be safely treated with benzodiazepines. When large doses of benzodiazepines are not effective, intravenous nitroprusside or phentolamine should be considered (3). B antagonists or compounds with partial β-blocking effects are contraindicated as the use of β antagonists in the setting of cocaine intoxication can lead to unopposed α stimulation, with resultant marked increases in hypertension and worsening coronary vasoconstriction (2,4).

Patients with suspected cocaine-induced ischemia or MI should be treated similarly to those with traditional acute coronary syndromes (ACS), with some notable exceptions (4). Aspirin, nitroglycerin, and heparin remain important initial therapies. Intravenous benzodiazepines should be provided as early management (1). They will decrease the central stimulatory effects of cocaine, thereby indirectly reducing the CV toxicity of cocaine (4). B antagonists are contraindicated, as they exacerbate cocaine-induced coronary artery vasoconstriction (2). Percutaneous interventions (angioplasty) are preferred over fibrinolysis, which has no proven efficacy in the setting of cocaine-associated MI and a possible reduced safety profile. There is an increased likelihood of interventions being performed in patients who are not sustaining an acute infarction because young patients have a high prevalence of early repolarization and "false-positive" ST-segment elevations on the ECG. Such therapy should, therefore, be used with caution. Finally, there are anecdotal reports of the safety and efficacy of phentolamine, an α antagonist, for treatment of cocaine-associated ACS (4,5). Verapamil reverses cocaine-induced vasoconstriction, but several animal experiments suggest that it exacerbates CNS toxicity. Thus, it may have a role in patients with continued ischemia who do not have signs of central stimulation from cocaine.

Supraventricular dysrhythmias due to cocaine toxicity may be difficult to treat. Adenosine can be administered, but its effects may be temporary. Use of calcium channel blockers in association with benzodiazepines appear to be most beneficial. Beta-blockers should be avoided (4).

Ventricular dysrhythmias may be a result of excess adrenergic tone or cocaine's sodium channel blocking effects. Management with benzodiazepines, lidocaine, and/or sodium bicarbonate appears to be most useful (7,8). Bicarbonate is preferred when patients have dysrhythmias directly after the use of cocaine. In this setting, the dysrhythmias are presumably related to the type I antidysrhythmic effects of cocaine. Bicarbonate reverses cocaine-associated QRS widening. Lidocaine can be used when dysrhythmias appear to be related to cocaine-induced ischemia. ECG evidence for the type I antidysrhythmic effects of cocaine has often disappeared by the time symptomatic ischemia develops.

Cocaine-induced seizures are typically brief and self-limited. For refractory cases, benzodiazepines and phenobarbital are the first- and second-line agents, respectively. Phenytoin is not recommended.

Patients with suspected cerebrovascular infarctions and hemorrhage should be treated the same as other patients with these conditions. Intracranial and systemic hypertension necessitating treatment is accomplished using standard therapies, except that β blockers should not be utilized.

The main concern in asymptomatic body packers is to eliminate the packages out of the gastrointestinal system. Whole-bowel irrigation with subsequent radiologic verification of passage of all drug-filled containers may be warranted.

Body stuffers who manifest clinical signs of toxicity should be treated similarly to other cocaine-exposed individuals. Additionally, activated charcoal should be administered liberally.

Symptomatic body packers should be treated more aggressively, because rapid deterioration and severe toxicity can result from their potentially massive exposures. Immediate surgical removal of the ruptured package(s) may be lifesaving. Aggressive supportive care with activated charcoal and benzodiazepines is warranted as preparations are made for surgery.

CRITICAL INTERVENTIONS

- Assess patients with cocaine toxicity for myocardial ischemia/MI, dysrhythmias, hyperthermia, and rhabdomyolysis.
- Administer intravenous benzodiazepines for CNS and cardiovascular toxicity.

DISPOSITION

Patients with severe agitation, hyperthermia, and possible rhabdomyolysis need to be admitted. Patients with cocaine-associated chest pain need to be assessed for risk of CV events. Criteria for patients with a low risk of CV events that are safe for ED discharge after a brief observation period include lack of ischemic changes on ECG; normal serial cardiac troponin I values; no dysrhythmias, or recurrent symptoms during a 9- to 12-hour observation period (9). Most patients with ED cocaine-associated chest pain (~70%) will meet these criteria (9).

The disposition of patients with neurologic complications is the same as for other patients with these conditions. The likelihood of compliance with outpatient follow-up should be considered when contemplating the discharge of patients who may need further evaluation. If definitive care cannot be provided at the site of presentation, transfer may be necessary. Personnel with advanced life-support training should accompany patients requiring transfer. All patients should be referred for substance abuse counseling and treatment.

Body stuffers who remain asymptomatic for 4 to 6 hours may be discharged after treatment with activated charcoal. Body packers need to be admitted until packets have been removed.

COMMON PITFALLS

- Failure to consider cocaine toxicity in the differential diagnosis of patients with chest pain, seizures, agitation, altered mental status, and dysrhythmias
- Failure to recognize the limitations of the ECG in the evaluation of cocaine-related chest pain
- Failure to appreciate the differences between the management of cocaine-related chest pain and traditional therapy for ACS
- Failure to recognize the dangers of using β-adrenergic antagonists to treat cocaine toxicity
- Failure to ensure the rectal passage of cocaine-filled packages in body stuffers and body packers prior to discharge

ICD9

970.8 Poisoning by other specified central nervous system stimulants

REFERENCES

1. Baumann DM, Perrone J, Hornig SF, et al. Randomized, double-blind, placebo-controlled trial of diazepam, nitroglycerin, or both for treatment of patients with potential cocaine-associated acute coronary syndromes. *Acad Emerg Med* 2000;7:878.
2. Hoffman RS: Cocaine and β-blockers: should the controversy continue? *Ann Emerg Med* 2008;51:127.
3. Hollander JE, Carter WC, Hoffman RS. Use of phentolamine for cocaine-induced myocardial ischemia. *N Engl J Med* 1992;327:361.
4. Hollander JE. Management of cocaine-associated myocardial ischemia. *N Engl J Med* 1995;333:1267.
5. Hollander JE, Hoffman RS, Burstein J, et al, and the Cocaine Associated Myocardial Infarction Study Group. Cocaine associated myocardial infarction. Mortality and complications. *Arch Intern Med* 1995;155:1081.
6. Hollander JE, Levitt MA, Young GP, et al. The effect of cocaine on the specificity of cardiac markers. *Am Heart J* 1998;135:245.
7. Shih RD, Hollander JE, Hoffman RS, et al, and the Cocaine Associated Myocardial Infarction Study Group. Clinical safety of lidocaine in cocaine associated myocardial infarction. *Ann Emerg Med* 1995;26:702.
8. Shih RD, Majlesi N, Hung O, et al. Cocaine-associated seizures and incidence of status epilepticus. *Ann Emerg Med* 2007;50:S27.
9. Weber JE, Shofer FS, Larkin GL, et al. Validation of a brief observation period for patients with cocaine-associated chest pain. *N Eng J Med.* 2003;348:510.

CHAPTER 51

Hallucinogens

PRE-HOSPITAL CONSIDERATIONS
- Consider sedation with benzodiazepines versus haloperidol versus physical restraints.
  - Benzodiazepines are greatly preferred.
  - Sedation masks symptoms and may limit history taking.
- Sedate or restrain the patient to ensure safe transport.
- For the hyperthermic patient:
  - Use sedation rather than physical restraint.
  - Begin cooling measures.

CLINICAL PRESENTATION

Unlike other drugs of abuse, most users of hallucinogens rarely present acutely to the healthcare provider (2,6). Hallucinogens in general have few significant adverse side effects, and patients generally present to the emergency department for secondary reasons (e.g., trauma) or for "bad trips." The unique nature of hallucinogens defines their clinical presentation. Unless combined with other drugs, patients should be alert and fully oriented and able to give a history of use. A clear sensorium is a key historical and examination point, suggesting the use of lysergic acid diethylamide (LSD). This finding contrasts with drug-induced delirium, such as that associated with phencyclidine (PCP), in which, by definition, the patient's orientation is altered.

Hallucinations or illusions are alterations in the perception of time and body image and changes in the interpretation of sensory information. Hallucinogenic experiences are commonly referred to as a "trip," and the experience tends to be an extremely personal one. The perceptual changes that users perceive can affect any of the senses: hearing, taste, smell, touch, or sight. The person can experience exaggeration, diminution, or mixing (synesthesias) of their sensory perception. The users' sense of time may be altered, generally slowed, as may their sense of space. Body dysmorphisms are common, in which personal physical features take on abnormal proportions. Events can be perceived as hyperreligious or evil (1,9). Additional clues to the diagnosis include the sympathomimetic effects of some of the compounds involved, although these effects may be mild. Common physical signs and symptoms of acute intoxication include mydriasis, diaphoresis, piloerection, tremors, and mildly elevated blood pressure, pulse, respiratory rate, and temperature. These findings may be masked by the coingestion of ethanol or other sedative-hypnotic agents.

Injury is the predominant adverse event related to hallucinogen use and generally results from the acute behavioral effect of the drug. There are few, if any, dangerous physiologic effects of the drugs themselves. The psychological effects can be overwhelming, and occasionally the hallucinations can be perceived as frightening or threatening ("bad trips"). These experiences can include or engender paranoia, acute psychosis, panic, and significant depression. Suicide and unintentional death have been reported (6,7,9). There is no reported withdrawal syndrome from hallucinogens, although tolerance and cross tolerance between compounds can occur.

Mescaline use is associated with significant, unpleasant side effects. Initial signs and symptoms include nausea, vomiting, abdominal pain, diaphoresis, nystagmus, and ataxia. These symptoms typically resolve within 1 to 2 hours of ingestion and precede the onset of the hallucinations, which begin within 4 to 6 hours. The effects typically last for 6 to 12 hours (6).

Hallucinogenic doses of nutmeg cause severe side effects, such as dizziness, flushing, tachycardia, nausea, vomiting, constipation, and panic. Because of the relative severity of the side effects, it is not a popular means of producing hallucinations. When ingested, the hallucinations begin within 1 to 4 hours and last 12 to 24 hours. Many users report an extended period of sleep after use (upward of 16 hours).

Ingestion of *Psilocybe* mushrooms is typically associated with nausea and sometimes vomiting. Onset of effect is approximately 30 minutes, and the duration is typically 4 to 6 hours. The effects are typically described as being "less intense" and more illusionary than those produced by LSD (1,3,5,7,8). α-Methyltryptamine (AMT) has a longer duration of effect (approximately 12–24 hours) than that of Foxy (between 3 and 6 hours). Toad licking has resulted in digoxin-like bradycardia and significant adverse effects from other components of toad secretions (3).

The hallucinogen persisting-perception disorder (HPPD), commonly known as "flashbacks," associated with the use of LSD should not be confused with prolonged sensory perception (afterimages), also known as palinopsia. Patients with HPPD characteristically experience, in the absence of the drug, recurrent perceptual disturbances similar to those encountered during acute intoxication. HPPD is often triggered by stress, illness, or other challenges. HPPD can occur after a single use of the drug and may last for a prolonged period (up to years) (3,4). HPPD is associated with the use of phenothiazine antipsychotics to control the acute behavioral symptoms of acute intoxication, suggesting that sedatives such as benzodiazepines, rather than antipsychotics, should be used for this purpose. Proposed therapies for HPPD include clonazepam, carbidopa, and psychotherapy (4). Another rare reported adverse effect of LSD is permanent psychosis (4,9).

The time of onset and duration of effect can help determine the identity of the hallucinogen (Table 51.1). Long-acting agents include LSD, mescaline, and nutmeg. Medium-acting agents include psilocybin, psilocin, Foxy, AMT, and

TABLE 51.1	Common Hallucinogenic Compounds		
Common Name	**Name**	**Onset (h)**	**Duration (h)**
DMT	*N, N*-dimethyl-tryptamine	Rapid	0.5 to 1
Salvia divinorum	Salvinorin A	Rapid	1 to 2
Foxy	5-methoxy-*N, N*-diisopropyltryptamine	Rapid	3 to 6
Psilocybin	4-phosphoryloxy-*N, N*-dimethyltryptamine	0.5	4 to 6
LSD	Lysergic acid diethylamide	Few	4 to 12
Mescaline	3,4,5-trimethoxyphenylethylamine	4 to 6	6 to 12
Nutmeg	5-allyl-1,2,3-trimethoxybenzene	1 to 4	12 to 24
AMT	α-Methyltryptamine	Rapid	12 to 24
Ibogaine	Ibogaine	4 to 8; 10 to 20	12 to 24

Bufo sp–toad toxins. Short-acting hallucinogens include DMT, ibogaine, and salvinorin A.

Smoking DMT leads to effects that typically begin within minutes and last between 30 and 60 minutes. Rapid onset and short duration of action has earned DMT the moniker "the businessman's lunch," because the user can experience a "trip" in the time allotted for a meal (2,3,6). Following the ingestion of ayahuasca, DMT also has a rapid onset of action and short duration of effect (3,5,7,8).

The ingestion of *Salvia divinorum* produces effects that begin in 5 to 10 minutes and last approximately 1 to 2 hours. When the vapor is inhaled or the plant is smoked, effects begin in seconds and last about 30 minutes (2,10). Ibogaine ingestion can cause both early (4–8 hours after ingestion) and late (10–20 hours after ingestion) hallucinations (2,5–8).

DIFFERENTIAL DIAGNOSIS

Other abused agents that can cause hallucinations include sympathomimetics, anticholinergics, and dissociative anesthetic agents and related compounds. Cocaine and amphetamines are associated with psychosis at high doses or following binges. Patients characteristically develop a delusional state that does not always involve clear hallucinations. Symptoms may last for several days but typically respond to antipsychotic medications. Anticholinergic agents (e.g., scopolamine and atropine) may produce dramatic epidemic hallucinations when teenagers discover Jimsonweed (*Datura stramonium*) and ingest the seeds. Patients generally have other manifestations of the anticholinergic syndrome and are always delirious. Dissociative anesthetic agents, such as PCP, ketamine, and the related compound dextromethorphan, produce hallucinations that are generally described as dysphoric. Clinical features include delirium and prominent nystagmus. Autonomic manifestations are usually more prominent than hallucinations in each of these conditions. In contrast, in traditional hallucinogens such as LSD, hallucinations are prominent, and autonomic effects are usually mild.

Hallucinations have been reported as idiosyncratic reactions to almost all medications. Street-drug adulterants (e.g., cyanide, local anesthetics, quinine, quinidine, caffeine, theophylline, and strychnine) should be considered in the differential of hallucinosis. Because central nervous system structural, infectious, and psychiatric conditions can cause hallucinations, exposure to a hallucinogenic agent should be a diagnosis of exclusion. With or without the history of hallucinogen exposure, these conditions should always be considered in the differential diagnosis.

ED EVALUATION

The history should include the name or description of the hallucinogen, the time of ingestion, amount(s) taken, the route of exposure, and the nature and time of onset of hallucinations and other symptoms. Slang names may provide a presumptive identity, if the chemical name is not known. A history of previous drug use, psychiatric problems, and medical conditions, particularly cardiovascular disease, should be documented. The clinician should specifically explore the possibility of concomitant traumatic injuries.

The physical examination should focus on the mental status, neurologic evaluation, and cardiovascular system. A full set of vital signs is documented and repeated frequently. The patient should be examined carefully for evidence of trauma, underlying disease, and heat-related illness.

Ancillary testing is neither necessary nor useful in patients with mild hallucinogen intoxication, except to rule out other diagnoses. Patients with moderate or severe symptoms (e.g., excessive agitation and significantly abnormal vital signs) should have a chest radiograph; cardiac monitoring and a 12-lead electrocardiogram; complete blood count; determination of electrolyte, glucose, blood urea nitrogen, creatinine, and creatine-kinase levels; and urinalysis performed to exclude other conditions or exposures. Significant psychomotor agitation can occur with a variety of perceived stimuli, and rhabdomyolysis should be considered. Routine toxicology screens are rarely sensitive or specific enough to provide confirmation or exclusion of another agent as the causative etiology of a specific clinical presentation. Quantitative blood (or urine) hallucinogen levels are not clinically useful or routinely available.

ED MANAGEMENT

Management is supportive. Standard life support measures should be instituted as needed. The focus of care should then be to provide a calm, quiet environment for the patient. Providers should attempt to reduce the patient's anxiety, help to provide a foundation for reality testing, and provide continued, empathetic reassurance. In cases in which the experience is causing the patient significant agitation or distress, pharmacologic sedation with a benzodiazepine should be provided. Phenothiazines should be avoided because they have been implicated in HPPD (4,9).

Although activated charcoal can bind most, if not all, of these compounds, the efficacy of this intervention is undefined. Because consequential morbidity is exceedingly rare and because GI decontamination may be particularly unpleasant for a patient who is hallucinating, its use should be limited to patients with significant coingestions.

CRITICAL INTERVENTIONS

- Provide a calm, quiet environment with continuous observation and repeated reassurance.
- Administer benzodiazepines for persistent or severe agitation or psychological distress.

DISPOSITION

For the majority of patients presenting after use of a hallucinogen, their disposition will be discharge. In the absence of any adverse sequelae (e.g., trauma, rhabdomyolysis, electrolyte abnormality, etc.), the patient should be watched until reality testing is assured, and appropriate referral to a psychiatrist or substance abuse program can be provided. Admission is warranted only for persistence of psychosis or if the patient has a concomitant medical or surgical issue that makes this necessary.

COMMON PITFALLS

- Failure to obtain a complete set of vital signs, especially an accurate core temperature
- Failure to differentiate between hallucinations and delirium; patients with drug-induced hallucinations have clear orientation with altered content
- Failure to make safety of the patient and staff a priority
- Failure to consider metabolic, structural, infectious, traumatic, and psychiatric etiologies of the hallucinatory state
- Failure to screen for occult conditions caused by the behavioral abnormalities of these compounds, such as rhabdomyolysis
- Failure to consider coingestants or nonclassical hallucinogen-producing compounds (i.e., anticholinergic agents) and their specific toxicities

ICD9

969.6 Poisoning by psychodysleptics (hallucinogens)

REFERENCES

1. De Rios MD, Grob CS, Baker JR. Hallucinogens and redemption. *J Psychoactive Drugs* 2002; 34(3):239–248.
2. Drug Enforcement Agency. DEA Web site. http://www.dea.gov/Accessed on November 30, 2007.

3. Goldrank LR, Flomenbaum NE, Lewin NA, et al., eds. *Goldfrank's Toxicologic Emergencies,* 8th ed. New York: McGraw Hill, 2006:1202–1211.

4. Halpern JH, Pope HG Jr. Hallucinogen persisting perception disorder: what do we know after 50 years? *Drug Alcohol Depend* 2003;69(2):109–119.

5. Halpern JH, Sewell RA. Hallucinogenic botanicals of America: a growing need for focused drug education and research. *Life Sciences* 2005;78:519–526.

6. National Institute on Drug Abuse. NIDA Web site. http://www.drugabuse.gov/drugpages/Accessed on November 30, 2007.

7. Richardson WH, Slone CM, Michels JE. Herbal drugs of abuse: an emerging problem. *Emerg Med Clin N Am* 2007;25:435–457.

8. Schultes RE. The plant kingdom and hallucinogens (part 1 & II). *Bull Narc* 1969;21(3,4):3–16, 15–27.

9. Taylor RL, Maurer JI, Tinklenberg JR. Management of "bad trips" in an evolving drug scene. *JAMA* 1970;213(3):422–425.

10. Vortherms TA, Roth BL. Salvinorin A: from natural product to human therapeutics. *Mol Interv* 2006;6(5):257–265.

CHAPTER 52

Methylxanthines

PRE-HOSPITAL CONSIDERATIONS
- Bring pills and pill bottles in cases of suspected overdose.

CLINICAL PRESENTATION

Initial symptoms of methylxanthine poisoning include nausea, vomiting, and abdominal pain. Diarrhea and gastrointestinal (GI) bleeding may develop later. Spontaneous vomiting may limit drug absorption, especially with caffeine ingestions, but serum drug levels may continue to rise despite vomiting, particularly when sustained-release preparations have been ingested. Additional signs and symptoms include headache, insomnia, agitation, delirium, tinnitus, tremors, motor hyperactivity and hypertonicity, jitteriness, hyperventilation, polyuria, seizures, coma, GI bleeding, hyperthermia, and ventricular and supraventricular tachydysrhythmias (2,7,9). At low doses, theophylline induces a mild and transitory hypertension. At high doses, the direct effect of theophylline on the β_2-adrenoreceptors reduces the total peripheral resistance, inducing hypotension. This effect may explain why hypotension is seen with acute but not chronic overdose. Laboratory abnormalities include leukocytosis, hyperglycemia, hypokalemia, hypophosphatemia, ketosis, metabolic acidosis, and respiratory alkalosis (2,7). Decreased serum calcium and magnesium levels, elevated serum amylase and uric acid levels, and evidence of dehydration (elevated blood urea nitrogen and creatinine levels) or rhabdomyolysis (elevated creatine phosphokinase level and myoglobinuria) may be noted.

The risk of tachydysrhythmias depends on the duration of exposure, drug concentration, and age. After an acute overdose (single ingestion), patients may develop life-threatening dysrhythmias or seizures when serum concentrations exceed 80 μg/mL (2). These same effects can occur with lower serum concentrations (>60 μg/mL) in chronic intoxication. Patients younger than 6 months of age or older than 60 years may experience serious toxicity with serum concentrations >30 μg/mL, in both acute and chronic overdose. Similarly, patients older than 40 years are at greater risk of serious cardiac dysrhythmias at lower serum concentrations than are healthy younger patients (3).

Seizures are usually generalized but can be focal. The risk of seizure seems to be greater in patients with a history of neurologic problems (e.g., seizures, cerebrovascular insufficiency) (7). Permanent neurologic damage after coma or intractable seizures appears to correlate with the duration of these toxic manifestations.

DIFFERENTIAL DIAGNOSIS

Because the clinical effects of methylxanthine poisoning can be characterized as a "β-adrenergic storm," poisoning by direct-acting β-agonists (e.g., albuterol, terbutaline, and related bronchodilators) can cause a similar clinical picture. Poisoning by amphetamines, sympathomimetics, anticholinergics, hallucinogens, monoamine oxidase inhibitors, and epinephrine should also be considered in the differential diagnosis. Agitated psychiatric states, drug withdrawal, and medical conditions such as central nervous system infection, electrolyte disturbance, hypoglycemia, hypocalcemia, pheochromocytoma, and thyroid storm may cause similar signs and symptoms.

ED EVALUATION

The history should include the time, amount, and formulation of theophylline or caffeine ingested; past or recent therapeutic use of these agents; and routine medical history. Symptoms before arrival should be noted. The maximum possible serum drug level (in micrograms per milliliter) can be estimated by doubling the acutely ingested dose (in milligrams per kilogram).

The physical examination should focus on vital signs, mental status and neurologic evaluation, cardiorespiratory status, and GI function. Vomitus and stool should be checked for overt or occult blood. Laboratory evaluation for symptomatic patients should include a quantitative theophylline or caffeine level; complete blood count; determination of electrolyte, glucose, blood urea nitrogen, and creatinine levels; and urinalysis. Drug levels should be repeated every 2 to 4 hours following acute ingestions, until the level is no longer rising. Patients with elevated theophylline levels and moderate or severe clinical toxicity should also have measurements of serum amylase; creatine phosphokinase and urine myoglobin; calcium, magnesium, and phosphorus levels; and arterial blood gas analysis, as appropriate.

Cardiac monitoring and an electrocardiogram (ECG) should be obtained on all patients. Patients with respiratory symptoms or an abnormal pulmonary examination or ECG should have a chest radiograph.

ED MANAGEMENT

Advanced life-support measures are instituted, as necessary. Activated charcoal (AC) significantly reduces the absorption of theophylline, and repeated administration enhances the total body clearance of theophylline (1). Because serum concentrations may not peak for many hours after ingestion (up to 24 hours with slow-release preparations), every patient with an oral theophylline overdose should receive AC, regardless of the time of ingestion. A dose of 0.5 to 1.0 g/kg of body weight should be given every 2 to 4 hours until drug levels are in the therapeutic range. If the patient cannot tolerate charcoal because of persistent vomiting, one should try to administer smaller but more frequent doses (continuous infusion by nasogastric tube, if necessary) and give an antiemetic such as metoclopramide, droperidol, or ondansetron (5).

Gastric drug bezoar formation has been reported after sustained-release theophylline overdose. Endoscopic evaluation and drug-mass removal should be considered in patients with rising drug levels and severe poisoning. Whole-bowel irrigation did not add to the benefit of multiple-dose AC in an experimental sustained-release theophylline overdose.

Seizures should be treated aggressively with diazepam or lorazepam. If seizures do not stop rapidly or if they recur, phenobarbital (15–20 mg/kg) should be administered intravenously. If this treatment is unsuccessful within 20 to 30 minutes, thiopental, in a loading dose of 3 to 5 mg/kg followed by an infusion of 2 to 4 mg/kg/h, is usually efficacious, but these doses can be increased, if necessary. Phenytoin or fosphenytoin are ineffective in controlling methylxanthine-induced seizures. Neuromuscular paralysis may be necessary to stop muscle contractions, facilitate ventilation, and prevent hyperthermia and rhabdomyolysis. Electroencephalographic monitoring and continued treatment of seizures are necessary during paralysis. Correction of accompanying acidemia may avoid dysrhythmias.

A β-adrenergic antagonist (e.g., esmolol, propranolol) is the drug of choice to treat supraventricular and ventricular dysrhythmias after acute overdose. Intravenous (IV) doses of propranolol (1 mg in adults or 0.02 mg/kg in children) should be given slowly and repeated every 5 to 10 minutes until dysrhythmias stop or to a maximal dose of 0.1 mg/kg. Although propranolol is normally contraindicated in patients with asthma or chronic obstructive pulmonary disease, it has been used without adverse effects in asymptomatic asthmatics with acute theophylline poisoning. In such patients, the short-acting β-antagonist esmolol (500 μg/kg IV in 1 min followed by an infusion of 50 μg/kg/min) may be preferable to propranolol (6). However, because esmolol is selective for β_1-receptors, it could theoretically worsen hypotension resulting from β_2 stimulation. Active bronchospasm is a contraindication to the use of β-blockers. Lidocaine (1–1.5 mg/kg IV in 2–3 min followed by an infusion of 1–4 mg/min [children: 0.02–0.05 mg/kg/min]) may be used for ventricular dysrhythmias. Verapamil has been effective in patients with atrial tachydysrhythmias associated with theophylline intoxication. Correction of hypoxemia, acidemia, hypokalemia, and other metabolic abnormalities is also important. Because hypokalemia is a result of an intracellular shift of potassium rather than a total-body deficit, overly aggressive therapy for this condition may result in hyperkalemia as toxicity resolves and should be avoided. Hyperglycemia is transient and well tolerated and usually does not necessitate insulin therapy.

Hypotension should be treated with IV fluid, followed with pressors as needed—e.g., phenylephrine (IV infusion at 100–180 μg/min [in children

0.1–0.5 μg/kg/min] and titrated to desired response) or norepinephrine (IV infusion at 4 μg/min [in children 0.05–0.1 μg/kg/min] and titrated to desired response). Hyperthermia and rhabdomyolysis should be treated with standard measures.

Hemodialysis should be considered for persistently unstable hemodynamic parameters; for seizures; and for theophylline serum concentrations >80 μg/mL after an acute ingestion, >60 μg/mL after chronic ingestion, and >40 μg/mL after an acute or chronic intoxication, if age is <6 months or >60 years or there is severe underlying cardiovascular disease (2,3,8). Similar parameters should be used in patients with caffeine poisoning. A tandem setup of in-line hemodialysis and hemoperfusion can be used for patients with severe metabolic abnormalities and high drug levels. Exchange transfusion has also been used in neonates with caffeine or theophylline intoxication when hemodialysis is technically difficult (4).

CRITICAL INTERVENTIONS

- Obtain quantitative drug levels every 2 to 4 hours following acute overdose, until the level is no longer rising.
- Administer AC to enhance drug clearance; give antiemetics if necessary.
- Administer benzodiazepines and barbiturates intravenously for seizures.
- Administer β-adrenergic antagonists (e.g., esmolol, propranolol) for supraventricular and ventricular tachydysrhythmias, unless bronchospasm is present.
- Arrange for hemodialysis and/or charcoal hemoperfusion for patients with seizures, hypotension, tachydysrhythmias, progressive clinical toxicity, or high theophylline serum levels.

DISPOSITION

Patients with a serum theophylline level <35 μg/mL and mild symptoms can usually be treated in the emergency department and discharged when they become asymptomatic. Patients with levels >35 μg/mL should be admitted to a monitored bed. Those patients with severe neurologic or cardiotoxic manifestations or serum concentrations >50 μg/mL should be admitted to an intensive care unit (ICU). A nephrologist should be consulted for patients who meet or are approaching criteria for extracorporeal elimination therapy. If ICU and extracorporeal treatment are not available, the patient should be transferred to a facility with these capabilities.

COMMON PITFALLS

- Failure to appreciate that patients with chronic exposures develop toxicity at lower drug levels than with acute overdose
- Failure to consider the patient's age, the type of intoxication (acute vs. chronic), and underlying diseases (previous neurologic or cardiac problems) when interpreting theophylline serum concentrations

- Failure to appreciate that hypotension (not hypertension) is characteristic of severe acute (but not chronic) caffeine or theophylline poisoning
- Failure to appreciate that seizures can result in acidemia, hyperthermia, rhabdomyolysis, and permanent neurologic damage
- When prescribing theophylline, failure to consider the effects of age, underlying disease, and potential drug interactions on drug kinetics and dosing

ICD9

974.1 Poisoning by purine derivative diuretics

REFERENCES

1. Berlinger WG, Spector R, Goldberg MJ, et al. Enhancement of theophylline clearance by oral activated charcoal. *Clin Pharmacol Ther* 1983;33:351–354.
2. Gaudreault P, Guay J. Theophylline poisoning: pharmacological considerations and clinical management. *Med Toxicol* 1986;1:169–191.
3. Olson KR, Benowitz NL, Woo OF, et al. Theophylline overdose: acute single ingestion versus chronic repeated overmedication. *Am J Emerg Med* 1985;3:386–394.
4. Osborn HH, Henry G, Wax P, et al. Theophylline toxicity in a premature neonate-elimination kinetics of exchange transfusion. *Clin Toxicol* 1993;31:639–644.
5. Sage TA, Jones WN, Clark RF. Ondansetron in the treatment of intractable nausea associated with theophylline toxicity. *Ann Pharmacother* 1993;27:584–585.
6. Seneff M, Scott J, Friedman B, et al. Acute theophylline toxicity and the use of esmolol to reverse cardiovascular instability. *Ann Emerg Med* 1990;19:671–673.
7. Sessler CN. Theophylline toxicity: clinical features of 116 consecutive cases. *Am J Med* 1990;88:567–576.
8. Shannon MW. Comparative efficacy of hemodialysis and hemoperfusion in severe theophylline intoxication. *Acad Emerg Med* 1997;4:674–678.
9. Shum S, Seale C, Hathaway D, et al. Acute caffeine ingestion fatalities: management issues. *Vet Hum Toxicol* 1997;39:228–230.

CHAPTER 53

Phencyclidine and Ketamine

PRE-HOSPITAL CONSIDERATIONS
- Use restraints and/or additional personnel to control a combative patient.

CLINICAL PRESENTATION

The effects of phencyclidine (PCP) and ketamine begin within minutes after administration, and they last 8 to 24 hours for PCP and 30 minutes to 4 hours for ketamine. Patients with impaired hepatic or renal function experience longer durations of toxicity. Psychological dependence and tolerance are described with both drugs. Despite sedative effects, neither drug diminishes respiratory drive significantly, and deaths resulting from direct drug toxicity are rare (3,6,7,11). Traumatic injuries from drug related behavior are common (7).

PCP use results in euphoria, severe auditory hallucinations, short-term memory impairment, and other neuropsychiatric toxicities. Patients may experience visual distortions, aggressiveness, and feelings of disconnection from reality. Severely poisoned patients display extreme behavioral swings between catatonia and excessive agitation, marked by severe violence, combativeness, and "superhuman strength" (6). Children exhibit primarily motor effects, with less aggressive behavior (9). Acute psychotic reactions to PCP may be clinically indistinguishable from schizophrenia.

Neurologic signs include ataxia, dystonia, hypertonia, and seizures. Prominent sympathomimetic findings include tachycardia, hypertension, diaphoresis, and agitation. Hypertension from PCP intoxication may lead to intracranial hemorrhage and focal neurologic symptoms with or without associated trauma (1). Less than 5% of cases develop hyperthermia from the excessive muscular rigidity, hyperactivity, or sustained seizures. Rhabdomyolysis and crush injury from struggling against hard leather restraints can occur (5). Pupils are paradoxically small, secondary to stimulation of opioid receptors. Excessive lacrimation and hypersalivation may occur, secondary to cholinergic stimulation (7). Nystagmus occurs in >50% of PCP overdoses and may be horizontal, vertical, or rotatory.

Ketamine intoxication is similar but less severe, characterized by dose-dependent disturbances in perception, with less agitation or violent behavior than with PCP intoxication (11). Patients often describe a "floating" feeling. Although signs and symptoms are more short-lived than those of PCP, severe overdoses may result in a prolonged effect, described as a numbing, out-of-body experience with the perception of paralysis (3). Smaller doses result in diminished attention span, pain perception, and memory. Mild tachycardia and hypertension may result from sympathomimetic effects. Miosis, nystagmus, ataxia, mumbling speech, delirium, and hallucinations are common. Although ketamine is a bronchodilator, it also induces bronchorrhea and sialorrhea (11).

DIFFERENTIAL DIAGNOSIS

PCP intoxication should be suspected in any patient with acute onset of schizophrenia or psychotic behavior, especially with fluctuating mental status. Violent behavior, indifference to painful stimuli, and difficulty restraining the patient are useful clues.

PCP and ketamine can mimic the effects of cocaine and other sympathomimetics, anticholinergic agents, and opiate derivatives. Patients with sympathomimetic and anticholinergic poisoning have tachycardia and hypertension, but miosis, nystagmus, and salivation are typically absent. Withdrawal from PCP or ketamine (violence, muscle rigidity, convulsions, coma, and psychosis) can mimic ethanol and sedative-hypnotic withdrawal (6,7).

Because PCP or ketamine may be taken with other drugs, additional signs or symptoms may also be present (10). Cyanide poisoning should be considered in PCP-intoxicated patients who have been smoking the drug. Occult traumatic injury should always be considered (7).

ED EVALUATION

The history should include the time, amount, and route of exposure, and the circumstances and events prior to arrival. Details should be obtained from police and sources other than the patient. A physical and mental status examination should focus on vital signs, including temperature, neurologic findings, evidence of trauma, aspiration pneumonia, and other complications of injection drug use.

Quantitative serum or urine levels for PCP or ketamine are not practical in the emergency department. Drug levels do not correlate with severity of symptoms and are unlikely to be available before symptoms have resolved. Qualitative rapid urine drug immunoassay may be useful to confirm the presence of PCP, although many hospital-based drug screens do not routinely test for PCP. False-negative results for PCP are quite common, because urinary PCP excretion often falls below the limit of detection. False-positive results for PCP have occurred from both ketamine and dextromethorphan (2). Ketamine detection is not a component of commercially available rapid drug screens. Urine sent for high performance liquid chromatographic analysis for PCP or ketamine can confirm the presence of the drug; however, symptoms resolve long before these results return (8). Urinalysis may be positive for hemoglobin, suggesting the presence of myoglobin and rhabdomyolysis (5). In lethargic, comatose, or extremely violent patients, serum electrolytes, complete blood count, arterial blood gas (ABG), renal function studies, creatinine phosphokinase, and serum ethanol level should be measured. Brain computed tomography is indicated with signs of head trauma (1).

ED MANAGEMENT

Security should be present. Advanced life-support measures should be instituted as necessary, followed by aggressive supportive care. Patients with coma should have rapid bedside glucose determination, thiamine, and naloxone. Because naloxone does not bind to σ-opioid receptors, the opioid effects of PCP and ketamine are not reversible.

Agitation and psychosis may require physical restraints. As soon as possible, intravenous (IV) diazepam (0.1 mg/kg/dose) or lorazepam (0.1 mg/kg/dose) should be given. The dose may be repeated every 5 to 10 minutes as necessary. Haloperidol 5 to 10 mg IV or intramuscular (0.5 mg for children) every 30 to 60 minutes is generally effective, but butyrophenones may exacerbate hypertonia (4,6). Anecdotally, agitation may be decreased by placing the patient into a darkened room with minimal sensory stimulation. Phenothiazines may lower the seizure threshold, exacerbate hyperthermia, contribute to systemic acidosis, or induce hypotension and are therefore not recommended. Neuromuscular paralysis may be necessary in refractory cases of violent psychosis (6).

Seizures should be treated with benzodiazepines: diazepam 0.1 to 0.2 mg/kg/dose IV, lorazepam 0.05 to 0.1 mg/kg IV, or midazolam 0.1 to 0.2 mg/kg IV. Refractory seizures may be treated with phenobarbital 10 to 15 mg/kg IV. Phenytoin does not effectively treat PCP or ketamine seizures.

Severe hypertension is generally transient. Severe and persistent hypertension may be treated with esmolol 0.025 to 0.1 mg/kg/min IV or nitroprusside 2 to 10 μg/kg/min IV. Hyperthermia should be treated with evaporative cooling, sedation, and chemical paralysis in refractory cases. Patients with rhabdomyolysis should be given IV saline to restore and maintain adequate urine flow. Mannitol 0.5 g/kg IV may be of benefit. Deposition of myoglobin renal tubules may be decreased by alkalinization with 100 mEq/L of sodium bicarbonate in 5% dextrose solution. Hemodialysis may be needed for myoglobin-induced oliguria or anuria (5).

Activated charcoal can be administered. Although PCP is secreted into the stomach, so little of the drug is actually secreted into the stomach that neither continuous gastric suctioning nor multiple dose activated charcoal increase drug clearance significantly nor shorten the duration of symptoms (6).

Although urinary acidification with ammonium chloride can theoretically enhance PCP (and ketamine) excretion, this practice is not recommended. Acidification does not shorten the duration of toxicity, can worsen acidemia, and may promote renal failure by increasing myoglobin precipitation in renal tubules. Hemodialysis and hemoperfusion do not enhance PCP or ketamine elimination, because of high protein binding and large volumes of distribution.

CRITICAL INTERVENTIONS

- Obtain a core temperature, ABG, and serum creatine kinase to assess for hyperthermia, acidosis, and rhabdomyolysis in patients with agitation, psychosis, and seizures.
- Administer IV benzodiazepines or haloperidol for agitation and psychosis requiring physical restraint.
- Administer IV benzodiazepines and barbiturates for seizures and neuromuscular hyperactivity resulting in hyperthermia or rhabdomyolysis.
- Treat hyperthermia with evaporative cooling, sedation, and neuromuscular paralysis, as needed.
- Administer saline, with or without mannitol and sodium bicarbonate, to patients with rhabdomyolysis.
- Administer IV esmolol or nitroprusside for persistent and severe hypertension.

DISPOSITION

Neurosurgical, orthopedic, and trauma consultation may be necessary for physical trauma associated with PCP or ketamine intoxication. Patients with altered mental status after 4 to 6 hours, major trauma, or hemodynamic instability should be admitted or transferred to a critical-care setting. Patients with persistent psychiatric symptoms after resolution of drug toxicity should be referred to a psychiatrist. All patients should be referred to substance-abuse counseling.

COMMON PITFALLS

- Failure to consider the possibility of intracranial hemorrhage and trauma in patients with altered mental status
- Exclusion of PCP or ketamine intoxication on the basis of a negative drug screen
- Failure to appreciate that ketamine and dextromethorphan can result in a false-positive PCP on immunoassays
- Exposure of healthcare personnel to harm by inadequate preparations for security, restraint, and sedation

ICD9

305.9 Nondependent other mixed or unspecified drug abuse
968.3 Poisoning by intravenous anesthetics

REFERENCES

1. Boyko OB, Burger PC, Heinz ER. Pathological and radiological correlation of subarachnoid hemorrhage in phencyclidine abuse. *J Neurosurg* 1987;67:446–448.
2. Budai B. Dextromethorphan can produce false positive phencyclidine testing with HPLC. *Am J Emerg Med* 2002;20(1):61–62.
3. Curran HV, Monaghan L. In and out of the K-hole: a comparison of the acute and residual effects of ketamine in frequent and infrequent ketamine users. *Addiction* 2001;96(5):749–760.
4. Giannini AJ, Underwood NA, Condon M. Acute ketamine intoxication treated by haloperidol: a preliminary study. *Am J Ther* 2000;7:389–391.

5. Lahmeyer HW, Stock PG. Phencyclidine intoxication, physical restraint, and acute renal failure: case report. *J Clin Psychiatry* 1983;44:184–185.

6. McCarron MM, Schulze BW, Thompson GA, et al. Acute PCP intoxication: clinical patterns, complications, and treatment. *Ann Emerg Med* 1981;10:290–297.

7. McCarron MM, Schulze BW, Thompson GA, et al. Acute PCP intoxication: incidence of clinical findings in 1000 cases. *Ann Emerg Med* 1981;10:237–242.

8. Moore KA, Sklerov J, Levine B, et al. Urine concentrations of ketamine and norketamine following illegal consumption. *J Anal Toxicol* 2001;25:583–588.

9. Schwartz RH, Einhorn A. PCP intoxication in seven young children. *Pediatr Emerg Care* 1986; 2(4):238–241.

10. Siegel RK. Phencyclidine and ketamine intoxication: a study of four populations of recreational users. *NIDA Res Monogr* 1978;21:119–147.

11. Weiner AL, Vieira L, McKay CA, et al. Ketamine abusers presenting to the emergency department: a case series. *J Emerg Med* 2000;18(4):447–451.

CHAPTER 54

Sympathomimetics

PRE-HOSPITAL CONSIDERATIONS

- Keep in mind that the patient may be uncooperative or violent.
- Secure intravenous access.
- Protect from self-induced trauma.

CLINICAL PRESENTATION

Patients presenting to the emergency department with acute sympathomimetic toxicity typically display tachycardia, hypertension, diaphoresis, and hyperactivity. Pupils may be normal or dilated. Some patients exhibit psychotic behavior. Tremor and hyperreflexia can progress to seizures. In cases of severe toxicity, hypertension can lead to cerebral ischemia or intracerebral hemorrhage (4). Because the hypertension is usually acute, it can cause neurologic injury at pressures lower than those typically seen in patients with chronic hypertension; this is presumably caused by the lack of autoregulatory mechanisms. Sustained increases in muscle activity and seizure may result in rhabdomyolysis with significant elevation in creatine kinase (CK) and myoglobinuric renal failure. Patients with continued untreated muscle activity are at risk for severe metabolic acidosis and hyperthermia. Hyperthermia is a late and ominous finding in patients suffering from sympathomimetic toxicity.

Common mental status changes include euphoria, agitation, psychosis, anxiety, and confusion. These changes are usually related to the expected drug effects, but other causes such as intracranial hemorrhage, ischemia, or cerebral edema must be considered. Hyponatremia related to markedly increased free water intake and elevated antidiuretic hormone levels may be seen in patients who have been "clubbing" or "raving" (2). Bruxism, or jaw clenching and teeth grinding, occurs with methylenedioxymethamphetamine (MDMA; ecstasy) ingestion (1).

Amphetamine and other sympathomimetics have been associated with acute myocardial infarction (MI), supraventricular and ventricular tachydysrhythmias, and cardiomyopathy with heart failure in a variety of age groups (1,4). Myocardial ischemia is thought to be related to vasospasm rather than occlusive disease. Chronic use of sympathomimetic drugs, even in therapeutic doses, has led to elevations in blood pressure and heart rate. Long-standing amphetamine abuse has also been associated with vasculitis that is responsive to treatment with immunosuppressants.

Sympathomimetic drug use and abuse can cause significant toxicity, disability, and death. Recognition of the disease process and rapid and aggressive treatment are necessary to prevent progression of symptoms.

DIFFERENTIAL DIAGNOSIS

Sympathomimetic toxicity should be considered in any patient with some or all of the clinical findings described previously. In particular, young patients with intracerebral hemorrhage, myocardial ischemia/MI, dysrhythmia, severe hypertension, or altered mental status should be interviewed with particular emphasis on legal and illegal drug use. However, a variety of toxicologic and organic disease processes may produce similar signs and symptoms. Toxicity from anticholinergic agents, cocaine, phencyclidine, monoamine oxidase inhibitor interactions, and serotonin syndrome may produce a similar clinical picture. Withdrawal syndromes, as seen with alcohol, clonidine, γ-hydroxybutyrate, or sedative-hypnotics, should also be considered.

The differential diagnosis of sympathomimetic toxicity also includes thyroid storm, pheochromocytoma, infection, non-drug induced intracerebral hemorrhage, ischemic stroke or seizure, brain tumor, MI, aortic dissection, and psychiatric disease.

ED EVALUATION

The initial evaluation should focus on the vital signs. The sympathomimetic poisoned patient develops tachycardia, hypertension, and hyperthermia. Hyperthermia is the most important determinant of mortality, and accurate temperature measurement should be a priority. An axillary temperature is not adequate for these patients, and a rectal or esophageal measurement is best. Once the vital signs have been addressed, a neurologic assessment is paramount. Hallucinations, agitation, dystonias, and seizures are noted in some patients. Choreoathetosis from excessive dopamine stimulation in the basal ganglia is often referred to as "crack dancing" but is seen with other sympathomimetic drugs. The constellation of findings depends upon the specific sympathomimetic drug involved.

Laboratory testing includes electrolytes, blood urea nitrogen, creatinine, total CK, and urinalysis. These tests are important for the assessment of hydration, hyponatremia from excessive hypotonic water intake during periods of excessive drug abuse, rhabdomyolysis, and signs of renal failure from myoglobinuria. An electrocardiogram (ECG) and troponin may be helpful in cases of severe toxicity or in patients who develop chest pain, but continuous ECG monitoring is important in all patients to help monitor the effect of pharmacotherapy. A head computed tomography (CT) scan may be important, if there are signs of trauma or intracranial hemorrhage, but is likely to be of low yield in most patients. A urine drug screen (e.g., EMIT assay) should not be considered a useful diagnostic test. A negative amphetamine screen on an EMIT assay does not eliminate a sympathomimetic as the cause of symptoms, because many sympathomimetic drugs do not produce positive tests. Similarly, a positive test does not mean the patient took an amphetamine or amphetaminelike drug immediately prior to arrival, because an amphetamine screen may remain positive for days after drug use. Clinical suspicion for sympathomimetic poisoning should be based on history and physical examination.

ED MANAGEMENT

The initial management of sympathomimetic poisoning should focus on treatment of the vital signs. Because hyperthermia is the most important determinant of mortality, aggressive cooling should be initiated early. Any elevation in temperature should be taken seriously, and a reasonable goal is to reduce temperature to below 38°C to 39°C. Because hyperthermia is a result of excessive muscle contraction or shivering, sedation or even paralysis should precede cooling measures for cooling to be more effective.

Chemical sedation treats hyperthermia and is also an effective treatment of other vital-sign abnormalities (e.g., tachycardia and hypertension) and agitation. Benzodiazepines are the best first-line agents in these cases. Benzodiazepines should be quickly titrated to the point of making the patient noticeably comfortable; when used by themselves, they rarely result in airway compromise. In addition, benzodiazepines treat possible seizures and other syndromes that may be included in the differential diagnosis (e.g., gamma-aminobutyric acid–agonist withdrawal or other drug-induced delirium). Reasonable intravenous (IV) starting doses in adults are diazepam 5 to 10 mg or lorazepam 2 to 4 mg every 5 to 10 minutes.

Hypertension is usually controlled by sedatives alone. However, when additional treatment is needed, nitroglycerin, phentolamine, and nitroprusside are good adjuncts. It is difficult to specify a target blood pressure for treatment, but a pressure <180/110 mm Hg is generally recognized as a reasonable goal. If there is evidence of hypertensive encephalopathy or intracranial hemorrhage, more aggressive treatment may be necessary. β-blockers should be avoided. Paradoxical hypertension may result from blockade of, β_2-mediated vasodilation and unopposed α_1-adrenergic vasoconstriction. Coronary-artery vasospasm has been noted when propranolol is used after cocaine administration in human volunteers (5). Besides benzodiazepines, sympathomimetic-induced delirium may also benefit from haloperidol (3). Antipsychotics like haloperidol antagonize central dopamine receptors and may offer additional benefit by a mechanism distinct from that of benzodiazepines. In particular, choreoathetosis associated with sympathomimetic poisoning will disappear after antipsychotic administration. Antipsychotics should be used with caution, because they can lower the seizure threshold, can lead to dysrhythmias from QT prolongation, and may alter temperature regulation. Haloperidol 5 mg IV, with increasing doses every 20 minutes, can be an effective addition to benzodiazepine pharmacotherapy.

Rhabdomyolysis requires aggressive fluid resuscitation, with a target urine output of 1 to 2 mL/kg/h. Sympathomimetic-poisoned patients are often volume depleted, and routine fluid administration is good practice in this population.

Gastrointestinal (GI) decontamination is rarely of benefit. In patients who present after the onset of symptoms, activated-charcoal administration is not expected to be helpful. The exception is in "body stuffers." Patients who have ingested poorly packaged stimulants to hide contraband from the police may benefit from activated charcoal because they may be subject to absorption (often erratic) of the drug. Body stuffers who present before the onset of symptoms should routinely receive activated charcoal. Other forms of GI decontamination are not routinely recommended for this patient population. "Body packers" are smuggling well-packaged stimulants and are treated differently.

CRITICAL INTERVENTIONS

- Measure the temperature in a timely manner in patients with agitation, hyperactivity, seizures, and abnormalities of other vital signs.
- Rapidly cool patients with hyperthermia while instituting core body temperature monitoring.
- Use benzodiazepines to treat hyperthermia, hypertension, and tachycardia from sympathomimetic poisoning.

DISPOSITION

Because the duration of toxicity is often brief, patients with mild signs or symptoms may be monitored in the emergency department. Observation and monitoring of vital signs is advised for a minimum of 6 hours or until symptoms abate. Patients with persistent headache or neurologic signs may require an urgent head CT. Patients with persistent central nervous system stimulation or vital-sign abnormalities should be admitted to an intensive care unit. The most ill patients, who present with hyperthermia, often require prolonged hospitalization for treatment of rhabdomyolysis and the associated renal failure. However, most cases require only short hospital stays for benzodiazepines, IV fluids, and monitoring of vital signs.

COMMON PITFALLS

- Failure to consider sympathomimetic toxicity in the differential diagnosis of tachycardia, hypertension, intracranial hemorrhage, and cerebral or myocardial ischemia.
- Failure to appreciate that headache, even without focal neurologic signs, may be the result of intracerebral hemorrhage.
- Failure to identify hyponatremia as a cause of cerebral edema and altered mental status.
- Failure to obtain a CK to check for rhabdomyolysis in patients with agitation and hyperthermia.

- Failure to appreciate that bradycardia in patients with hypertension as a result of sympathomimetic abuse is a normal reflex response. Treating bradycardia with atropine in this situation could aggravate hypertension.

ICD9

971.2 Poisoning by sympathomimetics (adrenergics)

REFERENCES

1. Appleby M, Fisher M, Martin M. Myocardial infarction, hyperkalemia and ventricular tachycardia in a young male body-builder. *Int J Cardiol* 1994;44:171–174.
2. Budisavljevic MN, Stewart L, Sahn SA, et al. Hyponatremia associated with 3,4-methylenedioxy-methylamphetamine ("Ecstasy") abuse. *Am J Med Sci* 2003;326:89–93.
3. Derlet RW, Albertson TE, Rice P. Antagonism of cocaine, amphetamine, and methamphetamine toxicity. *Pharmacol Biochem Behav* 1990;36:745–749.
4. Haller CA, Benowitz NL. Adverse cardiovascular and central nervous system events associated with dietary supplements containing ephedra alkaloids. *N Engl J Med* 2000;343:1833–1838.
5. Lange RA, Cigarroa RG, Flores ED, et al. Potentiation of cocaine-induced coronary vasoconstriction by β-adrenergic blockade. *Ann Intern Med* 1990;112:897–903.

CHAPTER 55

Thyroid Hormones

PRE-HOSPITAL CONSIDERATIONS

- Stabilize the patient and provide supportive care.
  - Airway, breathing, and circulation
  - Cardiac monitoring
  - Supplemental oxygen
  - Intravenous fluids

CLINICAL PRESENTATION

Acute oral overdose of thyroid hormones is typically asymptomatic on presentation, seldom produces serious toxicity, and has caused no deaths that have been reported. Thus, the minimal toxic and lethal doses are unknown, and there is no correlation between serum-T_4 concentration and clinical severity. Children are resistant to the effects of large overdoses (13). Elderly patients with compromised cardiovascular function may be more sensitive, but there are no data to support this speculation.

The few patients who manifest toxicity have the features of hyperthyroidism (fever; tachycardia; warm, moist skin; diarrhea; restlessness; and anxiety).

To assess toxic risk, it is important to differentiate between the different types of thyroid-hormone supplements. Because T_3 is the active thyroid hormone, acute toxicity would be expected with its ingestion, but only one such case has been reported (4). Although the onset of toxicity was within a few hours, it was minor and of brief duration (12 hours) despite a documented serum concentration 50 times normal. Although 80 tablets were ingested (or 80 therapeutic doses), this patient coingested significant amounts of an antidepressant and an antihistamine, which may have contributed to the observed toxicity. Significant early toxicity (at 6 hours) was seen in a 15-month-old boy who ingested 50 tablets of desiccated thyroid (combined T_3 and T_4 ingestion). Improvement was rapid and symptoms did not recur (7).

In contrast, T_4 overdose is relatively common (5,8,9,11). Ingestions of up to 30 mg have produced negligible toxicity (13), as have serum T_4 concentrations of 84.7 (11) and 90 μg/dL. Thus, there is a large tolerance for acute massive ingestion of levothyroxine. Several factors contribute to this inherent low toxicity. Conversion of T_4 to T_3 takes several days and is regulated by a negative-feedback loop. The presence of excess T_4 inhibits endogenous secretion of this hormone, inhibits the peripheral conversion of T_4 to T_3 (2), increases the disposal rates of both T_4 and T_3 (2), and downregulates the T_3 nuclear receptors. Also, elevation of serum concentrations of reverse T_3 (an inhibitor of thyroid hormones) has been observed in two T_4-overdose patients (6). Therefore, it is expected that the occurrence of toxicity would be less likely, and the onset of toxicity would occur later (in several days).

The only reported case of serious toxicity occurred in a 2-year-old boy who took 18 mg of levothyroxine (5). At about 6 hours after ingestion, his serum thyroxine concentration was 117.4 μg/dL, and he had two seizures 7 days later. There have been reports of minor toxicities such as asymptomatic tachycardia, low-grade fever, diarrhea, and hyperactivity (8,9).

The ingestion of products that contain both T_3 and T_4 may theoretically result in biphasic toxicity with early (within hours) and late (after several days) phases. However, there are no examples in the literature.

Chronic repeated ingestion of excessive amounts of thyroid hormones on a daily basis, rather than acute overdose, is more likely to produce this picture. Such patients may have virtually all the signs of hyperthyroidism except for exophthalmos. Overt hyperthyroidism and even death may occur (1,10). Such patients may be abusing thyroid hormones to lose weight or because of emotional instability or frank psychiatric illness. These patients often deny thyroid ingestion.

DIFFERENTIAL DIAGNOSIS

The differential diagnosis of chronic thyroid hormone abuse includes metabolic conditions (e.g., pheochromocytoma and hypoglycemia), central nervous system infection, organic brain syndrome, overdose with stimulants, psychoactive drugs (e.g., amphetamine, cocaine, anticholinergics, and hallucinogens), acute withdrawal states, and acute psychotic illness. For patients with elevated serum T_4 concentrations, the chief differentiation is from endogenous hyperthyroidism, in which the serum thyroglobulin concentration is elevated. The serum thyroglobulin concentration is depressed in patients with exogenous hyperthyroidism (10).

ED EVALUATION

The history includes the identity of the ingestant, the dose, the time of ingestion, the symptoms of hyperthyroidism, the reason for ingestion, and prior medical conditions. The identity of the hormone(s) involved is important because of their differing clinical courses after overdose. The physical examination is directed toward eliciting the findings of hyperthyroidism. For acute ingestions, the T4 concentration is measured 4 to 6 hours after overdose if the patient has ingested more than 2 mg of levothyroxine or its equivalent. This measurement should be done in all patients with chronic thyroid overdose. Patients with a level >25 μg/dL require follow-up.

ED MANAGEMENT

Supportive measures are instituted as necessary. Activated charcoal should be considered for patients who have ingested >2 mg of thyroxine or its equivalent (11). For the rare patient who develops symptoms after acute ingestion, acetaminophen for fever and propranolol (20–40 mg qid for adults and 0.25–0.5 mg/kg qid for children) for sympathetic hyperactivity may be necessary (8). The oral administration of iopanoic acid (Telepaque, 125 mg per day in a 2.5-year-old child), an iodine-containing radiocontrast agent that inhibits the conversion of T_4 to T_3, has also been used with apparent success (3). Prophylactic therapy (cholestyramine, prednisone, propylthiouracil, and propranolol) in asymptomatic patients has not been necessary (6,9,11). For the symptomatic patient with chronic thyroid ingestion, thyroid supplements should be discontinued, and the patient should be treated similar to endogenous hyperthyroidism and thyroid storm. Enhanced elimination by extracorporeal removal has not been shown to be of benefit (11).

CRITICAL INTERVENTIONS

- Admit or observe patients with large T_3 overdoses for 12 to 24 hours.
- Arrange for daily outpatient follow-up for a week after acute overdose of T_4 in patients with T_4 levels >25 μg/dL.
- Administer propranolol to patients with clinically significant sympathetic hyperactivity.

DISPOSITION

Patients with significant T_3 overdoses (20 therapeutic doses or more) should be admitted to an observation or inpatient unit. Vital signs, cardiac rhythm, and clinical status should be monitored for 12 to 24 hours. Because patients with acute T_4 overdose are at risk only for delayed toxicity, immediate inpatient observation is unnecessary. Toxicity after acute T_4 overdose has not been reported with serum concentrations <25 μg/dL; daily assessment for the next 10 days is required if this value is exceeded. Symptomatic patients should be treated as necessary. Patients who present with hyperthyroidism as a result of chronic abuse usually require admission. Consultation with an endocrinologist is advisable.

COMMON PITFALLS

- Failure to differentiate between T_3 and T_4 overdose
- Failure to differentiate between acute and chronic overdose
- Failure to appreciate that acute overdose can result in delayed toxicity
- Overzealous, unnecessary, and potentially harmful use of antithyroid drugs and extracorporeal removal in asymptomatic patients

ICD9

962.7 Poisoning by thyroid and thyroid derivatives

REFERENCES

1. Bhasin S, Wallace W, Lawrence JB, et al. Sudden death associated with thyroid hormone abuse. *Am J Med* 1981;71:887.
2. Braverman LE, Vagenakis A, Downs P, et al. Effects of replacement doses of sodium l-thyroxine on the peripheral metabolism of thyroxine and triiodothyronine in man. *J Clin Invest* 1973;52:1010.
3. Brown RS, Cohen JH, Braverman LE. Successful treatment of massive thyroid hormone poisoning with iopanoic acid. *J Pediatr* 1998;132:903.
4. Dahlberg PA, Karlsson FA, Wide L. Triiodothyronine intoxication. *Lancet* 1979;2:700.
5. Kulig K, Golightly LK, Rumack BH. Levothyroxine overdose associated with seizures in a young child. *JAMA* 1985;254:2109.
6. Lehrner LM, Weir MR. Acute ingestions of thyroid hormones. *Pediatrics* 1984;73:313.
7. Levy RP, Gilger WG. Acute thyroid poisoning. *N Engl J Med* 1957;256:459.
8. Lewander WJ, Lacouture PG, Silva JE, et al. Acute thyroid ingestion in pediatric patients. *Pediatrics* 1989;84:262.
9. Litovitz TL, White JD. Levothyroxine ingestions in children: an analysis of 78 cases. *Am J Emerg Med* 1985;3:297.
10. Mariotti S, Martino E, Cupini C, et al. Low serum thyroglobulin as a clue to the diagnosis of thyrotoxicosis factitia. *N Engl J Med* 1982;307:410.
11. Nystrom E, Lindstedt G, Lindbert PA. Minor signs and symptoms of toxicity in a young woman in spite of massive thyroxine ingestion. *Acta Med Scand* 1980;207:135.
12. Roesch C, Becker PG, Sklar S. Management of a child with acute thyroxine ingestion. *Ann Emerg Med* 1985;14:1114.
13. Tenenbein M, Dean HJ. Benign course after massive levothyroxine ingestion. *Pediatr Emerg Care* 1986;2:15.

Miscellaneous Agents and Conditions

CHAPTER 56

Biological Warfare Agents

PRE-HOSPITAL CONSIDERATIONS
* Use Universal Precautions with an N95 mask.

CLINICAL PRESENTATION

The clinical presentation of patients exposed to biological warfare (BW) agents will obviously vary depending on the agent.

Cutaneous anthrax results in a black eschar with significant surrounding edema at the site of skin entry. Most lesions will heal spontaneously, although 10% to 20% of untreated cases progress to septicemia and death. Cutaneous anthrax fatalities are rare with antibiotic therapy. Gastrointestinal anthrax causes nausea, vomiting, fever, abdominal pain, and mucosal ulcers, which can cause hemorrhage, perforation, and sepsis; mortality is high (8).

Inhalational anthrax has an incubation period of 1 to 6 days. Patients then develop fever, malaise, fatigue, nonproductive cough, and mild chest discomfort. Symptoms may abruptly progress to severe respiratory distress with dyspnea, diaphoresis, stridor, and cyanosis. Bacteremia, shock, metastatic infection (meningitis occurs in approximately 50% of cases), and death follow within 24 to 36 hours. Inhalational anthrax is a mediastinitis, rather than a pneumonia. Chest radiography and computed tomography typically shows mediastinal widening and pleural effusions, although pneumonic infiltrates are also reported (8).

Historically, the mortality rate from inhalational anthrax was nearly 100% once symptoms develop, even with antibiotics. Experience from the 2001 outbreak in the United States shows that more than half of the patients with inhalational anthrax survived with aggressive supportive care and antibiotic therapy. Earlier hospitalization appeared to correlate with improved outcome (2,9,12).

Bubonic plague has an incubation period of 2 to 10 days preceding the onset of fever, malaise, and painful, enlarged regional lymph nodes (buboes). Septicemia may occur and can be accompanied by disseminated intravascular coagulation (DIC) and acral gangrene. Necrosis of the digits and nose seen with septicemic plague is the likely origin of the term "black death" (7).

Pneumonic plague has an incubation period of 2 to 3 days. The onset of disease is acute and often fulminant. Patients develop fever, malaise, and cough productive of bloody sputum, rapidly progressing to dyspnea, stridor, cyanosis, and cardiorespiratory collapse. Plague pneumonia is almost always fatal unless treatment is begun within 24 hours of symptom onset.

Ulceroglandular tularemia is characterized by local skin ulceration and associated lymphadenopathy, fever, chills, headache, and malaise. Typhoidal tularemia presents with fever, prostration, and weight loss without adenopathy. Exposure to aerosolized bacteria should result in typhoidal tularemia with prominent respiratory symptoms like a nonproductive cough and substernal chest discomfort. Chest radiographs may show infiltrates, mediastinal lymphadenopathy, or pleural effusions. A temporarily incapacitating infection is most likely (4), but fatalities may occur.

Smallpox has a 12- to 14-day incubation period. Initial symptoms include fever, malaise, and prostration with headache and backache. Oropharyngeal lesions appear first, shedding virus into the saliva. Two to 3 days after the onset of fever, a papular rash develops on the face and spreads to the extremities. The fever continues as the rash becomes vesicular and then pustular. The pustules scab over and eventually separate, leaving pitted and hypopigmented scars. The mortality rate of smallpox can be as high as 30%, with death occurring during the second week of the illness (6).

Viral hemorrhagic fever (VHF) is characterized by fever, malaise, prostration, and hemorrhagic rash. Clinical features, such as the extent of renal, hepatic, and hematologic involvement, vary according to the agent involved. Mortality rates also vary, from <1% for Rift Valley fever up to 50% to 90% for the Ebola virus (3).

Botulism results in multiple bulbar nerve palsies and a symmetric descending paralysis, with death occurring from respiratory failure (see Chapter 59). Onset of symptoms can occur within 24 to 36 hours or take several days (1).

DIFFERENTIAL DIAGNOSIS

Familiarity with the expected clinical syndromes produced by BW agents will aid in the differential diagnosis. An acute respiratory syndrome with fever may occur with inhalational anthrax, pneumonic plague, Q fever, hantavirus, and exposure to several other bacterial, viral, and fungal agents, as well as several common, endemic respiratory tract infections (e.g., influenza, the common cold, bronchitis, and community-acquired pneumonia). Patients with inhalational anthrax are more likely to have nausea or vomiting, tachycardia, elevated transaminases, low sodium levels, high hematocrit, low albumin levels, and normal white blood cell counts than those with influenzalike illnesses and community-acquired pneumonia, and patients with an influenzalike illness are more likely to have myalgias, headache, and nasal symptoms (11). The presence of pulmonary infiltrates on chest radiographs does not rule out inhalational anthrax, although such patients are likely to also have an enlarged mediastinum and pleural effusions.

Agents producing cutaneous lesions include anthrax, plague, smallpox, tularemia, and many of the VHFs. Experience from the 2001 outbreak shows that cases of cutaneous anthrax may occur amidst other cases of inhalational anthrax. Small pustules or skin lesions may be found at the site of flea bites in cases of plague, whereas petechial rashes are common with VHFs. The individual lesions of smallpox closely resemble those from herpesvirus infections like chickenpox. Smallpox lesions will all be at the same stage of development, and they are found mostly in a centrifugal distribution (i.e., hand, feet, and face), in distinction from the typical centripetal pattern of chickenpox with patches of lesions at various stages of development.

An acute neurologic syndrome with fever suggests disease from a viral equine encephalitis, although other viral and bacterial BW agents (Q fever, smallpox, typhus) may also have prominent headache, photophobia, and myalgias. A neurologic syndrome without fever from BW agents is likely to be as a result of domoic acid, saxitoxin, tetrodotoxin, or botulism.

Botulism may resemble several other neurologic diseases, including myasthenia gravis, Guillain-Barré syndrome, tick paralysis, poliomyelitis, organophosphate poisoning, and so on. Although individual cases of such other diseases may occur uncommonly, the simultaneous presentation of multiple patients with progressive paralysis should immediately suggest an environmental exposure, either to botulinum toxin or an organophosphate chemical warfare agent.

ED EVALUATION

Historical data to collect include documentation of the time and place of BW agent exposure and if any other persons were potentially exposed and whether they are symptomatic. The time of onset, nature, progression, and severity of symptoms should be noted. The presence of any visualized suspect material (e.g., an unidentified white powder) should be determined, so that samples may later be taken by the proper authorities.

Physical examination should focus first on the vital signs and assessment of the patient's cardiopulmonary function and neuromuscular status to determine if emergent resuscitative efforts are necessary. Ideally, all patients should have continuous cardiac and oxygen saturation monitoring, although this may not be possible in a mass-casualty setting. A complete physical examination should be performed, with particular attention to detecting pulmonary rales, diminished breath sounds, the presence and characteristics of any rash, lymphadenopathy, meningismus, and any neurologic deficits.

Patients with pulmonary symptoms should have a chest radiograph, looking for pulmonary infiltrates, mediastinal widening, and pleural effusions. Chest computed tomography was also used in several patients with inhalational anthrax in 2001 (2,9,12). Arterial-blood-gas analysis should also be considered.

Ill patients should have a broad panel of other laboratory tests, which may include a complete blood count, comprehensive metabolic panel, DIC screening, serologies, blood cultures, and Gram staining, depending on the suspected agent and clinical status of the patient. Laboratory personnel should be informed of the suspected pathogen(s). Antibiotic-susceptibility testing should be performed on all bacterial isolates, as strains may be deliberately modified by terrorists to enhance antibiotic resistance. Patients with suspected smallpox should have vesicle fluid from lesions cultured, and scrapings should be sent for electron microscopic analysis. Spirometry and arterial blood gas analysis should be performed on patients with suspected botulism to establish their ventilatory capacity.

Plague can be diagnosed by various staining techniques, immunologic studies, or culturing the organism from blood, sputum, or lymph node aspirate. *Yersinia pestis* appears as a "safety-pin" bipolar coccobacillus. Chest radiographs in pneumonic plague show patchy or consolidated bronchopneumonia. Leukocytosis with bandemia is common, as are markers of low-grade DIC and elevations of bilirubin and the hepatic transaminases. Diagnosing tularemia is often difficult, as the organism is hard to isolate by culture and the symptoms are nonspecific.

ED MANAGEMENT

Advanced life-support measures are instituted as necessary for patients requiring resuscitation. Unlike with chemical weapons, patient decontamination is a minor issue with biological weapons. Most BW agents, with the notable exception of anthrax spores, are degraded by sunlight and desiccation and do not survive well in the environment for more than 1 to 2 days. In the scenario of a covert BW agent release, by the time patients present for medical care several days after exposure, decontamination is futile and will only delay care. Even with an acute, efficiently dispersed release of a biologic weapon via aerosol (including anthrax spores), little surface contamination is produced. Clothing removal and a soap-and-water shower will remove 99.99% of any remaining organisms on the skin (10), and this may occur in the patients' homes to reduce the strain on medical resources. Any grossly visible contamination with a BW agent, if present, should be removed by thorough water irrigation, sterilization of the skin with a sporicidal/bactericidal solution (e.g., 0.5% sodium hypochlorite, a 1:10 dilution of household bleach), and a final water rinse (10). If patient decontamination is performed at a healthcare facility, patients should be instructed to remove their clothing and place it into sealed and labeled plastic bags, wash their hands, and shower thoroughly with soap and water.

For patients who present with symptomatic illness after a covert attack, decontamination is unlikely to be helpful, but health care provider protection is critical. Standard infection-control measures (gloves, gown, mask with eye shield) provide adequate protection from most agents. However, unless the offending BW agent is already known, it must first be assumed that the patients have a potentially transmissible disease such as smallpox, pneumonic plague, or a VHF, which require airborne, contact, and droplet precautions. Patients with respiratory symptoms or a rash should be placed in a private negative-pressure room, and medical personnel caring for the patient should wear well-fitting N95 high-efficiency particulate air-filter masks pending the results of a more complete evaluation (10). If multiple casualties present at the same time, space limitations may mandate patient isolation in groups rather than individually.

Current treatment recommendations for anthrax rely primarily on ciprofloxacin and doxycycline (8) and are shown in Table 56.1. The currently recommended duration of therapy after bioterrorist exposure to anthrax is 60 days, as delayed development of inhalational anthrax might occur.

Effective vaccines against anthrax are available (5). Anthrax vaccine adsorbed (AVA) is used in the United States, which consists of a sterilized filtrate of an avirulent bacterial strain. As with any vaccine, local reactions to AVA occur in a minority of recipients (up to 20% with mild, local reactions), and self-limited systemic reactions occur more rarely (<1.5%); serious adverse events are rare. The

TABLE 56.1	Antibiotic Treatment of Anthrax, Plague, and Tularemia[a,b]
Condition	**Treatment**
Cutaneous anthrax or Postexposure anthrax prophylaxis	Ciprofloxacin 500 mg (10–15 mg/kg in children) PO twice daily, or Doxycycline 100 mg (2.2 mg/kg in children) PO twice daily. Amoxicillin 500 mg PO 3 times daily (80 mg/kg/d PO divided every 8 hours in children) may be substituted if unable to tolerate other drugs. Duration of treatment = 60 days with bioterrorism attacks.
Inhalational anthrax	Ciprofloxacin 400 mg (10–15 mg/kg in children) IV every 12 hours, or Doxycycline 100 mg (2.2 mg/kg in children) IV every 12 hours plus one or two additional antimicrobials with in vitro activity against *Bacillus anthracis;* IV treatment initially, then switch to oral when clinically appropriate. Duration of treatment = 60 days with bioterrorism attacks.
Active plague disease in contained casualty setting	Doxycycline 100 mg (2.2 mg/kg in children) IV every 12 hours, or Ciprofloxacin 400 mg (10–15 mg/kg in children) IV every 12 hours, or Chloramphenicol 25 mg/kg IV four times daily, or Streptomycin 1 g (15 mg/kg in children) IM twice daily, or Gentamicin 5 mg/kg IV once daily, or 2 mg/kg load and 1.7 mg/kg three times daily (2.5 mg/kg in children). Duration of treatment = 10 days.
Postexposure plague prophylaxis or mass-casualty setting	Doxycycline 100 mg (2.2 mg/kg in children) PO twice daily, or Ciprofloxacin 500 mg (20 mg/kg in children) PO twice daily. Duration of treatment = 7 days for postexposure prophylaxis; 10 days if disease present.
Tularemia	Identical to treatment for plague, except duration of therapy = 14 days.

[a]This table includes treatment regimens that are not FDA approved.
[b]References 4, 7, and 8 are reproduced with permission from *JAMA* 2001;285:2763–2773; *JAMA* 2000;283:2281–2290; *JAMA* 2002;287:2236–2252.
PO, by mouth; IV, intravenous; IM, intramuscular.

dosage schedule for AVA is 0.5 mL subcutaneously at 0, 2, and 4 weeks and 6, 12, and 18 months, with yearly boosters. For emergency use after confirmed exposure, the vaccine is given as soon as possible and again at 2 and 4 weeks, along with prophylactic antibiotics.

Respiratory droplet precautions are necessary in pneumonic plague until the patient has received antibiotics for at least 48 hours and shows clinical improvement. Antibiotic choices are similar to anthrax, with a high reliance on ciprofloxacin and doxycycline (see Table 56.1). Antibiotics must be initiated early after exposure, because waiting for symptoms will result in extremely high mortality (7). Antibiotic treatment for tularemia is virtually the same as for plague (4).

The treatment of smallpox is largely supportive. Persons exposed to smallpox but without clinical disease should also be isolated and observed for the development of fever and rash for 17 days; this observation period may occur at home. The antiviral drug cidofovir may be beneficial in preventing smallpox, if administered early after exposure, but is probably no better than postexposure vaccination (6).

Vaccination before smallpox exposure or within 4 days after exposure significantly ameliorates subsequent illness. Vaccination against smallpox carries some risk for adverse reactions. The two most serious reactions are postvaccinal encephalitis and progressive vaccinia. Postvaccinal encephalitis occurs in about three cases per million primary vaccinees. Forty percent of cases are fatal, and some survivors are left with permanent neurologic sequelae. Progressive vaccinia can occur in immunosuppressed individuals and is treated with vaccinia immune globulin.

Most VHF agents carry the risk of secondary infection through droplet aerosols, and careful patient isolation is critical. Ribavirin has been used for some VHFs, but supportive care is the mainstay of therapy (3).

The mainstay of botulism therapy is supportive care, with ventilation if necessary. An equine antitoxin for passive immunization is available in the United States from the Centers for Disease Control and Prevention (CDC) through contact with local and state health departments. The antitoxin prevents worsening of disease caused by the toxin serotypes responsible for foodborne illness (A, B, and E) but does not reverse established effects. An investigational heptavalent antitoxin against serotypes A through G is held by the U.S. Army. An investigational pentavalent toxoid for serotypes A through E has been used to actively immunize high-risk populations, such as laboratory workers, but would be ineffective as postexposure treatment (1).

CRITICAL INTERVENTIONS

- Wear gloves, gown, eye shield, and a N95 high-efficiency particulate air filter mask when evaluating and treating patients with possible BW agent exposure.
- If possible, place patients with respiratory symptoms or a rash in a private negative-pressure room.
- Contact appropriate local public health and law enforcement authorities in cases of suspected BW agent exposure.

DISPOSITION

All cases of suspected exposure to BW agents should be reported to local public health and law enforcement authorities. Unless the patient contracted their illness through unintentional exposure in a research laboratory, each case is potential evidence of a criminal bioterrorist act, requiring contact also with law enforcement agencies such as the local Federal Bureau of Investigation field office. Consultation with a physician familiar with BW agents, such as an infectious disease specialist, military physician, toxicologist, or poison center, is also recommended. Other potential resources include the CDC (770-488-7100) and the U.S. Army Medical Research Institute for Infectious Diseases (1-888-USA-RIID), which have 24-hour hotline services to assist physicians with biological agent inquiries.

Patients with known or suspected acute exposures to infectious BW agents are likely to be asymptomatic and require no emergent interventions. Such patients require initiation of appropriate postexposure prophylactic antibiotics and/or vaccinations, depending on the agent involved. Asymptomatic patients acutely exposed to anthrax or plague may be discharged home with antibiotic prescriptions, if adequate follow-up can be arranged through the local public health agency or their private physicians.

Patients exposed to smallpox may require quarantine, which should be coordinated with the assistance of public health and law enforcement agencies. Patients acutely exposed to toxin weapons might be asymptomatic at presentation but still require admission for a period of observation depending on the agent involved. Botulinum toxin exposure, for example, mandates admission to monitor for development of respiratory failure.

Unless part of a mass-casualty incident, all patients known or suspected to have illness from BW agent exposure should be admitted, with the level of care dependent on clinical severity. Outpatient management of cutaneous anthrax may be considered for patients without systemic toxicity, who can tolerate oral antibiotics, and in whom outpatient follow-up can be assured. Isolation precaution will be necessary for patients with pneumonic plague, smallpox, and many of the VHFs. In mass-casualty situations, admission may need to be more selective and reserved for patients who cannot tolerate outpatient therapy but who are not moribund.

COMMON PITFALLS

- Lack of familiarity with likely BW agents and the clinical syndromes they produce
- Failure to appreciate that some BW agents are transmissible and others are not and that isolation requirements may or may not be necessary
- Failure to institute appropriate postexposure prophylaxis among patients with plausible exposure scenarios

REFERENCES

1. Arnon SS, Schechter R, Inglesby TV, et al. Botulinum toxin as a biological weapon: medical and public health management. *JAMA* 2001;285:1059–1070.
2. Borio L, Frank D, Mani V, et al. Death due to bioterrorism-related inhalational anthrax: report of 2 patients. *JAMA* 2001;286:2554–2559.
3. Borio L, Inglesby T, Peters CJ, et al. Hemorrhagic fever viruses as biological weapons: medical and public health management. *JAMA* 2002;287:2391–2405.
4. Dennis DT, Inglesby TV, Henderson DA, et al. Tularemia as a biological weapon: medical and public health management. *JAMA* 2001;285:2763–2773.
5. Friedlander AM, Pittman PR, Parker GW. Anthrax vaccine: evidence for safety and efficacy against inhalational anthrax. *JAMA* 1999;282:2104–2106.
6. Henderson DA, Inglesby TV, Barlett JG, et al. Smallpox as a biological weapon: medical and public health management. *JAMA* 1999;281:2127–2137.
7. Inglesby TV, Dennis ST, Henderson DA, et al. Plague as a biological weapon: medical and public health management. *JAMA* 2000;283:2281–2290.
8. Inglesby TV, O'Toole T, Henderson DA, et al. Anthrax as a biological weapon 2002: updated recommendations for management. *JAMA* 2002;287:2236–2252.
9. Jernigan JA, Stephens DS, Ashford DA, et al. Bioterrorism-related inhalational anthrax: the first 10 cases reported in the United States. *Emerg Infect Dis* 2001;7:933–944.
10. Keim M, Kaufmann AF. Principles for emergency response to bioterrorism. *Ann Emerg Med* 1999;34:177–182.
11. Kuehnert MJ, Doyle TJ, Hill HA, et al. Clinical features that discriminate inhalational anthrax from other acute respiratory illnesses. *Clin Infect Dis* 2003;36:328–336.
12. Mayer TA, Bersoff-Matcha S, Murphy C, et al. Clinical presentation of inhalational anthrax following bioterrorism exposure: report of two surviving patients. *JAMA* 2001;286:2549–2553.

CHAPTER 57

Chemical Warfare Agents

PRE-HOSPITAL CONSIDERATIONS

- Avoid contamination of the environment and clinicians.
  - Use level A or level B personal protective equipment.
  - Carry out decontamination.
    - Dermal wet decontamination primarily for nerve and blistering agents
    - Dry decontamination (removal of clothing and jewelry) for other agents
- Administer atropine even if the patient is tachycardic because the condition may result from hypoxia.

CLINICAL PRESENTATION

Choking Agents. Clinical symptoms begin within minutes after significant chlorine exposure and include lacrimation, conjunctival irritation, rhinorrhea, cough, sore throat, chest burning, dyspnea, sputum production, nausea, headache, and respiratory failure. Corneal abrasions and cutaneous burns may result from eye and skin exposure, respectively. Following significant chlorine exposures, pulmonary edema develops within 2 to 4 hours and peaks at 12 to 24 hours (9). The chest x-ray may be normal or may show noncardiogenic pulmonary edema. Patients with significant phosgene exposure have a typical latency period of 4 to 6 hours (range, 1–24 hours) and then present with dyspnea, chest tightness, cyanosis, hemoptysis, hypotension, and pulmonary edema. Chest x-ray findings of pulmonary edema are rather late and nonspecific, occurring 6 to 8 hours after exposure. Diphosgene produces identical signs and symptoms. Following significant pulmonary agent exposure (e.g., chlorine gas), patients may subsequently develop reactive airways dysfunction syndrome, a chronic asthma-like condition.

Vesicating Agents. After mustard exposure, there is typically a latency period of 4 to 12 hours before the onset of symptoms. The latency period is shorter with high concentrations and long exposures, with increased ambient temperature and humidity, and in victims previously exposed to or innately susceptible to mustard (2,9). Sites of injury principally involve the skin, eye, and respiratory tract and may follow vapor or liquid exposure. Heavy exposure may lead to systemic effects such as bone marrow depression and sloughing of intestinal mucosa.

Cutaneous injury resulting from mustard exposure ranges from erythema to blisters and skin necrosis. The moist, thinner skin of the neck, axilla, and groin is more severely affected. After an asymptomatic period of 4 to 12 hours, erythema and edema develop. Vesication typically starts within 24 hours and evolves over several days. Vesicles coalesce into blisters, and skin necrosis occurs over 24 to 72 hours (9). Blister fluid does not contain active mustard and is not toxic (9). Skin denudation occurs over 6 to 9 days, and healing may take 4 to 10 weeks.

The eye is the organ most sensitive to sulfur mustard. Tissue injury occurs rapidly, but symptoms develop gradually over 4 to 8 hours and include eye pain, lacrimation, photophobia, and blurred vision (2,9). Physical findings include blepharospasm, eyelid edema, conjunctival injection and edema, chemosis, anterior chamber cellular infiltrates, and decreased vision. Corneal edema begins within 1 hour after exposure, and the corneal epithelium vesicates and sloughs within 4 to 36 hours (9). Resolution of injury depends on the severity of exposure and typically takes 1 to 2 weeks. About 90% of victims are visually disabled for 10 days with conjunctivitis, photophobia, and corneal swelling. The remaining 10% are severely affected and are at risk for permanent blindness from corneal opacification, scarring, and ulceration (9).

Respiratory epithelial damage occurs several hours after exposure. Victims may develop rhinitis, nasal bleeding, sinus discomfort, hoarseness, sore throat, cough, sputum production, and dyspnea of increasing severity. Hemorrhagic inflammation and erosions of the upper airway mucosa are followed by fibrinous pseudomembrane formation and sloughing of necrotic, ulcerated mucosa. Bronchospasm and partial airway obstruction result. After high-dose exposures, severe bronchitis, secondary bronchopneumonia, and respiratory failure may develop within 24 to 48 hours (2,9). Pulmonary edema is not a characteristic finding, as mustard does not typically affect the pulmonary parenchyma. The need for mechanical ventilation is a poor prognostic sign, and the majority of these patients subsequently die from progressive respiratory failure.

Bone marrow and gastrointestinal (GI) mucosal toxicity may occur with high concentration or prolonged exposure. Leukopenia develops within 5 to 7 days, with the white cell nadir occurring 10 days after exposure. Thrombocytopenia and anemia typically follow. The development of hematologic effects from mustard poisoning is a grave prognostic sign (9). Respiratory failure, bone marrow suppression, or superimposed bacterial infection are the most common causes of death from sulfur mustard poisoning (1,2).

The clinical manifestations of lewisite poisoning are similar to those of sulfur mustard, although lewisite causes immediate severe pain on contact with the skin, eyes, and nasal mucosa. Vapor condensing on the skin causes erythema within 30 minutes and blister formation within 2 to 3 hours (9). The eyes are very sensitive to lewisite, and permanent blindness from corneal destruction may result if decontamination is not initiated within 1 minute. Inhalation of lewisite vapor can result in death within 10 minutes from rapid respiratory mucosal sloughing and bleeding, leading to asphyxiation.

Nerve Agents. Clinical manifestations of nerve agent exposure are described in detail in Chapter 23. Toxicity may occur after inhalation of vapor, skin contact with vapor or liquid, or ingestion. The rate of onset and severity of effects are determined by the route of exposure and dose (9). At high ambient temperature, skin absorption is rapid and increasing amounts of the agent are volatilized, leading to increased inhalation (9). Small amounts of vapor cause miosis, rhinorrhea, mild dyspnea, cough, and wheezing (9). This can occur within seconds to minutes. Symptoms include eye pain, blurred and dim vision, headache, and dizziness (6). As the dose of vapor increases, nausea and vomiting, increased respiratory difficulty, progressive muscular weakness, and agitation develop. A high vapor concentration causes rapid loss of consciousness, seizures, flaccid paralysis, and respiratory arrest within seconds to minutes. Following sarin vapor exposure in the Tokyo incident, the most common manifestations were miosis (99%), headache (75%), dyspnea (63%), nausea (60%), eye pain (45%), blurred vision (40%), and vomiting (37%) (6). Tachycardia and hypertension were common, but bradycardia and bronchorrhea were not. Electrocardiographic manifestations include supraventricular and ventricular dysrhythmias, ischemic ST-T changes, atrioventricular conduction disturbances, and QTc interval prolongation (5). Seizures may be single and brief or multiple and persistent; status epilepticus will often occur in severely poisoned patients (5,6). Death is primarily a result of depression of the central respiratory drive (5,9). Respirations cease before significant neuromuscular blockade or bronchoconstriction occurs.

Victims of vapor exposure are unlikely to deteriorate once removed from exposure (6). In contrast, those with dermal exposure may subsequently worsen. Skin absorption of a lethal dose may occur within 1 to 2 minutes, yet symptoms are commonly delayed and develop after a latency period of 30 minutes to 18 hours (2,5,9). Skin exposure may produce local sweating and twitching or fasciculations before systemic toxicity (5,9). Conversely, serious effects may also occur abruptly, without antecedent local or mild symptoms after dermal exposure (5). In contrast to vapor exposure, miosis is absent early following skin exposure. Miosis may be present for weeks after exposure and is not readily responsive to systemic treatment (5).

Lacrimating Agents. Within seconds to minutes of exposure, lacrimating agents cause intense eye discomfort, blepharospasm, lacrimation, stinging and burning of the mouth and nose, salivation, rhinorrhea, irritation of the respiratory tract and stomach with coughing and vomiting, and skin irritation leading to burning pain and erythema (9). Because they are miscible in sweat, skin irritation is amplified in areas of increased sweat, such as the axilla, buttocks, and popliteal, antecubital, and inguinal regions. Skin effects increase with concentrated liquid spray or aerosol exposures, in warm, moist environments, and in those with pre-existing skin conditions. Toxic effects following exposure to tear agents typically resolve within 20 to 30 minutes (9). High-concentration, enclosed-space exposures, however, may result in significant respiratory effects that include acute laryngotracheobronchitis, pulmonary edema, and death. Pulmonary edema can be delayed 4 to 8 hours; peak effects should be evident by 12 hours.

Prolonged or repeated exposures to lacrimating agents may produce malaise, skin blistering, chest tightness, coughing, wheezing, hemoptysis, shortness of breath, and a feeling of suffocation. Reactive airways dysfunction and allergic contact dermatitis have been described in sensitized individuals. A severe dermatitis, labeled Hunan hand syndrome, has been described after prolonged skin exposure to capsaicin.

Incapacitating Agents. Manifestations of 3-quinuclidinyl benzilate (BZ) and fentanyl derivative poisoning are described in detail in Chapter 49 and Chapter 10, respectively. BZ poisoning may occur after inhalation of vapor or liquid aerosol, intravenous or intramuscular injection, or, to a small degree, skin contact with liquid. Following exposure by all routes (except skin), the onset of effects takes 1 hour, peaks at 8 hours, and gradually subsides over 24 to 72 hours (9). Effects may be delayed up to 24 hours after dermal exposure. Doubling the dose produces incapacitation within 1 hour and prolongs recovery an additional 48 hours. Wide variability in the onset, severity, and duration of effects should occur after BZ deployment by aerosol or vapor (9). The rate of onset and duration of clinical effects after inhalation of aerosolized fentanyl derivatives has not been fully elucidated (8). The gas mixture utilized in the Moscow hostage crisis produced effects within 15 minutes of exposure; toxicity lasted days in some survivors (8).

DIFFERENTIAL DIAGNOSIS

Deliberate release of chemicals by terrorists is likely to involve substances that cannot be immediately identified. Thus, the diagnosis is likely to be made by history, physical examination, and initial diagnostic testing (4,10). Diagnosis is also strongly suggested by the complete reversal of toxic effects following empiric antidotal therapy (6,8,10).

Chemical warfare agent (CWA) poisoning should be suspected when a group of patients present with the abrupt onset of a similar constellation of signs or symptoms, particularly if they involve the exposed mucosal or skin surfaces, the respiratory tract, or sudden systemic effects (4,10). Following a chemical attack, clinical effects will occur within minutes to hours, and large numbers of symptomatic patients will present to medical facilities within a short period of time (3,4,10). In contrast, following a bioagent attack, clinical effects are delayed as a result of the incubation period of the illness (see Chapter 56) (4,10). After several days, patients will present insidiously, often with nonspecific signs and symptoms. It is often difficult to identify the release site of the weapon, and the geographic distribution of patients may be wide by the time symptomatic disease develops.

Irritant or corrosive gas inhalation, hydrocarbon aspiration, and vesicating agent and high-dose lacrimating agent exposures may produce pulmonary signs and symptoms similar to those caused by choking agents. Exacerbations of asthma, chronic obstructive pulmonary disease, and allergic or infectious pneumonitis may present similarly. The vesiculobullous skin lesions that result from vesicating agents are most pronounced on exposed skin but may mimic those resulting from Stevens-Johnson syndrome, toxic epidermal necrolysis, pemphigus vulgaris, bullous pemphigoid, scalded skin syndrome, thermal and chemical burns, and hypersensitivity reactions. Nerve-agent poisoning is nearly identical to organophosphate and carbamate pesticide poisoning. Other agents and conditions that can produce similar clinical effects are botulism; nicotine; cholinergic drugs such as bethanechol, carbachol, edrophonium, methacholine, neostigmine, pilocarpine, physostigmine, pyridostigmine, and succinylcholine; and muscarine-containing mushrooms.

Nerve-agent, cyanide, or fentanyl-derivative exposure should be suspected if victims become comatose within minutes of exposure (4,9,10). Although the presence of coma, miosis, and respiratory depression is likely following exposure to both opioid and nerve agents, the additional presence of a seizure, fasciculations, and/or cholinergic findings strongly suggest intoxication with a nerve agent (10). Although a seizure may be present following exposure to both cyanide and nerve agents, the presence of intractable hypotension and acidemia despite adequate oxygenation suggests severe cyanide toxicity (4,9,10). BZ will produce effects identical to other anticholinergic agents (9). In the absence of history, unintentional atropine poisoning following use of a nerve-agent autoinjector cannot be differentiated from BZ toxicity. Lacrimating agents cause effects similar to those of irritant gas and lewisite exposure. Anxiety and hysterical reactions must also be considered in the differential diagnosis of patients exposed to warfare agents.

ED EVALUATION

An attempt should be made to document the amount, time, nature, and duration of exposure. The color and odor of the toxic agent may provide clues to its identity. The time of onset, nature, progression, and severity of symptoms should be noted. Ideally, all patients should have continuous cardiac and oxygen saturation monitoring, but priority must be given to the most severely affected patients in mass-casualty situations.

Physical examination should first focus on vital signs and an assessment of neuromuscular and cardiopulmonary function and then on the eyes, skin, and GI tract. If time allows, patients with eye symptoms should have fluorescein and slit-lamp examinations. If signs and symptoms of cyanide, choking, vesicating, or lacrimating agent toxicity are present, ancillary studies should include a chest radiograph, electrocardiogram (ECG), and arterial blood gas analysis, depending on the severity of symptoms. Additional laboratory evaluation after exposure to cyanide or a vesicating agent should include baseline complete blood count and serum electrolyte, blood urea nitrogen, creatinine, and glucose levels. Measurements of whole blood or plasma cyanide confirm cyanide poisoning but are rarely readily available. High blood lactate concentrations, a large anion gap metabolic acidosis, and high venous blood oxygen content suggest cyanide poisoning.

Patients with signs and symptoms of nerve agent toxicity should have a chest radiograph, ECG, arterial blood gas analysis, routine admission laboratory studies, and measurement of peak expiratory flow rate and plasma or red blood cell cholinesterase activity (see Chapter 23). Cholinesterase activity, however, will not be available in time to be useful in making treatment decisions, and it does not always correlate with the severity of disease (9,10). In the Tokyo sarin attack, 27% of patients with clinical manifestations of moderate poisoning had plasma cholinesterase levels in the normal range (6).

Routine toxicology testing will not identify CWAs. The diagnosis of CWA poisoning is confirmed by detecting chemical agents and their degradation products or cellular macromolecule adducts in environmental or body fluid samples. Unambiguous identification of CWAs should utilize gas or liquid chromatography in combination with mass spectrometry (GC or LC/MS). Rapid-detection kits may soon become available for clinical use.

ED MANAGEMENT

In the event of a chemical weapon attack, emergency field personnel will ideally be responsible for performing on-scene triage, decontamination, and initial treatment prior to patient transport. Although the nature of the exposure may not be immediately known, the release site of the weapon ("hot zone") is quickly discoverable and should be cordoned off. Emergency field personnel should wear appropriate personal protective equipment (PPE) until patients can be decontaminated and the threat of secondary exposure is no longer present. If the hazardous substance is unknown, this consists of an encapsulated, vapor-impermeable, and chemical-resistant suit; chemical-resistant gloves and boots; and a positive-pressure, self-contained breathing apparatus (level A PPE) (1,3,4,10). The importance of first-responder personal protection was illustrated in the Matsumoto and Tokyo sarin gas attacks in which 10% to 35% of rescuers developed mild toxicity (6). In each incident, patients were not decontaminated, and rescuers wore standard work clothing without respiratory protection. Mouth-to-mouth rescue breathing should be avoided as 10% of inhaled nerve agents are expired and could result in rescuer toxicity.

Initial management of victims includes establishing and maintaining the airway, breathing, and circulation, and gross decontamination (brushing off chemical powder, removal of clothing and jewelry, and removal of the patient from the contaminated environment). Rapid dermal decontamination is critical following exposure to the liquid or aerosolized formulations but less important following vapor exposure (3). Patient decontamination was inadequate in the Tokyo sarin gas exposure (vapor), yet secondary injury to hospital staff was minimal and did not necessitate treatment (6). Clothing should be removed and discarded in impervious plastic bags, particularly leather items (e.g., shoes, watchbands), which can absorb chemicals and act as depots. Clothing removal eliminates 85% to 90% of a contamination hazard (4,5,10). If time allows, skin should be decontaminated with a triple wash, which includes initial irrigation with tepid water, followed by 0.5% hypochlorite solution (household bleach diluted 1:10 with water) or alkaline soap, and then repeated, thorough water rinsing (3,9,10). The wastewater should be collected and isolated, if possible. If exposed, the eyes should be irrigated with copious amounts of water or saline. A topical anesthetic may be used, if available. For inhalation exposure, initial treatment includes administration of 100% humidified oxygen, assisted ventilation, as necessary, and removal from the vapor source.

Police, fire department, emergency medical, and HAZMAT (hazardous materials) personnel should inform hospital personnel of the nature and magnitude of exposure, the number and severity of casualties, and the manifestations of illness. On recognition of a mass-casualty incident, emergency physicians must implement the hospital disaster plan and establish a well-demarcated decontamination area outside the emergency department for patients that arrive without prior decontamination (3,10). Emergency department personnel treating a patient exposed to an unknown chemical agent should wear a chemical-resistant suit, gloves, and boots and an external self-contained breathing apparatus (SCBA) or positive-pressure supplied air respirator (level B PPE) until the threat of secondary exposure is cleared (1,3,10).

Choking Agents. Treatment of choking agent poisoning consists of copious irrigation of exposed skin and eyes, humidified oxygen, β-adrenergic agonist bronchodilators, ventilatory support, intravenous crystalloids for hypotension, and antibiotic administration for secondary infection (9). Nebulized 2% sodium bicarbonate may provide symptomatic relief following acute chlorine gas exposure (4,10). Although frequently recommended for chlorine and phosgene exposure, corticosteroids have no proven benefit. Animal studies suggest that tomelukast, a leukotriene-receptor antagonist, and N-acetylcysteine, an antioxidant and glutathione substitute, may limit the development of pulmonary edema following phosgene exposure.

Vesicating Agents. Because of rapid and irreversible binding to tissues, immediate decontamination is the best form of treatment for mustard agent exposure (2,9,10). Exposure to tissue or vesicle fluid will not produce secondary injury to healthcare personnel (1). The recommended method of decontamination is to wash with standard 5% household bleach, diluted 1:10, or copious amounts of soap and water (2). Water alone is ineffective, as mustard is relatively water-insoluble. Bleach produces "free" chlorine, which inactivates the mustard compound. Dry decontamination can be performed by applying absorbent powders (flour, baking soda [sodium bicarbonate], talcum powder, activated charcoal, or Fuller's earth) to the skin and wiping off with moist paper towels (2). Skin can also be decontaminated by irrigating with 10% sodium thiosulfate. Copious water or saline irrigation is the favored method for ocular decontamination.

Treatment is otherwise supportive. Skin burns should be treated with topical antibiotics such as silver sulfadiazine. Blisters and necrotic skin should be débrided. Ocular injury requires urgent ophthalmologic consultation. Treatment may include topical anesthetics, antibiotic ointment to prevent infection, and mydriatic or cycloplegic medication to prevent adhesions between iris and cornea (2,9,10). Respiratory care is the same as for choking agents.

Potential antidotes for sulfur mustard poisoning include mustard scavengers (glutathione, N-acetylcysteine, thiosulfate), antioxidants (vitamin E), NAD^+-level stabilizers (niacin and nicotinamide), anti-inflammatory drugs (corticosteroids, indomethacin), and nitric oxide synthase inhibitors (L-nitroarginine methyl ester) (9). Bone-marrow suppression may respond to granulocyte-colony-stimulating factor.

Treatment of lewisite exposure involves washing the skin with water, soap and water, solutions of dilute chlorine bleach (0.5%), or baking soda (sodium bicarbonate) (9). Dry decontamination may also be efficacious. Neither scrubbing nor hot water is appropriate, because both enhance lewisite absorption and toxicity. Blisters, shown to contain arsenic, should be opened and drained of fluid. Other treatment is identical to that of thermal burns.

Historically, systemic lewisite poisoning has been treated by intramuscular British antilewisite (BAL, 2,3-dimercapto-propanol, or dimercaprol), an arsenic chelator antidote, along with supportive care (see Chapter 31). BAL has also been used topically as a 5% ointment for skin lesions and as a 5% to 10% oil solution for ocular symptoms. Newer, less toxic dithiol analogs of BAL, meso-dimercaptosuccinic acid (DMSA, marketed as Succimer or Chemet), and 2,3-dimercapto-1-propansulfonic acid (DMPS) can be given orally (DMSA) or intravenously (DMPS) and have equal efficacy (see Chapters 31 and 41).

Nerve Agents.   Self-protection minimally involves a well-sealed respirator with a charcoal filter and heavy butyl rubber gloves (10). Victims of vapor exposure pose little threat to hospital personnel once clothing has been removed. Patients with liquid contamination of skin and clothing, however, pose a significant vapor and skin contact risk to rescuers (9). Skin should be decontaminated with a triple wash—irrigation with tepid water, followed by 0.5% hypochlorite solution or alkaline soap, and repeated, thorough water rinsing (3,9,10). U.S. military decontamination kits contain towelettes impregnated with a hypochlorite solution. Scrubbing should be avoided because abrading the skin can increase absorption. Water alone will not hydrolyze nerve agents, but it will dilute them. Eye decontamination involves copious saline irrigation. Hypochlorite should not be used in the eye.

Intubation, mechanical ventilation, and the use of muscarinic antagonists (e.g., atropine), oximes (e.g., pralidoxime), and benzodiazepines (e.g., diazepam) may be necessary. The use of succinylcholine to assist intubation may result in prolonged neuromuscular blockade as a result of nerve agent–induced plasma cholinesterase inhibition. If endotracheal intubation is necessary, a nondepolarizing neuromuscular blocker such as rocuronium (0.6–1.0 mg/kg IV) is recommended. Antidotal therapy is discussed in Chapter 23. Initially, atropine should be administered intravenously at a dose of 2 mg every 3 to 5 minutes (0.02–0.05 mg/kg in children) until respiratory secretions clear, bronchospasm resolves, and ventilation is normal (1,5,10). Heart rate and pupil size are poor endpoints for adequate atropinization (5,6,9,10). U.S. soldiers carry three atropine autoinjectors, each containing 2 mg, for rapid intramuscular self-injection. Cumulative atropine doses of 10 to 20 mg are usually adequate over the first 2 to 3 hours, with little or no therapy required thereafter (6,9). This differs from organophosphate pesticide poisoning, which may require significantly greater amounts of atropine and a longer duration of therapy. In the Tokyo sarin attacks, only 19% of poisoned patients required more than 2 mg of atropine; severely poisoned patients required 1.5 to 15.0 mg of atropine (mean, 6 mg) (6). Topical mydriatic cycloplegic eye drops (e.g., tropicamide) may be used for intractable eye pain as a result of ciliary spasm. Eye drops are not recommended for those patients with miosis as their only ocular finding.

Oxime therapy is recommended for all cases of nerve-agent poisoning. Because nerve agents age extremely rapidly, pralidoxime must be given as soon as possible after exposure to be effective. Initially, 1 to 2 g of pralidoxime should be administered as an intravenous bolus over 10 minutes (20–50 mg/kg in children), followed by a continuous infusion of 500 mg per hour (10–20 mg/kg/hr in children) (1,5,10). Side effects of pralidoxime includes hypertension and tachycardia. U.S. soldiers also carry three pralidoxime autoinjectors, each containing 600 mg of the oxime to be injected intramuscularly along with each atropine injection (9). Pralidoxime is dosed until signs and symptoms of intoxication have resolved (5). In the Tokyo sarin attacks, severely poisoned patients required 1 to 36 g pralidoxime (mean, 11 g) (6).

Seizure control protects against acute lethality and brain pathology (8–10). Seizures should be aggressively treated with high-dose benzodiazepines, such as intravenous diazepam 10 mg (0.2–0.4 mg/kg) or midazolam (0.1–0.3 mg/kg), in addition to standard therapy with an antimuscarinic and oxime agents (5,7,10). Both antimuscarinic agents and benzodiazepines are effective in treating nerve-agent seizures in experimental animals. Trihexyphenidyl and midazolam are the most potent and rapidly acting agents. Military physicians recommend diazepam prophylaxis for all severely exposed victims (9). U.S. soldiers carry 10-mg diazepam autoinjectors for intramuscular use following nerve agent exposure.

Conventional oximes (pralidoxime preparations, obidoxime, trimedoxime) are not clinically useful against soman. Newer H-series oximes (named after their inventor, Inge Hagedorn) are superior in their ability to reactivate unaged soman-inhibited acetylcholinesterase (AChE). They also have direct antimuscarinic and antinicotinic (ganglia-blocking and nondepolarizing neuromuscular-blocking) actions but do not protect from nerve agent–induced seizures (9). HI-6, a bisquaternary pyridinium oxide, is currently the most promising AChE reactivator for the treatment of nerve-agent poisoning; it is effective against all nerve agents and does not result in significant side effects in human studies (9,10). HI-6 is given at an adult dose of 250 to 500 mg IM every 6 hours. Efficacy is enhanced when it is used with atropine. Pretreating those at risk with a reversible AChE inhibitor, such as the carbamates physostigmine or pyridostigmine, is also effective against soman, in which enzyme aging is rapid and pralidoxime alone is unlikely to be effective (9). The intent is to carbamylate or bind 20% to 40% of AChE and limit subsequent nerve-agent binding. Carbamylated cholinesterase then spontaneously reactivates or is regenerated with oxime therapy, leaving the victim with enough AChE to function normally. Pyridostigmine pretreatment does not protect against sarin and VX, in which aging is slower and pralidoxime is effective. During the Persian Gulf war, U.S. soldiers were given pyridostigmine bromide in blister packs containing 21 30-mg tablets (5,9). Pyridostigmine was taken orally every 8 hours without causing impaired performance. Side effects were minimal, but they can mimic those of mild nerve gas poisoning.

Pyridostigmine does not cross the blood-brain barrier and offers no protection from central nervous system (CNS) toxicity. Other promising treatments include human monoclonal antibodies, for passive protection before exposure, and pretreatment with excess cholinesterase, which presumably scavenges the nerve agent.

A dermal topical protective agent containing a 50:50 mixture of perfluoroalkylpolyether and polytetrafluoroethylene has been developed for protection against all CWAs. It is known as *serpacwa* (skin exposure reduction paste against chemical warfare agents) and is applied to the skin of military personnel when chemical-agent exposure is deemed possible (5).

Lacrimating Agents. Treatment of lacrimating agent exposure is frequently unnecessary because effects resolve quickly. Symptomatic patients may require decontamination and supportive care. Healthcare personnel should wear rubber gloves; if contamination is heavy, airway protection may also be necessary. Skin should be washed thoroughly with soap and water or a mild alkaline solution such as 6% sodium bicarbonate or 1% benzalkonium chloride (9). Ambulatory patients can be bathed in a shower. Contact dermatitis may respond to topical corticosteroids and antipruritics. Tearing usually irrigates the eyes adequately, but topical anesthetics and saline irrigation may be helpful. Chemical conjunctivitis may require symptomatic treatment with topical vasoconstrictors. Corneal injuries are treated with cycloplegics, topical antibiotics, and ophthalmologic follow-up. Patients exposed to high concentrations of aerosols, as in enclosed spaces or near exploding tear-gas canisters, should be observed for 12 to 24 hours because of delayed pulmonary effects (9). Treatment of pulmonary toxicity consists of humidified oxygen, bronchodilators, and assisted ventilation, as needed.

Incapacitating Agents. Treatment of incapacitating-agent toxicity includes supportive care and the administration of antidotes. Standard doses of physostigmine (initial dose, 30 to 45 mcg/kg IV) are usually effective in reversing the anticholinergic effects of BZ (see Chapter 49) (9,10). For unclear reasons, however, physostigmine is ineffective if administered during the first 4 to 6 hours after the onset of clinical effects (9). The treatment of fentanyl-derivative poisoning is similar to that for other opioids (see Chapter 10). Because these agents bind with high affinity to opiate receptors, large doses of naloxone may be required for complete reversal of toxic effects. As a result of high lipophilicity, fentanyl derivatives will redistribute from tissue stores to the CNS and likely produce recurrent opioid effects (8). Based on animal studies, antagonist redosing will likely be necessary for a period of 2 to 24 hours (8).

CRITICAL INTERVENTIONS

- Decontaminate victims of CWA exposure by removing and discarding all clothing and washing the skin with copious amounts of soap and water.
- Wear level B PPE (e.g., chemical-resistant suit, gloves, boots, SCBA) when the CWA is unknown.
- Notify local law-enforcement authorities, the Federal Bureau of Investigation, and local or state health departments when CWA poisoning is suspected.
- Activate the hospital disaster plan and establish a decontamination area outside the emergency department for mass casualty incidents.
- Administer oxygen, bronchodilators, and artificial ventilation to patients with respiratory symptoms following choking, vesicating, and lacrimating agent exposure.
- Administer antidotal therapy to victims with cyanide, nerve agent, anticholinergic, and opioid poisoning.

DISPOSITION

Consultation with a regional HAZMAT specialist or experienced military physician is recommended for all CWA poisoning except civilian exposures to the lacrimating agents. Suspected CWA poisoning should prompt an immediate call to local law-enforcement authorities, the local Federal Bureau of Investigation field office, and local or state health department and laboratory. Patients with corneal or skin burns should have follow-up with an ophthalmologist or plastic surgeon.

Asymptomatic patients with choking agent exposure should be observed and monitored for at least 6 hours. Mild to moderately symptomatic patients may be discharged safely after several hours of observation if symptoms have improved or resolved with treatment. Some recommend that patients with a phosgene exposure should be admitted and closely observed because of phosgene's varying latency period and high potential morbidity. Asymptomatic patients with vesicating agent exposure should be observed and monitored for 12 hours. Following exposure to nerve agent vapor, patients with signs and symptoms confined to the eyes may be discharged safely after a short period of observation (6). Those with skin exposure to nerve agents (liquid or aerosolized droplets) should be observed for 24 hours. Victims of lacrimating agents may be treated and released if there is no significant pulmonary toxicity.

All patients with systemic symptoms, pulmonary toxicity, and severe or extensive dermal injury should be hospitalized. As a result of the long duration and recrudescent nature of clinical effects from incapacitating agents, all symptomatic victims should be observed for a minimum of 24 hours. The appropriate level of care will depend on clinical severity.

COMMON PITFALLS

- Failure to protect rescuers and medical personnel from secondary contamination
- Failure to decontaminate victims of chemical agent exposure in a timely fashion
- Failure to appreciate that effects can be delayed and progressive and to observe asymptomatic victims for appropriate periods of time
- Failure to administer antidotes in a timely manner

ICD9

989.9 Toxic effect of unspecific substance, chiefly nonmedicinal as to cause

REFERENCES

1. Borak J, Sidell FR. Agents of chemical warfare: sulfur mustard. *Ann Emerg Med* 1992;21:303–308.
2. Bozeman WP, Dilbero D, Schauben JL. Biologic and chemical weapons of mass destruction. *Emerg Med Clin North Am* 2002;20:975–993.
3. Brennan RJ, Waeckerle JF, Sharp TW, et al. Chemical warfare agents: emergency medical and emergency public health issues. *Ann Emerg Med* 1999;34:191–204.
4. Kales SN, Christiani DC. Acute chemical emergencies. *N Engl J Med* 2004;350:800–808.
5. Leikin JB, Thomas TGH, Walter R, et al. A review of nerve agent exposure for the critical care physician. *Crit Care Med* 2002;30:2346–2354.
6. Okumura T, Takasu N, Ishimatsu S, et al. Report on 640 victims of the Tokyo subway sarin attack. *Ann Emerg Med* 1996;28:129–135.
7. Shih T-M, Duniho SM, McDonough JH. Control of nerve agent-induced seizures is critical for neuroprotection and survival. *Toxicol Appl Pharmacol* 2003;188:69–80.
8. Wax PM, Becker CE, Curry SE. Unexpected "gas" casualties in Moscow: a medical toxicology perspective. *Ann Emerg Med* 2003;41:700–705.
9. Zajtchuk R, Bellamy RD, eds. *Textbook of military medicine: medical aspects of chemical and biological warfare, part I.* Washington, DC: Office of the Surgeon General, US. Department of the Army, 1997.
10. Zilker T. Medical management of incidents with chemical warfare agents. *Toxicology* 2005;214:221–231.

CHAPTER 58

Drug Withdrawal

PRE-HOSPITAL CONSIDERATIONS
- Assess vital signs.
- Assess capillary glucose.

CLINICAL PRESENTATION

The clinical presentation of drug withdrawal varies significantly among patients. Some patients underreport their substance use, although others overreport it. Patients who present with withdrawal symptoms (e.g., seizures) may or may not admit to drug use. Some patients may present with complications of drug abuse, such as pneumonia, endocarditis, and skin abscess, or an unrelated problem, such as a myocardial infarction or motor vehicle accident, and develop withdrawal symptoms while in the emergency department (ED) or after admission. Others present to the ED because they desire detoxification.

Sedative–hypnotic withdrawal may be indistinguishable from ethanol withdrawal except for differences in the time course (Table 58.1). Because many benzodiazepines have a much longer elimination half-life than ethanol and have active metabolites, withdrawal manifestations may be delayed after cessation of drug use. Lorazepam withdrawal may begin within 2 days of the last dose, whereas diazepam withdrawal may require a week or more before the onset of symptoms. More severe withdrawal is associated with high doses or short-acting benzodiazepines (9).

The clinical presentation of sedative–hypnotic withdrawal varies in intensity and duration. Mild withdrawal symptoms include anxiety, apprehension, irritability, dysphoria, and insomnia (9). Other symptoms may include anorexia, nausea, and vomiting. Mild autonomic and central nervous system (CNS) hyperactivity is characterized by tachycardia, hypertension, irritability, and hyperreflexia. Unlike patients with severe withdrawal, patients with mild withdrawal have a clear mental status. Most patients with mild withdrawal recover uneventfully after a few days, but some may develop more serious withdrawal manifestations.

Hallucinations, delusions, myoclonus, seizures, and agitation may appear with more severe withdrawal. Tachycardia, hypertension, tachypnea, hyperthermia, diaphoresis, and mydriasis may develop, as may tachyarrhythmias. At times, a new-onset seizure heralds the onset of sedative–hypnotic withdrawal. These

TABLE 58.1 Withdrawal Syndromes Seen in the Emergency Department

Type of Withdrawal	Onset of Symptoms
Ethanol	6–8 hr
Sedative-hypnotic (e.g., benzodiazepines, barbiturates)	3–7 d (long-acting drugs)
GHB	Hours to days
Baclofen	12–72 hr
Opioids	4–8 hr (heroin); 36–72 hr (methadone)
Cocaine	Within hours after binge
Antidepressants	Few days

patients may or may not have tremulousness and other sympathetic hyperactivity before seizure activity begins. Seizures tend to be generalized and tonic–clonic. They may occur singly or as a brief flurry with a normal sensorium between seizures. Status epilepticus is rare. Severe withdrawal symptoms, including seizures, may occur after the administration of flumazenil to patients chronically taking benzodiazepines. Withdrawal symptoms from long-acting benzodiazepines may persist for 3 weeks.

Withdrawal from γ-hydroxybutyrate (GHB), or its congeners γ-butyrolactone (GBL) or 1,4-butanediol, may also produce severe withdrawal manifestations (10). Frequent users ingest GHB multiple times per day. Autonomic and CNS abnormalities are the most common effects seen with GHB withdrawal. Initial symptoms may include anxiety and tremor. More severe GHB withdrawal is characterized by severe agitation, which may require physical restraints. Great variability in initial clinical presentation have even been reported in chronic users. Tachycardia, hypertension, insomnia, auditory and visual hallucinations, and delirium are the most common symptoms seen. The onset of symptoms may appear shortly after GHB intoxication clears, as early as 1 to 6 hours after the last dose, and the symptoms may persist for as long as 5 to 15 days. Few deaths from GHB withdrawal have been reported.

Withdrawal from oral or intrathecal baclofen may also be quite problematic (1). Withdrawal symptoms generally start 12 to 72 hours after the last dose. Typical symptoms of withdrawal include sleeplessness, confusion, agitation, hallucinations, delusions, hyperthermia, and hypertonia. Interestingly, seizures may occur in the setting of either baclofen toxicity or withdrawal. Abrupt withdrawal from intrathecal baclofen therapy, sometimes precipitated by unrecognized baclofen pump failure, may cause similar symptoms and may be life-threatening (4). In some cases, there is profound muscle rigidity resembling neuroleptic malignant syndrome or malignant hyperthermia.

Symptoms of mild opioid withdrawal include lacrimation, rhinorrhea, yawning, diaphoresis, anxiety, restlessness, and dysphoria. Piloerection is particularly characteristic. The patient may exhibit mild elevations in pulse, blood pressure, and respiratory rate, but these changes are usually not significant. More severe opioid withdrawal is characterized by vomiting, diarrhea, abdominal pain, and dehydration. Unlike sedative–hypnotic withdrawal, severe agitation, seizures (except in neonatal withdrawal), mental status changes, and hyperthermia are not seen with opioid withdrawal.

The severity and time course of the opioid withdrawal syndrome depends on the pharmacokinetics of the opioid. Shorter-acting agents (e.g., heroin) tend to have a more intense course than longer-acting agents (e.g., methadone). Heroin withdrawal usually begins within 4 to 8 hours after the last dose, peaking by 36 to 72 hours. In contrast, the onset of methadone withdrawal may be 36 to 72 hours after the last dose, and symptoms may persist for up to 2 weeks (8). At comparable doses, the severity and duration of withdrawal from injecting heroin appears greater than that from smoking heroin.

The sudden onset of opioid withdrawal may occur after an opioid antagonist such as naloxone is given to an unsuspected opioid-dependent patient. As a result of naloxone's short half-life, withdrawal symptoms do not usually persist beyond 20 to 60 minutes. Treatment with additional opioid to reverse these short-lived effects is not indicated. Giving opioids with agonist–antagonist properties, such as pentazocine (Talwin), nalbuphine (Nubain), and butorphanol (Stadol), to the opioid-dependent patient may also precipitate withdrawal symptoms. Opioid withdrawal from the long-acting opioid antagonists naltrexone and nalmefene may result in a markedly prolonged withdrawal period lasting upward of 1 to 2 days. Because the mixed agonist–antagonist buprenorphine is thought to cause a much less severe withdrawal syndrome, if any at all, it is increasingly used to treat opioid withdrawal.

Antidepressant withdrawal may result in anxiety, insomnia, lethargy, nausea, vomiting, headache, problems with balance, sensory abnormalities, and possibly aggressive and impulsive behavior. In most cases, these symptoms are mild and transient (5). Withdrawal from cocaine may result in lethargy, dysphoria, and depression.

DIFFERENTIAL DIAGNOSIS

The differential diagnosis of the withdrawal state is broad and includes many other serious conditions that may require different therapy (Table 58.2). Because drug-dependent patients are particularly prone to develop many of these conditions, careful exclusion of other etiologies is critically important. Examination of the skin, abdomen, eyes, and pulse rate may help to distinguish an anticholinergic toxidrome (dry skin, decreased bowel sounds, urinary retention, mydriasis, tachycardia) from a sympathomimetic toxidrome (moist skin, normal bowel sounds, no urinary retention, mydriasis, tachycardia).

Sedative–hypnotic withdrawal may be particularly difficult to distinguish from an underlying anxiety disorder. Differentiating withdrawal seizures from other

TABLE 58.2 Differential Diagnosis of Major Withdrawal Symptoms

Tremor	Seizures	Hallucinations	Delirium
Withdrawal	**Withdrawal**	**Withdrawal**	**Withdrawal**
Ethanol	Ethanol	Ethanol	Ethanol
Sedative– hypnotics	Sedative– hypnotics	Sedative– hypnotics	Sedative– hypnotics
Intoxications	**Intoxications**	**Intoxications**	**Intoxications**
Theophylline	Cocaine	LSD	Cocaine
Caffeine	Anticholinergics	Mescaline	Amphetamine
B-Agonists	Phenothiazines	Mushrooms	Phencyclidine
Mercury	TCAs	Peyote	Anticholinergics
Lithium	Theophylline	Phencyclidine	LSD
TCAs	Camphor	Anticholinergics	**Infectious**
Phenytoin	Isoniazid	Ergot	Meningitis
Metabolic	Phencyclidine	Nutmeg	Encephalitis
Hypoglycemia	Lidocaine	**Infectious**	Sepsis
Thyrotoxicosis	Organophosphates	Meningitis	**Metabolic**
Structural	**Infectious**	Encephalitis	Thyrotoxicosis
Cerebellar disease	Meningitis	Sepsis	Hypoglycemia
Other	Encephalitis	**Metabolic**	Hyperglycemia
Parkinsonism	**Metabolic**	Hypoglycemia	Hypocalcemia
	Hypoglycemia	Hypoxia	Hypoxia
	Hypoxia	**Structural**	Thiamine deficiency
	Hypothyroidism	CNS hemorrhage	**Structural**
	Thyrotoxicosis	Tumor	Head trauma
	Hypocalcemia	**Psychiatric**	CNS hemorrhage
	Hyperosmolar state	Schizophrenia	Tumor
	Hepatic failure	Bipolar disorder	Psychiatric
	Uremia	**Other**	**Other**
	Structural	Seizures	Seizures
	Head trauma	Heat-related illness	Heat-related illness
	CNS hemorrhage		
	Tumor		
	CVA		
	Other		
	Idiopathic epilepsy		
	Posttraumatic epilepsy		
	Degenerative disease		

LSD, lysergic acid diethylamide; CNS, central nervous system.

types of seizures may also be difficult. Other common causes include pre-existing idiopathic epilepsy, posttraumatic epilepsy, and other complications of drug abuse (e.g., hypoglycemia, hypomagnesemia, hyponatremia, head trauma). Poor anticonvulsant compliance with underlying seizure disorders may add to the diagnostic confusion. In the setting of baclofen use, a seizure could result from either overdose or withdrawal.

Opioid withdrawal must be distinguished from ethanol and other sedative–hypnotic withdrawal because of the significant differences in therapy. Symptoms of significant sedative–hypnotic withdrawal, such as confusion, agitation, and seizures, are not generally seen with opioid withdrawal; opioid withdrawal symptoms such as piloerection, yawning, lacrimation, and rhinorrhea are not seen with ethanol and sedative–hypnotic withdrawal. Some patients, however, may be withdrawing from both substances. Gastrointestinal (GI) manifestations of opioid withdrawal must be differentiated from other causes of gastroenteritis.

ED EVALUATION

Patients presenting with drug withdrawal require a comprehensive assessment. Patients initially should have cardiac monitoring and a fingerstick glucose and oxygen saturation analysis. The physician should obtain a complete history of substance abuse, previous withdrawal episodes, and all current and former medications. If possible, family, friends, and prehospital personnel are interviewed to gain additional information.

Physical examination should focus on vital signs, including rectal temperature; cardiovascular, neurological, and pulmonary systems; the skin; the abdomen; and the eyes. Close attention should be directed to any stigmata of chronic liver disease or evidence of intravenous (IV) drug use. There should be assessment for obvious and occult traumatic injury and complications of drug abuse, such as pneumonia, skin abscesses, bacterial endocarditis, acquired immunodeficiency syndrome, pancreatitis, liver disease, and GI bleeding.

Laboratory studies should include a complete blood count; electrolytes, glucose, blood urea nitrogen, and creatinine levels; liver function tests; coagulation profile; and ethanol level. A urine drug screen may be positive or negative for the offending agent. Rapid urine drug screens may not detect synthetic opioids such as methadone or propoxyphene. In patients with significant agitation, a creatine phosphokinase determination may detect rhabdomyolysis.

An elevated temperature requires a full sepsis workup, including urine and blood cultures, chest radiograph, and, often, a lumbar puncture. Obtaining a head computed tomography (CT) scan before lumbar puncture is critical in patients presenting with either focal neurologic deficits or high risk for intracranial hemorrhage. Patients with a first-time seizure in the setting of withdrawal should be evaluated in the same manner as any other patient with a new seizure. Subsequent withdrawal seizures do not necessarily require extensive re-evaluation.

ED MANAGEMENT

Drug withdrawal syndromes, particularly sedative–hypnotic withdrawal, must be recognized and treated in a timely fashion because early treatment can prevent withdrawal from progressing to a more serious stage. A successful treatment strategy must address several basic goals: alleviating symptoms, preventing progression, avoiding complications, and recognizing and treating coexisting medical problems. Planning for long-term rehabilitation and drug independence is usually better done as part of inpatient management.

Initial treatment should be directed at readily correctable causes of altered mental status. Oxygen should be given if the oxygen saturation is low, and an IV line should be established. Glucose and thiamine should be administered if there is evidence of hypoglycemia and malnutrition respectively. Volume resuscitation is often necessary, particularly in patients with severe withdrawal manifestations and dehydration.

Significantly agitated patients may initially need to be physically restrained to prevent injury, establish IV access, and facilitate sedation. Soft restraints should be used. Prolonged use of restraints is discouraged, because continued struggling against them may lead to rhabdomyolysis, hyperthermia, and metabolic acidosis. Once IV access is obtained and chemical sedation has achieved behavioral control, physical restraints should be discontinued.

Achieving adequate sedation is the cornerstone of successful treatment of sedative–hypnotic withdrawal. It may prevent progression to a severe agitated delirium state with its attendant complications. Reinstitution of therapy with the withdrawn drug or a cross-tolerant one is required for proper sedation. Many agents have been used over the years, but benzodiazepines have proven to be the most effective. Compared with other sedative–hypnotic agents, benzodiazepines are safer and produce less respiratory depression. Their dosage is easier to titrate, and the effects are more predictable.

Diazepam (Valium), chlordiazepoxide (Librium), and lorazepam (Ativan) are the most commonly used agents for ethanol withdrawal and can also be used for sedative–hypnotic withdrawal. These agents are eliminated over several days and are preferred over benzodiazepines with shorter half-lives. Compared with short-acting agents, long-acting agents may be more effective in preventing withdrawal seizures and contribute to smoother withdrawal with fewer rebound symptoms. Active metabolites of diazepam and chlordiazepoxide prolong their therapeutic effect. In elderly patients and those with hepatic dysfunction, lorazepam, which has no active metabolites, may be preferred. In other cases, lorazepam does not appear to offer any distinct advantage over diazepam or chlordiazepoxide.

IV dosing is preferred in all but the mildest cases of sedative–hypnotic withdrawal. Agitation may preclude oral administration, and GI dysfunction may impair drug absorption. IV therapy can be readily titrated. Lorazepam (but not diazepam or chlordiazepoxide) is predictably absorbed intramuscularly and may be useful in the wildly agitated patient before IV access is established.

The dose of benzodiazepines required to achieve proper sedation must be individualized and varies considerably, depending on the patient's tolerance to the drug. Symptom-triggered therapy is as efficacious as fixed-schedule therapy and decreases both the amount of benzodiazepine used and treatment duration (2). Frequent IV boluses should be given until the patient has achieved a restful state. Diazepam, 5 to 20 mg, can be given every 5 to 15 minutes until the patient is sleepy but arousable. Usually, sedation is obtained before respiratory depression develops, but close airway observation is always required.

Failure to obtain immediate sedation need not prompt switching to an alternative agent. Mixing different drugs or different routes of administration may increase the risk of adverse effects, particularly respiratory depression. However, if a patient does not respond completely to the chosen benzodiazepine, the use of another cross-tolerant agent may be valuable. Intermediate-acting or long-acting barbiturates such as pentobarbital, secobarbital, or phenobarbital are recommended in these situations. Doses of 100 mg of pentobarbital may be given intravenously every 5 to 10 minutes until sufficient sedation is achieved or a total dose of 600 mg is given.

Phenobarbital may also be used, although its onset of action may be delayed. Phenobarbital's long duration of effect, however, requires less frequent dosing and allows gradual self-tapering. Phenobarbital may be particularly helpful in withdrawal patients with idiopathic or posttraumatic epilepsy who require maintenance anticonvulsant levels. With GHB and GBL withdrawal, pentobarbital has been used with reported quicker resolution of symptoms, especially in patients with benzodiazepine-resistant withdrawal. The barbiturates are more likely to cause excessive sedation and respiratory depression.

The use of midazolam (a short-acting benzodiazepine) by continuous IV infusion has been suggested. This approach, however, requires more vigilant monitoring, especially in the patient who is not intubated, and does not provide the advantages of a long-acting agent. Propofol boluses (20 mg/dose) and infusions have also been used for refractory delirium tremens in ethanol withdrawal and should be also considered for refractory sedative–hypnotic withdrawal (7).

Withdrawal seizures should also be treated with benzodiazepines or barbiturates. Phenytoin is ineffective in treating or preventing withdrawal seizures. It should be reserved for patients with a history of an underlying chronic seizure disorder who require maintenance phenytoin therapy.

Neuroleptics such as the phenothiazines and butyrophenones (e.g., haloperidol) should not be used alone for sedative–hypnotic withdrawal. Although used for severe agitation, these neuroleptics are not cross-tolerant with ethanol or sedative–hypnotics, do not prevent or suppress withdrawal, and may result in hypotension, impaired thermoregulation, a lowered seizure threshold, and dystonic reactions. Uncontrolled clinical experience suggests that neuroleptics may be considered as adjunctive therapy for patients with refractory agitation and hallucinations and may also be useful in treating concomitant nausea, vomiting, and GI cramps.

Sympatholytic therapy with β-blockers (e.g., propranolol) and central adrenergic agonists (e.g., clonidine) has been used for sedative–hypnotic withdrawal, but these have certain disadvantages. Sympatholytics are not cross-tolerant with sedative–hypnotics and do not prevent agitation, confusion, or seizures. Moreover, their ability to normalize vital signs may mask a deteriorating clinical situation.

Once withdrawal is controlled, the dose of sedative–hypnotic should be gradually reduced over a period of 3 weeks to 3 months, depending on the dosage and duration of prior use. To avoid precipitating another episode of withdrawal, the dose should generally be tapered by no more than 10% a day, or 25% every 3 days.

The approach to GHB withdrawal is similar to that for other sedative–hypnotic withdrawal. Severe cases are often resistant to benzodiazepine treatment and require barbiturates or propofol. Neuroleptics should be avoided if possible (10).

Reinstitution of baclofen is the initial step in the management of baclofen withdrawal. For patients exhibiting symptoms and signs of more significant withdrawal, high-dose IV benzodiazepine treatment in addition to resumption of baclofen may be required (1). For patients refractory to benzodiazepines, dantrolene (for muscle relaxation) and cyproheptadine have also been recommended, although this approach has not been subjected to clinical trials.

For acute opioid withdrawal, clonidine may offer symptomatic relief because it decreases sympathetic activity in the locus ceruleus (8). An initial oral dose of 0.1 to 0.2 mg is recommended. Because hypotension may be particularly problematic after the first dose, the blood pressure should be monitored for 2 hours while the patient remains in the ED. A dose of 0.1 to 0.2 mg every 4 to 6 hours may help prevent recurrence of opioid-withdrawal symptoms. Nonspecific sedation with benzodiazepines can decrease anxiety and is also an option.

For patients who will be hospitalized with other medical problems, methadone may be given to relieve the symptoms of significant opioid withdrawal. A dose of 5 to 25 mg intramuscularly or orally blocks most manifestations of physiologic withdrawal. Parenteral administration guarantees absorption in the vomiting patient. Symptomatic improvement usually occurs within 30 to 60 minutes. Daily maintenance doses average 50 mg and range from 25 to more than 150 mg. Shorter-acting opioids such as morphine or meperidine are not recommended.

The implementation of a detoxification program is generally not initiated in the ED and requires referral to an appropriate facility. Federal regulations restrict the use of methadone to Food and Drug Administration–designated programs. Although this legislation does not prohibit the use of methadone in opioid addicts who are admitted for other reasons, unless the facility has an approved treatment program, the use of methadone solely for the treatment of opioid withdrawal is prohibited. Similarly, legislation prohibits prescribing methadone for the outpatient treatment of withdrawal without a specific license.

Buprenorphine, a partial μ-opioid agonist, has recently been approved for treatment of opioid dependence (3). Similar to methadone, buprenorphine suppresses opioid withdrawal symptoms and decreases use of illicit drugs. It is used both to manage heroin withdrawal and detoxification as well as to prevent relapse in maintenance therapy. Studies have suggested it is more effective than clonidine in reducing signs and symptoms of opioid withdrawal. Buprenorphine appears to have a ceiling effect on respiratory depression at low doses, although respiratory depression and deaths from buprenorphine have been reported. Special credentialing is required to use buprenorphine in the treatment of opioid detoxification.

Rapid and ultrarapid opioid detoxifications for inpatients followed by naltrexone maintenance therapy have also been used in recent years (6). These controversial techniques utilize antagonist-precipitated opioid withdrawal as a quick "cure" for opioid dependence. Complications include persistent withdrawal symptoms, pulmonary edema, and death.

Reinstitution of drug therapy and gradual tapering of the dose is recommended for antidepressant withdrawal. Benzodiazepines can be used for signs and symptoms of adrenergic hyperactivity. The treatment of cocaine withdrawal is supportive.

CRITICAL INTERVENTIONS

- Administer diazepam or other long-acting benzodiazepine to patients with sedative–hypnotic withdrawal, adding barbiturates or propofol for refractory cases.
- Administer clonidine and benzodiazepines if necessary to patients with opioid withdrawal.
- Administer methadone to patients with opioid withdrawal who require admission for other conditions.

DISPOSITION

Patients with moderate-to-severe sedative-hypnotic withdrawal should be admitted. Because withdrawal usually persists for several days, admitted patients should be closely monitored for signs of progression and treated as necessary. The level of care necessary depends on clinical severity. Because of potential complications, patients requiring IV sedation are best managed in an intensive or intermediate care unit. Patients with less severe withdrawal may be managed and observed on a medical floor, psychiatric floor, hospital-based detoxification unit, or detoxification unit outside of the hospital. Patients with mild withdrawal may also need to be admitted for the evaluation and treatment of concomitant medical problems that have not been adequately addressed. The inpatient setting also provides a protected environment away from the temptations of illicit drug use.

Outpatient management should be attempted only if the patient can be discharged home with a supportive family member or friend and appropriate outpatient follow-up can be arranged. Supervised withdrawal in the home setting, under the direction of a visiting nurse, may be appropriate in some of these circumstances.

Patients who present to the ED with opiate withdrawal may be discharged home if they do not have other concomitant medical problems that require hospital admission and they can tolerate oral fluids. Offering the patient a limited supply of clonidine (if tolerated in the ED) may help prevent further withdrawal symptoms. Prescriptions for opioids should not be given. Referral to a detoxification program is strongly recommended.

Social service, detoxification, or substance-abuse counseling and psychiatric referrals should be offered to all patients with a history of substance abuse.

COMMON PITFALLS

- Failure to consider the possibility of drug withdrawal in patients with signs and symptoms of adrenergic hyperactivity
- Failure to appreciate that sedative–hypnotic withdrawal is potentially life-threatening, whereas opioid withdrawal, although uncomfortable, does not cause significant morbidity
- Failure to appreciate that neuroleptics do not cross-react with sedative–hypnotics and are not indicated as the primary treatment of sedative–hypnotic withdrawal
- Failure to appreciate that GHB withdrawal may begin within hours of the last dose and be relatively resistant to treatment
- Failure to appreciate that baclofen withdrawal may occur in the setting of intrathecal baclofen pump dysfunction

ICD9

292.0 Drug withdrawal

REFERENCES

1. Coffey RJ, Edgar TS, Francisco GE, et al. Abrupt withdrawal from intrathecal baclofen: recognition and management of a potentially life-threatening syndrome. *Arch Physical Med Rehab* 2002;83: 735–741.
2. DeCarolis DD, Rice KL, Ho L, et al. Symptom-driven lorazepam protocol for treatment of severe alcohol withdrawal delirium in the intensive care unit. *Pharmacotherapy* 2007;27(4):510–518.
3. Gowing L, Ali R, White J. Buprenorphine for the management of opioid withdrawal. *Cochrane Database of Systematic Reviews* 2006;2:CD002025.
4. Greenberg MI, Hendrickson RG. Baclofen withdrawal following removal of an intrathecal baclofen pump despite oral baclofen replacement. *J Toxicol Clin Toxicol* 2003;41:83–85.
5. Haddad P. Newer antidepressants and the discontinuation syndrome. *J Clin Psychiatry* 1997;58: 23–27.
6. Hamilton RJ, Olmedo RE, Shah S, et al. Complications of ultrarapid opioid detoxification with subcutaneous naltrexone pellets. *Acad Emerg Med* 2002;9:63–68.
7. McCowan C, Marik P. Refractory delirium tremens treated with propofol: a case series. *Crit Care Med* 2000;28:1781–1784.
8. O'Connor PG, Fiellin DA. Pharmacologic treatment of heroin-dependent patients. *Ann Intern Med* 2000;133:40–54.
9. Petursson H. The benzodiazepine withdrawal syndrome. *Addiction* 1994;89:1455–1459.
10. Wojtowicz JM, Yarema MC, Wax PM. Withdrawal from gamma-hydroxybutyrate, 1,4-butanediol, and gamma-butyrolactone: a case report and systematic review. *Cand J Emerg Med* 2008;10(1): 69–74.

CHAPTER 59

Botulism

PRE-HOSPITAL CONSIDERATIONS

- Intubate as soon as respiratory insufficiency is notes, clinically or based on an arterial blood gas.
- Use transcutaneous pacing for unstable type II second or third-degree heart block.
- Attempt to prevent increases in vagal tone.

CLINICAL PRESENTATION

The initial symptoms of *foodborne botulism* are predominantly gastrointestinal, including nausea, vomiting, abdominal pain, and distention, and are likely a result of pathogenic agents or toxins in the contaminated food other than *Clostridium botulinum*. Symptoms usually develop within 12 to 36 hours but may develop as early as 4 hours or as late as 10 days. Other initial symptoms are often mild and include fatigue, weakness, and vertigo. Additional symptoms include sore throat, dry mouth, and poor visual accommodation. If the toxin exposure is minimal, patients gradually recover. Otherwise, symmetric, descending flaccid paralysis with prominent bulbar palsies such as diplopia, dysarthria, dysphonia, and dysphagia develops. Physical examination may reveal weakness or paralysis of the upper extremities; dilated, nonreactive pupils; and ophthalmoplegia. The patient may be drooling secondary to dysphagia and may have difficulty phonating. Deep tendon reflexes are preserved, and ataxia is absent. Weakness of the extremities and paralysis of respiratory muscles are the most concerning symptoms. Patients maintain a normal mental status and are afebrile. Autonomic instability, such as orthostatic hypotension, may also occur and may be the predominant or only symptom on presentation, confounding the diagnosis.

Infant botulism is characterized by constipation followed by neuromuscular paralysis. Cranial nerves are affected first, and paralysis may progress to peripheral and respiratory musculature. The term "floppy infant syndrome" may best describe the presentation. Symptoms can vary from mild lethargy with poor feeding to hypotonia with respiratory compromise. Since its description in 1976, infant botulism has been the most common form of botulism reported in the United States. It follows the ingestion of *C. botulinum* with toxin formation and absorption in the gut lumen (1). The gastrointestinal tracts of infants lack some of the bile acids and gastric acids that normally inhibit clostridial growth. Honey and corn syrup have been identified as sources of *C. botulinum* spores. Vacuum cleaner dust and soil have also been implicated. In the food samples tested, no preformed toxin has been identified, only clostridium spores. About 70% of cases are in breast-fed infants; presumably these infants have different gut flora when compared with their formula-fed counterparts.

The neurological symptoms of *wound botulism* are identical to that of food-borne botulism; however, gastrointestinal symptoms are absent. Wounds are typically in avascular areas, with crush injuries, and more recently, in patients injecting black tar heroin subcutaneously ("skin popping"). In one report, only 1 out of 102 cases of wound botulism did not occur in a drug user (9). As black tar heroin is made in Mexico, most cases are from the western United States with the preponderance from California. Iatrogenic cases may vary from mild symptoms to profound respiratory compromise requiring intubation. The history of recent botulinum toxin injection will help make the diagnosis. Botulinum toxin is used therapeutically for spasticity, cervical dystonia, blepharospasm, and hyperhidrosis, as well as for cosmetic purposes.

DIFFERENTIAL DIAGNOSIS

Regardless of the type of botulism, the neurological manifestations are similar. The diagnosis is easy when large outbreaks occur. However, the majority of cases involve only one patient. As a result, the diagnosis is often missed. Botulism should be considered in a patient presenting with gastrointestinal, autonomic, and cranial nerve dysfunction or in an infant with diminished sucking, feeding, and crying ability. The differential diagnosis for foodborne and infant botulism is listed in Table 59.1. Psychiatric illness should be a diagnosis of exclusion. Misdiagnosis as such has been fatal.

The gastrointestinal symptoms of botulism are nonspecific and do not demonstrate a distinctive pattern. Patients at this stage of the disease are often discharged with a diagnosis of food poisoning. Fever is absent in patients with botulism but can be present in certain types of food poisoning. A history of the consumption of canned foods, especially home-canned foods, may be helpful in arriving at the diagnosis.

Landry-Guillain-Barré syndrome is an acute, inflammatory, postinfectious, demyelinating polyradiculoneuropathy that usually results in ascending weakness or paralysis. In the Miller-Fisher variant of this syndrome, patients have bulbar palsies (diplopia, dysarthria, dysphonia, and dysphagia) and descending weakness or paralysis, making it extremely difficult to distinguish clinically from botulism. Lumbar puncture may reveal elevated protein without pleocytosis in the former. However, early in Landry-Guillain-Barré syndrome, the spinal fluid may be normal, and a slightly elevated spinal fluid protein may be seen in botulism. Of note, gastrointestinal symptoms are lacking in Landry-Guillain-Barré syndrome, unless part of the associated antecedent viral syndrome.

TABLE 59.1 Differential Diagnosis for Botulism

Foodborne Botulism	Infant Botulism
Cerebrovascular ischemia (CVA)	Electrolyte abnormalities
Chemical intoxication	Leigh disease[a]
Carbon monoxide	Meningitis
Barium carbonate	Metabolic encephalopathy
Methyl chloride	Myopathy (congenital)
Methyl alcohol	Reye syndrome
Cholinergic (organophosphate) agents	Sepsis
Diphtheria	Werdnig-Hoffman disease[b]
Elapidae envenomation (coral snake)	
Food poisoning	
Landry-Guillain-Barré syndrome	
Miller-Fisher variant	
Medication reactions (esp. aminoglycosides)	
Multiple sclerosis	
Myasthenia gravis	
Eaton-Lambert syndrome	
Paralytic shellfish poisoning	
Poliomyelitis	
Polymyositis	
Psychiatric disorders	

[a] Subacute necrotizing encephalomyelopathy.
[b] Spinal muscular atrophy.

Myasthenia gravis may present as weakness, ptosis, and ophthalmoplegia; however, gastrointestinal symptoms will be absent. A Tensilon (edrophonium) test may be necessary to differentiate myasthenia gravis from botulism. In this test, 10 mg of edrophonium, an acetylcholinesterase inhibitor, is administered slowly as a 1- to 2-mg intravenous bolus, followed by 8 mg given over 5 minutes. Within a minute, patients with myasthenia gravis should demonstrate improved strength that should last up to 5 minutes. As this drug blocks the metabolism of acetylcholine in the synapse, it is less effective in botulism in which there is decreased neurotransmitter release, although some smaller degree of clinical improvement may occasionally be seen.

The Centers for Disease Control and Prevention (CDC) have established definitive criteria for the diagnosis of botulism. It requires a patient who presents with descending paralysis to have one of the following: *C. botulinum* isolated from stool or wound specimens; botulinum toxin in serum, stool, or implicated food samples; or a compatible illness in a person who is epidemiologically linked to a case confirmed by the previous methods (2). Currently, a mouse bioassay is used to detect the presence of botulinum toxin. It is complicated, and results are often delayed. However, rapid assays have been developed and are undergoing further testing to be validly applied clinically and in the field (4). These assays potentially would allow for rapid confirmation of any suspected botulism diagnosis and thereby expedite treatment.

Although not included in the CDC diagnostic criteria, electromyography demonstrating findings typical of botulism may be required prior to the release of antitoxin. Botulism demonstrates a typical pattern on repetitive stimulation test (20–50 Hz) (8). Although this pattern is not pathognomonic for botulism, when it is combined with other clinical data it can be used to make the diagnosis.

ED EVALUATION

The history should include the time of onset; nature, progression, and severity of symptoms; and questions concerning diet, crush injuries, skin wounds, and injections as noted previously. The physical examination should focus on neurological evaluation with attention to assessment of cranial nerve function, muscle strength, and deep tendon reflexes. Abnormalities of pupil size and reactivity, extraocular motor function, swallowing, and phonation should be documented. As death from botulism is usually the result of respiratory insufficiency, patients should have frequent assessments of vital capacity and negative inspiratory force.

Routine laboratory evaluation of cell counts, serum electrolytes, and plain radiographs are usually normal in patients with botulism but may be helpful to exclude other diagnoses. Normal cerebrospinal fluid distinguishes botulism from other disease states such as meningitis or Landry-Guillain-Barré. Similarly, brain imaging (computed tomography or magnetic resonance imaging) is normal in patients with botulism but may yield the diagnosis of cerebral or cerebellar infarct.

As noted previously, the Tensilon test can help differentiate myasthenia gravis from botulism.

When the diagnosis of botulism is suspected, electromyography should be performed as soon as possible.

Stool, serum, or wound cultures should be sent for *C. botulinum*. Serum and stool samples and wound tissue should also be sent for detection of botulinum toxin. In one study, at least one of these laboratory tests was positive in 65% of patients diagnosed with botulism. Stool and sera should be refrigerated but not frozen. Wound specimens should be placed in an anaerobic device. Suspected food should be left in their original containers and placed in sterile unbreakable containers if possible.

ED MANAGEMENT

Supportive care is the mainstay of treatment. Endotracheal intubation with mechanical ventilation is recommended for patients with a vital capacity <30% of predicted (or <12 mL/kg). Fluids should be given to replete any gastrointestinal losses, and parenteral analgesics can be given for the pain associated with abdominal distention.

Despite the delay from ingestion of contaminated food to presentation, gastric decontamination should be considered in cases of foodborne botulism. Gastric lavage may help remove any remaining toxin or contaminated food from the stomach. Activated charcoal has been shown to reduce morbidity and mortality in an animal model (6). Only sorbitol-based cathartics should be used, as magnesium may exacerbate neuromuscular blockade. Although whole bowel irrigation can aid in removal of toxin from the gut, this theory has not been evaluated in a formal study.

Multiple antitoxin preparations are available for treatment. The equine-derived antitoxins are available in monovalent (types A, B, or E), bivalent (type AB), and trivalent (type ABE) formulations. A heptavalent (types A–G) antitoxin is held by the U.S. Army. The trivalent antitoxin is recommended when the exact botulinum serotype has not been identified (3). It is distributed by the CDC to nine local repositories in the United States and is available by contacting the state health department. Antitoxin is most effective when given within 24 hours of symptom onset and should be administered as soon as the diagnosis of botulism is suspected, without waiting for confirmatory testing. The antitoxin does not reverse symptoms already present on administration. It can only prevent symptom progression, further stressing the necessity of early administration.

The initial dose of antitoxin is one vial given intravenously, slowly over several minutes. Each vial contains 10 mL of trivalent antitoxin and should be diluted in a 1:10 ratio with normal saline. Subsequent doses can be given at 2- to 4-hour intervals based on symptom progression. The benefits of antitoxin therapy must be weighed against the potential adverse effects. Because antitoxin is an animal-derived biologic product, its use can result in anaphylaxis, hypersensitivity reactions, and serum sickness. The rate of adverse reactions is 9% to 17% with a 1.9% incidence of anaphylaxis. It is not recommended to administer a test dose to assess hypersensitivity, because botulism can be fatal and antitoxin is the only available therapy. Clinicians should be prepared to handle any adverse reactions and should have appropriate medications (e.g., epinephrine) readily available.

A human botulism immune globulin (BIG) is available for infant botulism. BIG is harvested from human donors previously immunized with the pentavalent (A–E) toxoid developed by the army for laboratory personnel who work with *C. botulinum*. It is only available from the California Department of Health Services Infant Botulism Treatment and Prevention Program. BIG has been shown to be more effective than antitoxin for the treatment of infant botulism (5).

Antibiotics should be administered for wound botulism. Penicillin G is usually the first-line agent, although many antibiotics have been shown to be effective against *C. botulinum*. Early surgical consultation should also be obtained for cases of wound botulism because débridement is considered a primary therapeutic intervention (7).

In contrast, antibiotic use in infant botulism is not generally recommended. The use of aminoglycosides has been demonstrated both clinically and experimentally to potentiate neuromuscular blockade. Use of antibiotics in infant botulism can exacerbate the condition as lysis of intraluminal *C. botulinum* may increase the amount of toxin absorbed (3). The benefit of antibiotic therapy for foodborne botulism has not been demonstrated and is not recommended.

CRITICAL INTERVENTIONS

- Consider adult botulism when there is a history of ingestion of smoked, salted, or canned food; consider infant botulism in a floppy baby with respiratory insufficiency.
- Consult a surgeon regarding débridement in cases of suspected wound botulism.
- Assess the vital capacity in patients with suspected botulism and perform endotracheal intubation on those with a vital capacity <30% of predicted (<12 mL/kg).
- Contact your state Department of Health or the CDC (770-488-7100) and administer botulism antitoxin as soon as possible.

DISPOSITION

Any patient suspected of having botulism should be admitted to a critical-care setting. This allows for observation, frequent neurological examinations, assessments of respiratory status, and monitoring for anaphylaxis, which is a risk with the administration of the antitoxin.

Consultations can be obtained not only to aid in diagnosis but also to render treatment or assume care. Infectious disease, toxicology, and neurology consultants can help confirm the diagnosis. A pulmonary and critical care specialist should be consulted because patients need frequent respiratory evaluations and should be admitted to an intensive care unit. Early surgical consultation should be obtained for cases of wound botulism because débridement is considered a primary therapeutic intervention (7). Contact with the state health department or CDC Emergency Operations Center (770-488-7100), available 24 hours a day is also required as soon as possible to allow for early administration of antitoxin.

Prolonged admission is the usual course, as the recovery period can last from weeks to months and occasionally up to a year. Patients who receive early and aggressive supportive care usually do well. Although patients can make a complete recovery, long-term sequelae are not uncommon and can range from fatigue to persistent muscle weakness and dyspnea.

COMMON PITFALLS

- Failure to consider the diagnosis of botulism in patients with diplopia, dysphagia, dysphonia, and weakness or in infants with constipation, feeding problems, and hypotonia
- Failure to adequately monitor respiratory function as death usually results from respiratory insufficiency
- Failure to appreciate that electromyography is the most rapidly available diagnostic test

- Failure to appreciate that early antitoxin administration is the best therapy
- Failure to administer antitoxin pending results of a test dose to assess for hypersensitivity

ICD9

005.1 Botulism food poisoning

REFERENCES

1. Arnon SS, Midura TF, Clay SA, et al. Infant botulism. Epidemiological, clinical, and laboratory aspects. *JAMA* 1977;237(18):1946–1951.
2. Centers for Disease Control and Prevention. Case definitions for infectious conditions under public health surveillance. *MMWR Recomm Rep* 1997;46(RR-10):1–55.
3. Centers for Disease Control and Prevention. *Botulism in the United States 1899–1996: handbook for epidemiologists, clinicians and laboratory workers.* Atlanta, GA: Centers for Disease Control and Prevention, 1998.
4. Cai S, Sing Cai S, Singh BR, Sharma S. Botulism diagnostics: from clinical symptoms to in vitro assays. *Crit Rev Microbiol* 2007;33(2):109–125.
5. Frankovich TL, Arnon SS. Clinical trial of botulism immune globulin for infant botulism. *West J Med* 1991;154(1):103.
6. Gomez HF, Johnson R, Guven H, et al. Adsorption of botulinum toxin to activated charcoal with a mouse bioassay. *Ann Emerg Med* 1995;25(6):818–822.
7. Hikes DC, Manoli A II. Wound botulism. *J Trauma* 1981;21(1):68–71.
8. Valli G, Barbieri S, Scalato G. Neurophysiological tests in human botulism. *Electromyogr Clin Neurophysiol* 1983;23(1–2):3–11.
9. Werner SB, Passaro D, McGee J, et al. Wound botulism in California 1951–1998: recent epidemic in heroin injectors. *Clin Infect Dis* 2000;31(4):1018–1024.

CHAPTER 60

Oral Hypoglycemic Agents

PRE-HOSPITAL CONSIDERATIONS
- Transport all medications, pills, and pill bottles involved in overdose for identification in the emergency department.

CLINICAL PRESENTATION

Symptoms from hypoglycemia fall into two main categories, autonomic and neuroglycopenic. Autonomic symptoms are a result of excessive adrenergic tone, resulting from the release of counterregulatory hormones. Anxiety, palpitations, diaphoresis, irritability, and tremor are seen at serum glucose levels near 60 mg/dL in nondiabetic volunteers. Neuroglycopenic symptoms such as dizziness, tingling, blurred vision, difficulty thinking, and faintness begin at glucose levels near 50 mg/dL. However, there is a wide variation in the glucose level at which symptoms develop. Some individuals, particularly women and children, can be asymptomatic with glucose levels <50 mg/dL, and diabetics can develop symptoms of hypoglycemia at a "normal" or elevated glucose level when the level rapidly falls from a higher one. Additionally, concurrent therapy with β-adrenergic blockers or underlying diabetic neuropathy may mask the autonomic symptoms of hypoglycemia.

Focal neurologic deficits can occur with hypoglycemia, and, in severe cases, coma or seizures can be seen. Mild hypothermia may develop with prolonged hypoglycemia. Hypokalemia may result from intracellular potassium shifting.

Metformin-associated lactic acidosis (MALA) presents with nonspecific signs and symptoms. Patients may have nausea, vomiting, anorexia, epigastric pain, diarrhea, somnolence, or lethargy. Kussmaul respirations (hyperpnea and tachypnea) represent increased ventilation in response to the metabolic acidosis. Hypotension, hypothermia, and respiratory failure have also been reported. Various cardiac dysrhythmias, including premature ventricular contractions, bradycardia, asystole, and ventricular fibrillation have been reported, probably secondary to severe acidemia.

DIFFERENTIAL DIAGNOSIS

Hypoglycemia is a potential etiology for any patient with altered mental status, neurologic findings, or signs of sympathetic stimulation such as diaphoresis or tremor. The differential diagnosis of patients with such findings is large and includes trauma, stroke, brain tumors, central nervous system infections, severe metabolic disorders, and a wide variety of drug intoxications. Hypoglycemia should be considered as the potential cause for patients presenting with trauma or seizures. Patients particularly at risk are those with a personal or family history of noninsulin-dependent diabetes, as a result of their access to oral hypoglycemic drugs.

Diabetics presenting with an elevated anion-gap metabolic acidosis may have MALA or diabetic ketoacidosis. These conditions may be differentiated based on the history (e.g., intercurrent illness, recent oral intake, intentional ingestion) and the presence or absence of hyperglycemia, ketosis, and hyperlactatemia. The thiazolidinediones and α-glucosidase inhibitors have no significant acute toxicity in overdose, although hepatic dysfunction may occur with chronic use.

ED EVALUATION

Assessment of the patient's airway, breathing, and circulation is the first priority. The history should determine whether the patient has taken an overdose or only therapeutic doses, the type of medication(s), the amount ingested, and the time and course of symptoms. Physical examination should pay particular attention to the neurologic status, as hypoglycemia may present with subtle cognitive changes, such as irritability, distractibility, or even focal motor deficits. A rapid bedside glucose test should be performed early in patients with altered mental status.

Laboratory evaluation should include a confirmatory quantitative glucose determination. A serum chemistry panel is also indicated to check for electrolyte abnormalities and renal insufficiency. Repeat bedside glucose determinations should be performed at least every 1 to 2 hours during the initial evaluation and immediately whenever the patient shows signs of any altered mental status.

Patients with suspected metformin toxicity need a chemistry panel to evaluate for an anion-gap metabolic acidosis and renal insufficiency as well as a serum lactate level. If an elevated anion-gap is present, an arterial blood gas analysis will help define the degree of acidosis.

ED MANAGEMENT

Gastrointestinal decontamination with activated charcoal should be considered for patients presenting early after oral hypoglycemic agent ingestion. The first-line treatment for hypoglycemia is intravenous (IV) dextrose. Adults should be given 1 to 2 mL/kg of 50% dextrose (typically 1–2 ampules D50W); children should receive 2 to 4 mL/kg of 25% dextrose. Repeat dextrose boluses may be necessary, as determined by serial serum glucose determinations, and an infusion of 5% to 10% dextrose can be initiated to maintain euglycemia (60–110 mg/dL). If higher dextrose concentrations are required, the infusion should be given via a central venous catheter. The transient hyperglycemia that occurs with bolus dextrose therapy can cause reflex secretion of additional insulin (3), exacerbating the underlying problem and increasing the overall dextrose requirements. Hence, excessive dosing of dextrose should be avoided.

Diazoxide and octreotide are two options for treating refractory or recurrent hypoglycemia as a result of sulfonylurea poisoning. Diazoxide is a direct arterial vasodilator that also inhibits pancreatic insulin release by opening potassium channels, but this drug is mostly an "antidote" of historical interest only. Octreotide, a synthetic somatostatin analog that inhibits pancreatic insulin secretion, is becoming the standard therapy for refractory sulfonylurea-induced hypoglycemia (1,3,4). Octreotide is superior to diazoxide plus glucose and to glucose alone in volunteer sulfonylurea overdose by decreasing hypoglycemia, glucose requirements, and circulating-insulin levels (1). In clinical experience, octreotide use significantly decreases recurrent hypoglycemic episodes in patients with sulfonylurea toxicity (4). Dosing of octreotide has not been standardized, and it has been given both subcutaneously (SC) and IV for this indication. Suggested dosing is 50–100 μg SC or IV every 6 to 12 hours for adults and 4 to 5 μg/kg/day divided every 6 hours in children.

No specific therapy exists for MALA. Endotracheal intubation and correction of hypotension with IV fluids and vasopressors are likely to be needed in severe cases. Severe cases can be treated with hemodialysis, which will correct the acidosis as well as remove lactate and metformin.

CRITICAL INTERVENTIONS

- Obtain serial serum-glucose levels on patients with potential sulfonylurea and meglitinide overdose.
- Administer IV dextrose for hypoglycemia, but avoid inducing hyperglycemia.
- Administer octreotide to patients with recurrent hypoglycemia.
- Obtain a serum-lactate level on patients with metabolic acidosis who are taking metformin.

DISPOSITION

Patients developing hypoglycemia from sulfonylurea drugs should be treated with dextrose and admitted to the hospital. The half-lives of the sulfonylureas are long enough that recurrent episodes of hypoglycemia should be expected. Admission to a critical care unit is often necessary, as the frequency of glucose determinations (at least every 1–2 hours) may preclude observation on a general medical ward. Also, patients may require frequent adjustments in dextrose infusions or treatment with octreotide. Extended observation in an emergency department holding unit may be considered, depending on local capabilities, if the patient does not suffer from recurrent hypoglycemia requiring repeat dextrose boluses or infusions. Hypoglycemia from meglitinide toxicity theoretically should be of shorter duration than from sulfonylureas; however, as a result of a lack of published evidence that short-term observation is safe, such patients should currently be managed like sulfonylurea-toxic patients and be admitted for serial glucose determinations.

Considerable controversy remains regarding the optimal management of asymptomatic patients exposed to oral hypoglycemic medications (2,5,6). This controversy stems from the fact that many of the patients evaluated for sulfonylurea toxicity are children in whom the history of actual ingestion (vs. mere exposure to the pills) is not entirely clear, who present with normal mental status and glucose levels, and who generally have a benign outcome. Nevertheless, because rapid drug detection to confirm actual exposure is not commonly available, these patients need a period of observation to monitor for hypoglycemia; the duration of this observation period is the crux of the controversy. Published evidence generally supports an observation period of 8 hours (6). Patients who develop hypoglycemia are treated and admitted, although those who do not manifest hypoglycemia may be discharged home or referred for psychiatric evaluation as appropriate. Prophylactic treatment of asymptomatic euglycemic patients with glucose should be avoided, as this may mask the development of hypoglycemia and lead to an inappropriate disposition. Cases of delayed hypoglycemia from sulfonylurea agents have occurred when the patients have been given parenteral glucose (6). Oral food intake is acceptable and seems less likely to mask hypoglycemic agent toxicity. Because of the required length of observation and the potentially dire consequences of discharging a patient who later becomes hypoglycemic, some authors recommend medical admission and at least 24 hours of observation for all patients with a known or suspected overdose of sulfonylurea drugs (5).

Patients with MALA also require admission, usually to an intensive care unit, because the associated mortality is so high and these patients often have significant comorbidities. Patients with an acute biguanide overdose, but without lactic acidosis, should be admitted and have serial serum-chemistry determinations.

Patients overdosing with the other oral agents for diabetes are unlikely to require admission, unless concerning coingestants or comorbidities are present. In all cases, consultation with a poison control center or medical toxicologist can assist in determining the optimal patient disposition.

COMMON PITFALLS

- Failure to appreciate that hypoglycemia can result in focal neurological deficits and focal seizures
- Failure to observe patients with sulfonylurea and meglitinide overdose for at least 8 hours
- Administering prophylactic dextrose to patients with sulfonylurea and meglitinide overdose who are asymptomatic or euglycemic
- Failure to appreciate that excessive glucose administration promotes insulin secretion and can lead to recurrent hypoglycemia in sulfonylurea and meglitinide poisoning

ICD9

962.3 Poisoning by insulins and antidiabetic agents

REFERENCES

1. Boyle PJ, Justice K, Krentz AJ, et al. Octreotide reverses hyperinsulinemia and prevents hypoglycemia induced by sulfonylurea overdoses. *J Clin Endocrinol Metab* 1993;76:752–756.
2. Burkhart KK. When does hypoglycemia develop after sulfonylurea ingestion? *Ann Emerg Med* 1998;31:771–772.
3. Harrigan RA, Nathan MS, Beattie P. Oral agents for the treatment of type 2 diabetes mellitus: pharmacology, toxicity, and treatment. *Ann Emerg Med* 2001;38:68–78.
4. McLaughlin SA, Crandall CS, McKinney PE. Octreotide: an antidote for sulfonylurea-induced hypoglycemia. *Ann Emerg Med* 2000;36:133–138.
5. Quadrani DA, Spiller HA, Widder P. Five year retrospective evaluations of sulfonylurea ingestion in children. *J Toxicol Clin Toxicol* 1996;34:267–270.
6. Spiller HA, Villalobos D, Krenzelok EP, et al. Prospective multicenter study of sulfonylurea ingestion in children. *J Pediatr* 1997;131:141–146.

CHAPTER 61

Mushrooms

PRE-HOSPITAL CONSIDERATIONS
- Bring any unconsumed mushrooms or mushroom pieces to the hospital to aid in diagnosis. Refrigerate specimens, if possible, and place in a brown paper bag.

CLINICAL PRESENTATION

Patients often present within several hours of a mushroom meal with nonspecific gastrointestinal (GI) symptoms, including nausea, vomiting, and diarrhea. Fortunately, the majority of these patients are suffering from GI irritants and require only supportive care. Patients who have consumed the more toxic mushrooms containing cyclopeptides, orellanine, or monomethylhydrazine generally have a delay of 8 to 12 hours before symptom onset. A short time to symptom onset gives the clinician some reassurance that patients presenting early are likely to have a benign clinical course. A notable exception is with *Amanita smithiana* ingestion; patients ingesting this mushroom are likely to have GI symptoms within hours of ingestion but subsequently develop renal failure over the next 48 hours to several weeks. Fortunately, *A. smithiana* ingestions are rare, and the only cases reported in the United States have been in the Pacific Northwest. Another caveat applies to those who have consumed a "mushroom salad" that contained both cytotoxic and GI irritant species and thus present with symptoms earlier than 6 to 8 hours.

Each class of toxic mushroom has a distinctive constellation of presenting symptoms, signs, laboratory abnormalities, and end-organ involvement (Table 61.1). Patients who have ingested cyclopeptide- or amatoxin-containing mushrooms will typically present 6 to 12 hours after ingestion with nausea, vomiting, abdominal pain, and severe watery diarrhea. Hypovolemia and electrolyte disturbances may occur from GI losses. Symptoms may improve 24 to 48 hours into the illness, followed by hepatic injury marked by elevated transaminases, bilirubin, and often renal dysfunction. Within 2 to 6 days, fulminant hepatic and renal failure may develop, with subsequent hepatic encephalopathy, coagulopathy, seizures, and death. With intensive supportive therapy, survival may be as high as 90% (2); however, with fulminant hepatic failure, orthotopic liver transplant may be required (1).

TABLE 61.1 Presenting Symptoms/Signs, Toxin, Laboratory Abnormalities, and Treatment after Mushroom Ingestion

Presenting Symptoms or Laboratory Abnormality	Associated Features	Mushroom Class/Toxin	Species	Treatment[a]
Hallucinations	Mydriasis, tachycardia, coma, seizures Mild hallucinations, coma, myoclonus, seizures	Psilocin Ibotenic acid/muscimol	*Psilocybe* and *Conocybe* sp *Amanita muscaria, pantheria, gemmata*	Benzodiazepines Low-stimulus environment
Cholinergic signs	DUMBELS[c]	Muscarine	*Clitocybe* and *Inocybe* sp	Atropine for pulmonary symptoms
Disulfiram reaction	N/V/D, flushing, ↑HR assoc. with ethanol use	Coprine	*Coprinus* sp	Antihistamines
Renal failure	Delayed GI symptoms	Orellanine[b]	*Cortinarius* sp	Supportive/hemodialysis
Renal failure	Early GI symptoms	Allenic norleucine[b]	*Amanita smithiana*	Supportive/hemodialysis
Rhabdomyolysis	Myalgias, fatigue	Unknown myotoxin[b]	*Tricholoma equestre*	Maintenance of urine output, ± urinary alkalinization
Early gastrointestinal symptoms (2–3 hr)	N/V/D	GI irritants	*Chlorophyllum* sp, many others	Supportive care only Antiemetics
Delayed gastrointestinal symptoms (>6 hr)	Delayed hepatotoxicity	α-Amanitin[b]	*A. phalloides, virosa, Lepiota* sp	Multidose activated charcoal Penicillin N-Acetylcysteine Silitinin? Consider transplant
Delayed gastrointestinal symptoms	Delayed nephrotoxicity N/V/D, CNS, hepatic	Orellanine[b] Gyromitrin[b] (monomethyl hydrazine)	*Cortinarius* *Gyromitra* sp	Supportive/hemodialysis Pyridoxine

[a]In addition to supportive care, including IV fluids and antiemetics, and decontamination if appropriate.
[b]Mushrooms that lead to potentially lethal poisoning.
[c]Diarrhea, urination, miosis, bradycardia, bronchorrhea, bronchospasm, emesis, lacrimation, salivation.

Mushrooms containing coprine are typically edible and cause no symptoms. If ethanol is consumed between several hours to 3 days after the ingestion, however, a disulfiram-like reaction may be seen. Symptoms include nausea, vomiting, facial flushing, hypotension, tachycardia, headache, vertigo, and metallic taste. Symptoms typically last up to several hours (5).

Mushrooms containing GI irritants cause symptoms similar to gastroenteritis, usually beginning 30 minutes to 6 hours after ingestion. Vomiting and diarrhea, sometimes bloody, may last for 48 hours and are typically self-limited. With severe diarrhea, patients may become significantly dehydrated.

Patients consuming mushrooms containing ibotenic acid and muscimol can have a varied presentation as a result of both γ-aminobutyric acid–ergic and glutamate effects. Symptoms usually begin within 30 to 180 minutes of ingestion and may include a combination of euphoria, mild hallucinations, obtundation, agitation, myoclonus, and seizures.

The "false morel" *Gyromitra esculenta* is often confused with the edible true morel or *Morchella* species and results in significant toxicity. The severity of symptoms depends on the amount ingested and method of preparation. Parboiling or drying may eliminate the gyromitrin toxins. Patients often become symptomatic 5 to 8 hours after ingestion and present with nausea, vomiting, and diarrhea. These symptoms may last up to several days before resolving. Central nervous system (CNS) effects, including fatigue, headache, ataxia, tremor, and (rarely) seizures, may be seen. After 24 to 72 hours, there may be evidence of hepatic and/or renal damage, as well as hemolysis and methemoglobinemia. In more severe cases, coma and death may result (6).

The onset of symptoms following ingestion of muscarine-containing mushrooms is rapid, usually within 30 minutes. Cholinergic signs and symptoms include those identified by the commonly used mnemonic DUMBELS: diaphoresis, urination, miosis, bronchorrhea, emesis, lacrimation, and salivation. With supportive treatment, patients typically recover with no long-term effects.

Rhabdomyolysis with myalgias, weakness, and fatigue begins 24 to 72 hours after ingesting *Tricholoma equestre* mushrooms. Symptoms usually improve over the following 2 weeks, but death can occur. Fatal cases have had persistent creatine kinase elevations and evidence of myocardial damage on autopsy.

Toxicity from orellanine-containing *Cortinarius* sp is most often seen in Europe and is relatively uncommon in the United States. GI symptoms, including nausea, vomiting, diarrhea, and abdominal or flank pain, begin 2 to 14 days after ingestion, at which time renal damage has already occurred. Progression to end-stage renal failure may ensue.

Similar to poisoning by *Cortinarius* sp, the ingestion of alienic norleucine-containing *A. smithiana* produces renal damage 2 to 4 days after ingestion. One distinguishing feature is that *A. smithiana* often causes GI symptoms within 2 to 12 hours.

Abuse of psilocin-containing mushrooms is common among young adults, frequently in combination with alcohol and other drugs. Patients often present to the emergency department as a result of severe anxiety from unpleasant hallucinations ("bad trips"). Other signs and symptoms may include mydriasis, tachycardia, GI symptoms, coma, and seizures. Another important feature (as with lysergic acid diethylamide [LSD] and similar drugs) is the association with high-risk behavior and poor decision making, which may lead to traumatic injuries.

DIFFERENTIAL DIAGNOSIS

Toxic mushroom ingestion should be considered in the differential diagnosis of patients presenting with GI symptoms, hepatic or renal damage, delirium or hallucinations, disulfiram-like reactions, seizures, or rhabdomyolysis. The GI symptoms from both GI-irritant and the more toxic mushrooms will often be indistinguishable from gastroenteritis. Eliciting a history of recent ingestion of wild mushrooms may be the only clue to the diagnosis.

Hepatotoxicity similar to that caused by *Amanita* ingestion can occur with overdose of acetaminophen and iron, chronic isoniazid therapy, and many non-toxicologic etiologies, including viral hepatitis. In addition to coprine-containing mushrooms, a large number of chemicals and pharmaceuticals can cause a disulfiram-like reaction when ethanol is consumed (see Chapter 2). Other hallucinogens, CNS depressants, γ-hydroxybutyrate (GHB), or withdrawal syndromes may cause symptoms similar to those seen after the ingestion of mushrooms containing ibotenic acid and muscimol. Agents causing toxicity similar to hydrazine-containing mushrooms include isoniazid and some types of rocket fuel. Direct muscarinic agonists or acetylcholinesterase inhibitors produce cholinergic toxicity similar to that seen with muscarine-containing mushrooms. Some of these agents include organophosphate or carbamate pesticides, nerve agents, physostigmine, and pilocarpine. The differential diagnosis of renal failure includes prerenal causes, intrinsic nephrotoxins, and postrenal causes. Conditions that may be confused with psilocin intoxication include use of LSD, mescaline, morning glory, hallucinogenic amphetamines (e.g., methylenedioxymethamphetamine [MDMA]), or hallucinogenic tryptamines (e.g., dimethyltryptamine [DMT]); alcohol withdrawal; or medical causes of delirium. Other causes of rhabdomyolysis include various metabolic disorders or increased muscular activity from myoclonus, rigidity or seizures, trauma, or prolonged immobilization.

ED EVALUATION

Of greatest importance is species identification, and the key history is the time interval between ingestion of the mushroom and the onset of symptoms. Other information that may be helpful includes the quantity consumed, cooked versus raw, fresh versus dried, and if ethanol was consumed within 3 days of the meal. Positive identification of the mushroom involved can be difficult but may be possible if the patient brings a sample of the offending mushroom. One method used by the Illinois Poison Center involves the physician taking digital images of the mushroom in three planes, sending the images electronically to the poison center, and obtaining consultation from a mycologist (3). Contacting a regional poison center (800-222-1222) can be helpful in this regard.

The physical examination should focus on vital signs, assessment of hydration status, and evaluation of eyes, skin, abdomen, and neurologic status. Patients with prolonged GI symptoms or clinical evidence of dehydration should have measurement of serum electrolyte, blood urea nitrogen, creatinine, and glucose as well as a urinalysis. Evaluation of patients presenting with weakness or myalgias should include a serum creatine phosphokinase. Those with possible amatoxin poisoning should have liver function tests, chemistries, and coagulation studies. A serum creatinine >1.2 mg/dL with an international normalized ratio (INR) >2.5 may predict mortality (7). Except for muscarine, which can be identified by thin-layer chromatography, other mushroom toxins are not easily detected by routine toxicology screening. Thus, the best strategy is to have the mushroom in question identified by a mycologist.

ED MANAGEMENT

Supportive care is the mainstay of management for any toxic mushroom ingestion. Most patients will need no treatment other than intravenous (IV) fluids and antiemetics. Those exhibiting significant CNS effects, dehydration, seizures, or cardiovascular effects should have an IV line placed and noninvasive monitoring instituted. Benzodiazepines should be administered for seizures, severe agitation, or hallucinations. Activated charcoal should be considered for patients presenting within 1 to 2 hours of ingestion.

The search for a potential antidote for amatoxin-containing mushrooms has been extensive. Because of the infrequent nature of exposures, there are no prospective studies that conclusively demonstrate that any single agent is effective. Multiple-dose activated charcoal has been recommended because amatoxins are enterohepatically recirculated. Continuous nasoduodenal suctioning has also been used for this purpose. Charcoal hemoperfusion may also enhance toxin elimination if performed in the first 24 hours. High-dose IV penicillin (1 million units per kilogram per day for the first day, followed by 0.5 million units per kilogram per day for 2 more days) appears to have variable efficacy. The mechanism is unknown, but it is postulated to prevent or reduce hepatic uptake of amatoxins. Silibinin is thought to reduce hepatic uptake and interrupt enterohepatic circulation of amatoxins, but a pharmaceutical preparation is not available in the United States. Oral silymarin (1.4 to 4.2 g/d), a dietary supplement that contains silibinin, has been used as an alternative to IV silibinin, but the efficacy of this formulation is unknown. N-Acetylcysteine (NAC), traditionally used for the treatment of acetaminophen poisoning, may also be effective for nonspecific causes of hepatic injury. A large retrospective review and small case series suggest that NAC may be an effective adjunct (2). However, one comparative animal model demonstrated no benefit from NAC, penicillin, cimetidine, thioctic acid, or silymarin

(8). When fulminant hepatic failure occurs, orthotopic liver transplantation is the only successful therapy (1,4).

Patients with coprine-containing mushroom ingestion should be counseled to avoid alcohol. Antihistamines may provide symptomatic relief.

Monomethylhydrazine-containing mushrooms (*Gyromitra spp*) may cause seizures. If benzodiazepine therapy is not immediately successful, the patient should be given IV vitamin B_6 (pyridoxine). Gyromitrin causes an inhibition of glutamic acid decarboxylase, similar to isoniazid, and B_6 is effective in this setting. Suggested doses are 1 g for children and 5 g for adults.

Muscarine-containing mushrooms (e.g., *Clitocybe* sp) will generally respond well to supportive care alone. Atropine may be used for severe cholinergic symptoms. Atropine dosing should be targeted to reverse pulmonary symptoms of bronchorrhea and bronchospasm.

Patients with hallucinations should be placed in a quiet, low-stimulus environment, if possible. Haloperidol and lorazepam have also been reported to be effective for severe agitation and hallucinations.

The treatment of rhabdomyolysis includes maintenance of urine output by infusion of IV fluids, consideration of urinary alkalinization, and possibly dialysis.

CRITICAL INTERVENTIONS

- Determine the time of onset of symptoms with respect to the time of ingestion.
- Consult a regional poison center, toxicologist, or mycologist to assist with mushroom identification and management.
- Administer IV fluids and antiemetics to patients with GI symptoms and dehydration.
- Admit patients with symptoms that begin 6 to 8 hours after ingestion and monitor for liver and renal dysfunction.

DISPOSITION

Patients who present with GI symptoms that begin within 2 hours after ingestion, have not had a mixed mushroom ingestion, and have low likelihood of *A. smithiana* ingestion may be considered for discharge after favorable response to IV fluids and oral challenge. Patients who have ingested hallucinogenic mushrooms may be safely discharged when their mental status returns to normal. Those who develop GI symptoms 6 to 8 hours after ingestion or whose ingestion is identified as a possible cyclopeptide-containing species should be admitted to the hospital, and liver and renal function should be followed. In the case of hepatotoxicity from *Amanita phalloides* or other cyclopeptide-containing mushroom, consultation with a gastroenterologist and transfer to a transplant center is prudent.

COMMON PITFALLS

- Failure to include wild mushroom ingestion in the differential diagnosis of gastroenteritis, altered mental status, and liver or renal dysfunction of unknown cause

- Assuming that a potentially lethal mushroom has not been ingested along with less toxic species because symptoms began soon after ingestion
- Failure to appreciate that therapy is based primarily on clinical symptoms and should not be delayed or withheld because the mushroom has not been identified

ICD9

988.1 Toxic effect of mushrooms eaten as food

REFERENCES

1. Broussard CN, Aggarwal A, Lacey SR, et al. Mushroom poisoning—from diarrhea to liver transplantation. *Am J Gastroenterol* 2001;96(11):3195–3198.
2. Enjalbert F, Rapior S, Nouguier-Soule J, et al. Treatment of amatoxin poisoning: 20-year retrospective analysis. *J Toxicol Clin Toxicol* 2002;40(6):715–757.
3. Fischbein CB, Mueller GM, Leacock PR, et al. Digital imaging: a promising tool for mushroom identification. *Acad Emerg Med* 2003;10(7):808–811.
4. Ganzert M, Felgenhauer N, Zilker T. Indication of liver transplantation following amatoxin intoxication. *J Hepatol* 2005;42(2):202–209.
5. Michelot D. Poisoning by *Coprinus atramentarius*. *Nat Toxins* 1992;1(2):73–80.
6. Michelot D, Toth B. Poisoning by *Gyromitra esculenta*—a review. *J Appl Toxicol* 1991;11(4):235–243.
7. Saviuc P, Danel V. New syndromes in mushroom poisoning. *Toxicol Rev* 2006;25(3):199–209.
8. Tong TC, Hernandez M, Richardson WH III, et al. Comparative treatment of alpha-amanitin poisoning with N-acetylcysteine, benzylpenicillin, cimetidine, thioctic acid, and silybin in a murine model. *Ann Emerg Med* 2007;50(3):282–288.

CHAPTER 62

Plants

PRE-HOSPITAL CONSIDERATIONS

- Collect seeds, leaves, flowers, and/or spores in a paper bag.
- Contact a local botanist.
- Do not give syrup of ipecac. It is not recommended in the setting of severe gastrointestinal (GI) distress and/or altered mental status.

CLINICAL PRESENTATION

There is no single physical characteristic that differentiates a poisonous plant (Table 62.1) from a nonpoisonous one (Table 62.2). Nontoxic plant parts can lodge in the throat and cause choking and gagging. Large amounts of nontoxic plant material may cause vomiting. Alkaloid content of plants can vary by year and by location as a result of factors that affect growth such as soil conditions, fertilizer, and amounts of rainfall and sunshine. It is often impossible to make a definite association between symptoms and severity on one hand and specific plant and amount of material ingested on the other. In general, houseplants are less toxic than outdoor plants (1). Small accidental tastes of plants by young children are very common and are less likely to cause severe problems than are intentional use or misuse of plants by adolescents and adults.

Patients arriving at the emergency department (ED) after a plant exposure may present as a puzzle, depending on the age of the patient, the type of plant involved, amount of exposure, and the reason for the exposure. A young child who tasted some red berries is clinically different from an adolescent who smoked a plant in hopes of becoming intoxicated. In turn, the adult patient who has brewed a concentrated tea to attempt suicide is also clinically different. Each case will present different diagnostic and management challenges.

Almost all categories of toxic plants include some degree of GI symptoms as a result of ingestion. The mechanism of action and toxic concentration differ by genus (see Table 62.1). Plant toxins can cause nausea, vomiting, abdominal cramping, and diarrhea in addition to systemic effects such as fluid and electrolyte depletion, GI bleeding, tissue sloughing, and shock. Many plants that cause epithelial irritation and dermatitis also cause GI irritation. The degree of severity depends on the amount ingested (1,5,6,8).

TABLE 62.1   Toxic Plants

Common Name	Botanical Name	Toxins/Effects
Absinth	*Artemisia* sp	Stimulants/depressants
Abutilon	*Abutilon* sp	Dermatitis
Acacia, black	*Robinia pseudoacacia*	Toxalbumins
Aconite	*Aconitium napellus*	Aconitum
Acorn	*Quercus* sp	Tannic acid/dermatitis
Adam-and-Eve	*Arum maculatum*	Calcium oxalates/dermatitis
African lily	*Agapanthus africanus*	Dermatitis
Agapanthus	*Agapanthus* sp	Dermatitis
Agapanthus, pink	*Nerine bowdenii*	Gastrointestinal
Akee	*Blighia sapida*	Stimulants/gastrointestinal
Alder, American	*Alnus crispus*	Dermatitis
Allamanda, pink or purple	*Cryptostegia grandiflora*	Cardiac glycosides
Allamanda, wild	*Urechitis* sp	Cardiac glycosides
Allium	*Allium sativum*	GI/dermatitis/hypoglycemia
Almond, bitter	*Prunus dulcis*	Cyanogenic glycosides
Alocasia	*Alocasia* sp	Calcium oxalates
Aloe vera	*Aloe* sp	Anthraquinones
Aloe, Indian	*Aloe* sp	Anthraquinones
Alstroemeria	*Alstroemeria aurantiaca*	GI/dermatitis
Amaryllis	*Amaryllis* sp	GI
Amaryllis	*Hippeastrum* sp	GI/allergen
Amaryllis belladonna	*Amaryllis belladonna*	GI
Anemone	*Anemone* sp	Protoanemonin
Angel wings	*Caladium* sp	Calcium oxalates/dermatitis
Angelica	*Angelica archangelica*	Photodermatitis
Angel's trumpet	*Datura* sp	Anticholinergic
Angel's trumpet	*Brugmansia* sp	Anticholinergic
Anthurium	*Anthurium* sp	Calcium oxalates
Apple (chewed seeds)	*Malus* sp	Cyanogenic glycosides
Apricot (chewed pits)	*Prunus armeniaca*	Cyanogenic glycosides
Archangel	*Angelica archangelica*	Photodermatitis
Arnica	*Arnica* sp	Arnica
Arrowhead vine	*Syngonium podophyllum*	Calcium oxalates
Arum	*Arum* sp	Calcium oxalates/dermatitis
Arum lily	*Zantedeschia aethiopica*	Calcium oxalates
Asarum	*Asarum* sp	Aristolochic acid
Ash tree	*Fraxinus* sp	Dermatitis
Aspen tree	*Populus tremuloides*	Dermatitis
Asthma plant or weed	*Euphorbia* sp	Dermatitis
Asthma weed	*Lobelia inflata*	Lobeline/dermatitis
Aucuba	*Aucuba japonica*	GI
Australian pine	*Araucaria heterophylla*	Dermatitis
Autumn crocus	*Colchicum autumnale*	Colchicine
Azalea	*Rhododendron genus*	Grayanotoxins
Balsam pear	*Memordica charantia*	Gastrointestinal
Baneberry	*Actaea* sp	Protoanemonin
Barbados nut	*Jatropha curcas*	Toxalbumins
Barberry	*Berberis* sp	Berberine
Bayberry	*Myrica pennsylvanica*	Dermatitis

TABLE 62.1   Toxic Plants (*Continued*)

Common Name	Botanical Name	Toxins/Effects
Be still tree	*Thevetia peruviana*	Cardiac glycosides
Bearberry	*Arctostaphylos uva-ursi*	Hydroquinones
Bear's foot	*Helleborus* sp	Hellebore
Bear's grape	*Arctostaphylos uva-ursi*	Hydroquinones
Beaver poison	*Cicuta maculata*	Stimulants
Beaver tail cactus	*Opuntia* sp	Contact dermatitis, wound injury from thorns
Belladonna	*Atropa belladonna*	Anticholinergic
Bellyache bush	*Jatropha gossypifolia*	Toxalbumins
Bindweed	*Alystegia sepium*	GI/dermatitis
Bindweed	*Calystegia sepium*	GI/dermatitis
Bird of paradise	*Poinciana gilliesii*	GI
Bird of paradise flower	*Strelitzia reginae*	GI
Bittersweet	*Solanum* sp	Solanine
Bittersweet, American	*Celastrus scandens*	GI
Black acacia	*Robinia pseudoacacia*	Toxalbumins
Black cohosh	*Cimicifuga racemosa*	Cimicifuga
Black-eyed Susan	*Rudbeckia hirta*	Dermatitis
Black-eyed Susan	*Abrus precatorius*	Toxalbumins
Black henbane	*Hyoscyamus niger*	Anticholinergic
Black lily	*Dracunculus vulgaris*	Calcium oxalates
Black locust	*Robinia pseudoacacia*	Toxalbumins
Black nightshade	*Solanum nigrum*	Solanine
Black snakeroot	*Cimicifuga racemosa*	Cimicifuga
Black snakeroot	*Zygadenus venenosus*	Veratrum alkaloids
Blackwort	*Symphytum officinale*	Pyrrolizidine alkaloids
Blazing star	*Chamaelirium luteum*	GI
Blood flower or lily	*Haemanthus coccineus*	GI
Blood root	*Sanguinaria canadensis*	GI/depressant
Blue bonnet	*Lupinus* sp	Acute: anticholinergic Chronic: permanent neurotoxicity
Blue cohosh	*Caulophyllum thalictroides*	Cytisine
Blue flag	*Iris versicolor*	GI/dermatitis
Blue gum tree	*Eucalyptus* sp	GI
Blue star	*Ipomoea tricolor*	Lysergic acid amides
Bog heather	*Erica* sp	Grayanotoxins
Boneset	*Symphytum officinale*	Pyrrolizidine alkaloids
Boston ivy	*Parthenocissus tricuspidata*	Soluble oxalates/calcium oxalates
Bottlebrush buckeye	*Aesculus parviflora*	GI/depressant
Bougainvillea	*Bougainvillea* sp	Dermatitis
Box elder	*Acer negundo*	Dermatitis
Boxwood	*Buxus sempervirens*	GI/dermatitis
Bracken fern	*Pteridium aquilinum*	Carcinogen
Bradford pear	*Pyrus calleryana*	Cyanogenic glycosides
Broom bush	*Retama raetam*	Depressants
Broom tops	*Cytisus scoparius*	Cytisine
Broom tops	*Spartium scoparium*	Cytisine
Broom, Scotch	*Cytisus scoparius*	Cytisine

(continued)

TABLE 62.1 Toxic Plants (*Continued*)

Common Name	Botanical Name	Toxins/Effects
Broom, Spanish	*Spartium junceum*	Cytisine
Buckeye	*Aesculus* sp	GI/depressant
Buckhorn	*Osmunda cinnamonea*	Raw or undercooked: GI
Buckthorn	*Karwinski humboltiana*	Progressive ascending paralytic neuropathy
Buckthorn	*Rhamnus cathartica*	Anthraquinones
Buckwheat	*Fagopyrum esculentum*	Allergic asthma-like symptoms
Buddhist pine	*Podocarpus macrophylla*	GI
Bull nettle	*Solanum carolinense*	Solanine
Burn plant	*Aloe* sp	Anthraquinones
Burning bush	*Dictamnus* sp	Photodermatitis
Burning bush	*Euonymus* sp	GI
Burning bush	*Kochia* sp	Photodermatitis/soluble oxalates
Buttercup	*Ranunculus* sp	Protoanemonin
Butterfly weed	*Asclepias* sp	Cardiac glycosides
Button	*Lophophora williamsii*	Hallucinogen
Cactus (thorns)	*Cactus* sp	Injury from thorn wounds
Caladium	*Caladium* sp	Calcium oxalates/dermatitis
Caladium	*Colocasia esculenta*	Calcium oxalates
Calla lily	*Zantedeschia* sp	Calcium oxalates
Calla, black	*Arum palestinum*	Calcium oxalates
Camphor tree	*Cinnamomum camphora*	Camphor
Camus, death	*Zygadenus* or *Zigadenus* sp	Veratrum alkaloids
Candle plant	*Senecio* sp	Pyrrolizidine alkaloids
Candleberry	*Myrica* sp	Dermatitis
Candleberry tree	*Aleurites* sp	GI/dermatitis
Candlenut tree	*Aleurites* sp	GI/dermatitis
Candytuft	*Iberis amara*	Dermatitis
Cape leadwort	*Plumbago capensis*	Dermatitis
Cape plumbago, blue	*Plumbago capensis*	Dermatitis
Cardinal flower	*Lobelia cardinalis*	Lobeline/dermatitis
Carnation	*Dianthus* sp	Dermatitis
Carolina allspice	*Calycanthus* sp	Stimulants
Carolina jasmine or jessamine	*Gelsemium* sp	Gelsemium
Carolina moonseed	*Cocculus carolinus*	Stimulants
Carolina wild woodbine	*Gelsemium* sp	Gelsemium
Carolina yellow jessamine	*Gelsemium* sp	Gelsemium
Carrot, wild	*Cicuta maculata*	Stimulants
Cascara	*Rhamus purshiana*	Anthraquinones
Cassava	*Jatropha manihot*	Cyanogenic glycosides
Cassava (raw root)	*Manihot esculenta*	Cyanogenic glycosides
Castor bean	*Ricinus communis*	Toxalbumins
Catnip	*Nepeta cataria*	Hallucinogen (subjective)
Cayenne pepper	*Capsicum* sp	Capsaicin
Cedar	*Juniperus virginia*	GI/dermatitis
Celandine	*Chelidonium majus*	GI/hepatotoxicity/dermatitis

TABLE 62.1   Toxic Plants (*Continued*)

Common Name	Botanical Name	Toxins/Effects
Celery	*Apium graveolens*	Photodermatitis
Century plant	*Agave* sp	Contact dermatitis/thorn injury/GI
Chamomile	*Anthemis cotula*	Dermatitis/allergen
Chapparal leaf	*Larrea tridentate*	Hepatotoxicity
Cherry (chewed pits)	*Prunus* sp	Cyanogenic glycosides
China tree	*Melia azedarach*	Chinaberry
Chinaberry	*Melia azedarach*	Chinaberry
Chinese elm	*Ulmus parvifolia*	Dermatitis/allergic reactions
Chinese hackberry	*Celtis sinensis*	Dermatitis
Chinese lantern	*Abutilon* sp	Dermatitis
Chinese lantern plant	*Physalis* sp	Solanine
Chinese tallow tree	*Sapium sebiferum*	GI/dermatitis
Chinese yew (do not confuse with *Taxus*)	*Podocarpus macrophylla*	GI
Choke cherry	*Prunus* sp	Cyanogenic glycosides
Cholla	*Opuntia* sp	Contact dermatitis, wound injury from thorns
Christmas berry	*Photinia arbutifolia*	Cyanogenic glycosides
Christmas berry	*Schinus terebinthifolius*	Dermatitis
Christmas candle	*Euphorbia tithymaloides*	GI
Christmas candle	*Pedilanthus tithymaloides*	GI
Christmas rose	*Helleborus niger*	Hellebore
Chrysanthemum	*Chrysanthemum* sp	Pyrethrums
Cineraria	*Senecio cruentus*	Pyrrolizidine alkaloids
Citronella grass	*Cymbopogon nardus*	Dermatitis
Clematis	*Clematis* sp	Protoanemonin
Clivia	*Clivia miniata*	Gastrointestinal
Clover, sweet	*Melilotus alba*	Warfarin
Clover, white	*Melilotus alba*	Warfarin
Cocklebur	*Xanthium orientale*	Dermatitis
Coffee bean	*Sesbania* sp	GI/hepatotoxicty
Coffee tree	*Polyscias guilfoyei*	Dermatitis/GI/depressant
Coffeeberry	*Rhamnus californica*	Anthraquinones
Cohoba	*Anadenanthera peregrina*	Hallucinogens
Cohosh, black	*Cimicifuga racemosa*	Cimicifuga
Cola nut	*Cola nitida*	Caffeine
Colchicine	*Colchicum autumnale*	Colchicine
Colic root	*Asarum* sp	Aristolochic acid
Colocasia	*Colocasia esculenta*	Calcium oxalates
Comfrey	*Symphytum officinale*	Pyrrolizidine alkaloids
Conqueror root	*Exogonium purga*	GI
Coral beads	*Cocculus carolinus*	Stimulants
Coral bean	*Erythrina* sp	Cyanogenic glycosides
Coral berry	*Actaea spicata*	Protoanemonin
Coral berry	*Rivina humilis*	GI
Coral berry	*Symphoricarpos* sp	GI
Coral plant	*Jatropha multifida*	Toxalbumins
Coriaria	*Coriaria* sp	Stimulants

(*continued*)

TABLE 62.1 Toxic Plants (*Continued*)

Common Name	Botanical Name	Toxins/Effects
Corn lily	*Veratrum* sp	Veratrum alkaloids
Cotoneaster	*Cotoneaster* sp	Cyanogenic glycosides
Cottonwood	*Populus deltoides*	Dermatitis
Coyotillo	*Karwinski humboltiana*	Progressive ascending paralytic neuropathy
Crabapple (chewed seeds)	*Malus baccata*	Cyanogenic glycosides
Creeping charlie	*Glechoma hederacea*	GI
Creosote bush	*Larrea tridentate*	Hepatotoxicity
Crocus, prairie	*Anemone* sp	Protoanemonin
Crocus, wild	*Anemone* sp	Protoanemonin
Crotalaria	*Crotalaria* sp	Pyrrolizidine alkaloids
Croton	*Codiaeum* sp	Dermatitis
Croton	*Croton tiglium*	GI/dermatitis
Crown of thorns	*Euphorbia milii*	GI/dermatitis
Crown plant	*Calotropis gigantea*	Cardiac glycosides
Crown vetch	*Coronilla varia*	Photodermatitis
Cruel plant	*Araujia sericifera*	GI/dermatitis
Cukoo pint	*Arum maculatum*	Calcium oxalates/dermatitis
Cup of gold	*Solandra* sp	Solanine/anticholinergic
Curlilocks	*Hedera helix*	GI/dermatitis
Curly dock	*Rumex crispus*	Soluble oxalates/dermatitis
Cut-leaf philodendron	*Monstera deliciosa*	Calcium oxalates
Cycas	*Cycas* sp	Cyanogenic glycosides
Cycas or cycads	*Zamia* sp	Cyanogenic glycosides
Cyclamen	*Cyclamen* sp	GI
Daffodil (bulb)	*Narcissus* sp	GI/dermatitis
Dagga, wild	*Leonotis leonurus*	Intoxicant/mild sedative
Daisy	*Chrysanthemum* sp	Pyrethrums
Daphne	*Daphne mezereum*	Daphne
Datura	*Datura* sp	Anticholinergic
Dead man fingers	*Oenanthe crocata*	Stimulant/respiratory failure
Deadly nightshade	*Atropa belladonna*	Anticholinergic
Death camus	*Zygadenus* or *zigadenus* sp	Veratrum alkaloids
Delphinium	*Delphinium* sp	Aconitum
Desert rose	*Adenium obesum*	Cardiac glycosides
Devil weed	*Datura stamonium*	Anticholinergic
Devil's apple	*Datura stramonium*	Anticholinergic
Devil's backbone	*Euphorbia tithymaloides*	GI
Devil's backbone	*Pedilanthus tithymaloides*	GI
Devil's bit	*Chamaelirium luteum*	GI
Devil's darning needle	*Clematis virginiana*	Protoanemonin
Devil's ear	*Arisaema triphyllum*	Calcium oxalates/dermatitis
Devil's ivy	*Epipremnum aureum*	Calcium oxalates
Devil's ivy	*Scindapsus aureus*	Calcium oxalates
Devil's plague	*Daucus carota*	Dermatitis
Devil's tomato	*Solanum eleagnifolium*	Solanine
Devil's tongue	*Amorphophallus rivieri*	Calcium oxalates/dermatitis
Devil's trumpet	*Datura stramonium*	Anticholinergic

TABLE 62.1   Toxic Plants (*Continued*)

Common Name	Botanical Name	Toxins/Effects
Dieffenbachia	*Dieffenbachia* sp	Calcium oxalates
Dog buttons	*Strychnos nux-vomica*	Strychnine
Dog parsley	*Aethusa cynapium*	Stimulants/coniine
Dogbane	*Apocynum* sp	Cardiac glycosides
Dogwood, bloodtwig	*Cornus sanguinea*	Dermatitis
Dolls-eyes	*Actaea spicata*	Protoanemonin
Donkeytail	*Euphorbia myrsinites*	GI/dermatitis
Dragon lily or plant	*Dracunculus vulgaris*	Calcium oxalates
Dragon root	*Arisaema triphyllum*	Calcium oxalates/dermatitis
Dumbcane or plant	*Dieffenbachia* sp	Calcium oxalates
Dusty miller	*Senecio* sp	Pyrrolizidine alkaloids
Dwarf bay	*Daphne mezereum*	Daphne
Easter flower	*Anemone patens*	Protoanemonin
Easter rose	*Helleborus niger*	Hellebore
Eggplant (green parts)	*Solanum melongena*	Solanine
Elderberry (green parts)	*Sambucus* sp	GI
Elephant garlic	*Allium ampeloprasum*	GI/dermatitis/hypoglycemia
Elephant's ear	*Alocasia, colocasia, caladium* sp	Calcium oxalates
Elephant's ear	*Caladium* sp	Calcium oxalates/dermatitis
Elephant's ear	*Colocasia esculenta*	Calcium oxalates
Elephant's ear philodendron	*Philodendron hastatum*	Calcium oxalates
Elephant's foot	*Elephantopus* sp	Mucous membrane irritant/allergen
Elm tree	*Ulmus* sp	Dermatitis/allergic reactions
Emerald idol	*Opuntia* sp	Contact dermatitis/wound injury from thorns
English ivy	*Hedera helix*	GI/dermatitis
English laurel	*Prunus laurocerasus*	Cyanogenic glycosides
Eucalyptus	*Eucalyptus* sp	GI
Euonymus	*Euonymus* sp	GI
Euonymus, winged	*Euonymus alata*	GI
Evening trumpet flower	*Gelsemium sempervirens*	Gelsemium
Eye balm or root	*Hydrastis canadensis*	GI/stimulant/cardiac
Eye bright	*Euphorbia* sp	Dermatitis
Eyebane	*Euphorbia maculata*	Dermatitis
Eye-bright	*Chamaesyce nutans*	Dermatitis
Eye-bright	*Lobelia inflata*	Lobeline/dermatitis
Fairy wand	*Chamaelirium luteum*	GI
False hellebore	*Veratrum* sp	Veratrum alkaloids
False Jerusalem cherry	*Solanum capsicastrum*	Solanine
False parsley	*Aethusa cynapium*	Stimulants/coniine
False parsley	*Cicuta maculata*	Stimulants
False Queen Anne's lace	*Ammi majus*	Dermatitis
Fava bean	*Vicia faba* (not to be confused with *Vicia sativa*)	Favism: GI, hemolytic anemia, jaundice, hemoglobinuria, vascular collapse
Fennel, dog	*Anthemis cotula*	Dermatitis/allergen

(*continued*)

TABLE 62.1 Toxic Plants (*Continued*)

Common Name	Botanical Name	Toxins/Effects
Fennel, wild	*Nigella damascena*	Protoanemonin
Fever root	*Cicuta maculata*	Stimulants
Feverfew	*Tanacetum* sp	Allergic contact dermatitis
Ficus	*Ficus benjamina*	Dermatitis
Fiddleheads	*Osmunda cinnamonea*	Raw or undercooked: GI
Filbert	*Corylus* sp	Dermatitis
Fire cracker plant	*Aesculus pavia*	GI/depressant
Firebush or weed	*Kochia scoparia*	Photosensitivity/soluble oxalates
Fire-on-the-mountain	*Euphorbia cyathophora*	GI/dermatitis
Five-fingered root	*Oenantha crocata*	Stimulant/respiratory failure
Flag	*Iris* sp	GI/dermatitis
Flax	*Linium* sp	Cyanogenic glycosides
Flax olive	*Daphne* sp	Daphne
Fleabane	*Erigeron* sp	Dermatitis
Flowering maple	*Abutilon* sp	Dermatitis
Flying saucers	*Ipomoea tricolor*	Lysergic acid amides
Fool's parsley	*Aethusa cynapium*	Stimulants/coniine
Four o'clock (seeds)	*Mirabilis jalapa*	GI/dermatitis/hallucinogen
Foxglove	*Digitalis purpurea*	Cardiac glycosides
Fragrance of the night	*Cestrum nocuturnum*	Anticholinergic/solanine
Fraxinella	*Dictamnus* sp	Photodermatitis
Gaillardia	*Gaillardia* sp	Dermatitis
Garden sorrel	*Rumex acetosa*	Soluble oxalates
Garlic	*Allium sativum*	GI/dermatitis/hypoglycemia
Garlic, elephant	*Allium ampeloprasum*	GI/dermatitis/hypoglycemia
Gelsemium	*Gelsemium* sp	Gelsemium
Geranium	*Pelargonium* sp	Mild dermatitis may occur
Ginger, variegated	*Alpina sanderae*	Dermatitis
Ginkgo	*Ginkgo biloba*	Dermatitis Chronic: prolonged bleeding times
Ginseng	*Panax pseudoginseng*	Chronic: diarrhea/CNS stimulation/hypertension
Gladiola	*Gladiola* sp	GI/possible dermatitis
Gloriosa lily	*Gloriosa* sp	Colchicine
Gloriosa superba	*Colchicum autumnale*	Colchicine
Glory lily	*Gloriosa* sp	Colchicine
Gold cup	*Solandra* sp	Solanine/anticholinergic
Golden chain tree	*Laburnum* sp	Cytisine
Golden pothos	*Epipremnum aureum*	Calcium oxalates
Golden rain	*Cassia fistula*	GI
Golden seal	*Hydrastis canadensis*	GI/stimulant/cardiac
Golden shower	*Cassia fistula*	GI
Golden slipper	*Cypripedium calceolus*	Dermatitis
Golden trumpet	*Allamanda cathartica*	GI/dermatitis
Good luck leaf	*Oxalis deppei*	Soluble oxalates
Gopher plant	*Euphorbia lathyrus*	GI/dermatitis
Gordolobo	*Achillea millefolium*	GI/dermatitis
Gotu kola	*Hydrocotyle* sp	Depressant/dermatitis

TABLE 62.1   Toxic Plants (*Continued*)

Common Name	Botanical Name	Toxins/Effects
Grapefruit (peels and thorns)	*Citrus paradisii*	Photodermatitis
Greasewood	*Larrea tridentate*	Hepatotoxicity
Green dragon	*Datura stramonium*	Anticholinergic
Green trumpet	*Datura stramonium*	Anticholinergic
Ground lemon	*Podophyllum peltatum*	Severe dermatitis/GI/depressant/alopecia
Groundsel	*Senecio* sp	Pyrrolizidine alkaloids
Habanero pepper	*Capsicum* sp	Capsaicin
Hawaiian baby woodrose	*Argyreia nervosa*	Lysergic acid alkaloids
Hawaiian poppy	*Argemone glauca*	GI/depressant
Hawaiian prickly poppy	*Argemone glauca*	GI/depressant
Hawaiian woodrose	*Merremia tuberose*	Lysergic acid amides
Hazelnut	*Corylus* sp	Dermatitis
Healing onion	*Ornithogalum caudatum*	Cardiac glycosides
Heart leaf philodendron	*Philodendron* sp	Calcium oxalates
Heath, berry	*Erica* sp	Grayanotoxins
Heath, heather	*Calluna vulgaris*	Grayanotoxins
Heather, bog	*Erica* sp	Grayanotoxins
Heather, Scotch	*Calluna vulgaris*	Grayanotoxins
Heavenly blue	*Ipomoea* sp	Lysergic acid alkaloids
Heliotrope	*Heliotropium* sp	Pyrrolizidine alkaloids
Hellebore	*Helleborus niger*	Hellebore
Hellebore	*Veratrum viride*	Veratrum alkaloids
Hells bells	*Datura stramonium*	Anticholinergic
Hemlock	*Conium maculatum*	Coniine
Hemlock, poison	*Conium maculatum*	Coniine
Hemlock, spotted	*Cicuta maculata*	Stimulants
Hemlock, water	*Cicuta maculata*	Stimulants
Henbane	*Hyoscyamus* sp	Anticholinergic
Holly	*Ilex* sp	GI
Hop, common	*Humulus lupulus*	Allergen/dermatitis/conjunctivitis
Hops, wild	*Bryonia* sp	GI
Horse chestnut	*Aesculus* sp	GI/depressant
Horseradish	*Armoracia rusticana*	GI
Horsetail	*Equisetum* sp	Chronic: suspected carcinogen
Hyacinth (bulb)	*Hyacinthus orientalis*	GI/dermatitis
Hydrangea	*Hydrangea* sp	Cyanogenic glycosides
Hydrocotyle	*Hydrocotyle* sp	Depressant/dermatitis
Hypericum	*Hypericum perforatum*	Photodermatitis/GI/depressant/serotonin syndrome
Incense cedar	*Calocedrus* sp	Dermatitis
Inch plant	*Tradescantia* sp	Dermatitis
Indian currant	*Symphoricarpos* sp	GI/depressant
Indian ginger	*Asarum* sp	Aristolochic acid
Indian hemp	*Apocynum* sp	Cardiac glycosides
Indian kale	*Xanthosoma* sp	Calcium oxalates
Indian lilac	*Melia azedarach*	Chinaberry

(continued)

TABLE 62.1 Toxic Plants (*Continued*)

Common Name	Botanical Name	Toxins/Effects
Indian medicine aloe	*Aloe* sp	Anthraquinones
Indian paint	*Hydrastis canadensis*	GI/stimulant/cardiac
Indian poke	*Veratrum* sp	Veratrum alkaloids
Indian tobacco	*Lobelia inflata*	Lobeline/dermatitis
Indigo weed	*Baptisia tinctoria*	Cytisine
Indigo weed	*Sophora tinctoria*	Cytisine
Inkberry (pokeweed)	*Phytolacca americana*	GI/headache
Iris	*Iris* sp	GI/dermatitis
Irish shamrock	*Oxalis acetosella*	Soluble oxalates
Irish tops	*Cytisus scoparius*	Cytisine
Irish tops	*Spartium scoparium*	Cytisine
Iron weed	*Elephantopus* sp	Mucous membrane irritant/ allergen
Iron wood	*Cassia siamea*	Sedative/hepatitis
Italian arum	*Arum italicum*	Calcium oxalates
Ivy	*Hedera* sp	GI/dermatitis
Ivy arum	*Epipremnum aureum*	Calcium oxalates
Ivy bush	*Kalmia latifolia*	Grayanotoxins
Jack-in-the-pulpit	*Arisaema triphyllum*	Calcium oxalates/dermatitis
Jalapeno peppers	*Capsicum annuum*	Capsaicin
Japanese evergreen	*Euonymus japonica*	GI
Japanese lantern	*Physalis* sp	Solanine
Japanese yew (do not confuse with *Taxus*)	*Podocarpus macrophylla*	GI
Jasmine, Carolina	*Gelsemium sempervirens*	Gelsemium
Jasmine, night blooming	*Cestrum nocuturnum*	Anticholinergic/solanine
Jasmine, poet's	*Jasminum officinale*	Dermatitis
Jasmine, yellow	*Gelsemium* sp	Gelsemium
Jaundice berry	*Berberis vulgaris*	Berberine
Jaundice root	*Hydrastis canadensis*	GI/stimulant/cardiac
Jequirity bean	*Abrus precatorius*	Toxalbumins
Jerusalem cherry	*Solanum pseudocapsicum*	Solanine
Jessamine, day or night	*Cestrum diurnum*	Anticholinergic/solanine
Jessamine, night blooming	*Cestrum nocuturnum*	Anticholinergic/solanine
Jessamine, poet's	*Jasminum officinale*	Dermatitis
Jessamine, yellow	*Gelsemium* sp	Gelsemium
Jimson weed	*Datura stramonium*	Anticholinergic
Johnny jump up (seeds only)	*Viola cornuta*	GI
Jumping cactus	*Opuntia* sp	Thorn injury
Juniper	*Juniperus* sp	Dermatitis/berries: urinary tract irritant
Kaffir lily	*Clivia miniata*	Gastrointestinal
Kaht or Kat or Khat	*Catha edulis*	Stimulant
Kava	*Piper methysticum*	Mild sedative
Kentucky coffee tree	*Gymnocladus dioica*	Cytisine
Kola nut	*Cola nitida*	Caffeine
Kratom	*Mitragyna* sp	Psychoactive/opium substitute

TABLE 62.1 Toxic Plants (*Continued*)

Common Name	Botanical Name	Toxins/Effects
Laburnum	*Laburnum anagyroides*	Cytisine
Lady laurel	*Daphne mezereum*	Daphne
Lady's lace	*Ammi majus*	Dermatitis
Lady's slipper	*Cypripedium* sp	Dermatitis
Lady's slipper	*Pedilanthus tithymaloides*	GI
Lady-of-the-night	*Brunfelsia americana*	Stimulants
Lantana	*Lantana camara*	Anticholinergic-like symptoms
Larkspur	*Delphinium* sp	Aconitum
Leather wood or bush	*Dirca palustris*	GI/dermatitis
Leek, wild	*Allium ampeloprasum*	GI/dermatitis/hypoglycemia
Lemon (peels and thorns)	*Citrus limon*	Photodermatitis
Lenten rose	*Helleborus* sp	Hellebore
Leopard's bane	*Arnica* sp	Arnica
Licorice	*Glycyrrhiza glabra*	Hypermineralcorticoidism: hypertension, hypokalemia
Licorice, wild	*Abrus precatorius*	Toxalbumins
Licorice, wild	*Glycyrrhiza* sp	Hypermineralcorticoidism: hypertension, hypokalemia
Lilac, Indian	*Melia azedarach*	Chinaberry
Lilac, Persian	*Melia azedarach*	Chinaberry
Lily of the Incas	*Alstroemeria aurantiaca*	GI/dermatitis
Lily of the Nile	*Agapanthus* sp	Dermatitis
Lily-of-the-valley	*Convallaria majalis*	Cardiac glycoside
Lily-of-the-valley bush or shrub	*Andromeda japonica*	Grayanotoxins
Lily-of-the-valley bush or shrub	*Pieris japonica*	Grayanotoxin
Lime (peels and thorns)	*Citrus aurantifolia*	Photodermatitis
Linseed	*Linium* sp	Cyanogenic glycosides
Lion's tail	*Leonotis leonurus*	Intoxicant/mild sedative
Lobelia	*Lobelia berlandieri*	Lobeline/dermatitis
Locoweed	*Datura stramonium*	Anticholinergic
Locoweed	*Astragalus* sp	Pyrrolizidine alkaloids
Locoweed	*Cannabis sativa*	Euphoriant
Locoweed, stemless	*Oxytropis lambertii*	Pyrrolizidine alkaloids
Locoweed, white	*Oxytropis lambertii*	Pyrrolizidine alkaloids
Locust, black or yellow	*Robinia pseudoacacia*	Toxalbumins
Lombardy poplar	*Populus* sp	Dermatitis
Loquat (seeds)	*Eriobotrya japonica*	Cyanogenic glycosides
Lord and ladies	*Arum maculatum*	Calcium oxalates/dermatitis
Love apple	*Solanum aculeatissimum*	Solanine
Love apple (green parts)	*Lycopersicon lycopersicum*	Solanine
Love bean	*Abrus precatorius*	Toxalbumins
Lucky bean	*Abrus precatorius*	Toxalbumins
Lupine	*Lupinus* sp	Acute: anticholinergic Chronic: permanent neurotoxicity
Ma Huang	*Ephedra* sp	Stimulants
Mace	*Myristica fragrans*	Hallucinogen/anticholinergic

(*continued*)

TABLE 62.1 Toxic Plants (*Continued*)

Common Name	Botanical Name	Toxins/Effects
Mad apple	*Datura stramonium*	Anticholinergic
Madagascar periwinkle	*Cantharanthus roseus*	Vincristine/vinblastine
Mad-dog skullcap	*Calotropis gigantea*	Cardiac glycosides
Maidenhair tree	*Ginkgo biloba*	Dermatitis Chronic: prolonged bleeding times
Mandrake	*Podophyllum peltatum*	Severe dermatitis/GI/depressant/alopecia
Marble queen pothos	*Epipremnum aureum*	Calcium oxalates
Marguerite	*Chrysanthemum frutescens*	Pyrethrums
Marigold, African	*Tagetes sp*	Dermatitis
Marigold, French	*Tagetes sp*	Dermatitis
Marijuana	*Cannabis sativa*	Euphoriant
Marsh marigold	*Caltha palustris*	Protoanemonin
Mate	*Ilex paraguariensis*	Caffeine
Matrimony vine	*Lycium halimifolium*	Anticholinergic
Mauna loa	*Spathiphyllum floribundum*	Calcium oxalates
Mayapple	*Podophyllum peltatum*	Severe dermatitis/GI/depressant/alopecia
Meadow crocus	*Colchicum autumnale*	Colchicine
Meadow saffron	*Colchicum autumnale*	Colchicine
Medicinal aloe	*Aloe sp*	Anthraquinones
Medicine plant	*Aloe sp*	Anthraquinones
Melaleuca	*Melaleuca sp*	Dermatitis
Mescal bean	*Sophora secundiflora*	Cytisine
Mescal button	*Lophophora williamsii*	Hallucinogen
Mesquite	*Prosopis sp*	Dermatitis/allergen
Mexican bird of paradise	*Caesalpinia mexicana*	Tannins/GI
Mexican fire plant	*Euphorbia cyathophora*	GI/dermatitis
Mexican fireweed	*Kochia scoparia*	Photosensitivity/soluble oxalates
Mexican prickle poppy	*Argemone mexicana*	Berberine
Milk thistle	*Silybum marianum*	GI/diaphoresis after chronic use
Milkweed	*Asclepias sp*	Cardiac glycosides
Military herb	*Achillea millefolium*	GI/dermatitis
Miner's tea	*Ephedra sp*	Stimulants
Mistletoe, American	*Phoradendron flavescens*	GI
Mistletoe, European	*Viscum album*	GI
Mistletoe, European	*Viscum album*	GI
Moccasin flower	*Cypripedium calceolus*	Dermatitis
Mock azalea	*Adenium obesum*	Cardiac glycosides
Mock orange	*Poncirus trifoliata*	GI
Mock orange	*Prunus caroliniana*	Cyanogenic glycosides
Mole plant	*Euphorbia lathyrus*	GI/dermatitis
Monkshood	*Aconitum napellus*	Aconitum
Moon	*Lophophora williamsii*	Hallucinogen
Moon weed	*Datura stramonium*	Anticholinergic

TABLE 62.1 Toxic Plants (*Continued*)

Common Name	Botanical Name	Toxins/Effects
Moonflower	*Datura inoxia*	Anticholinergic
Moonflower	*Ipomoea alba*	Lysergic acid alkaloids
Moonseed	*Menispermum* sp	Stimulants/dermatitis
Moonseed, Carolina	*Cocculus carolinus*	Stimulants
Mormon tea	*Ephedra* sp	Stimulants
Morning glory (seeds)	*Ipomoea* sp	Lysergic acid alkaloids
Morning glory, wild	*Convolvulus arvensis*	GI/dermatitis
Morning-noon-and-night	*Brunfelsia* sp	Stimulants
Mosquito plant	*Pelargonium* sp	Mild dermatitis may occur
Mother-in-law plant	*Caladium* sp	Calcium oxalates/dermatitis
Mother-in-law plant	*Dieffenbachia sequine*	Calcium oxalates
Mother-in-law's tongue	*Dieffenbachia* sp	Calcium oxalates
Mountain box	*Arctostaphylos uva-ursi*	Hydroquinones
Mountain ivy	*Kalmia latifolia*	Grayanotoxins
Mountain laurel	*Kalmia latifolia*	Grayanotoxins
Mountain pasque-flower	*Anemone montana*	Protoanemonin
Mountain tobacco	*Arnica* sp	Arnica
Mum	*Chrysanthemum* sp	Pyrethrums
Muskrat weed	*Cicuta maculata*	Stimulants
Mustard, wild	*Brassica kaber*	Dermatitis
Myrtle	*Vinca minor*	Vincristine/vinblastine
Naked boys	*Colchicum autumnale*	Colchicine
Naked lady	*Amaryllis belladonna*	GI
Naked lady	*Colchicum autumnale*	Colchicine
Narcissus	*Narcissus* sp	GI/dermatitis
Nectar of the gods	*Allium sativum*	GI/dermatitis/hypoglycemia
Nectarine (chewed pits)	*Prunus persica*	Cyanogenic glycosides
Needlepoint ivy	*Hedera helix*	GI/dermatitis
Nephthytis	*Syngonium podophyllum*	Calcium oxalates
Nerve root	*Cypripedium calceolus*	Dermatitis
Nettle, spurge	*Cnidoscolus stimulosus*	Dermatitis
Nettle, stinging	*Urtica* sp	Dermatitis
Nicotiana	*Nicotiana* sp	Nicotine
Nicotine, ornamental	*Nicotiana longiflora*	Nicotine
Nightshade, American	*Phytolacca americana*	Gastrointestinal/headache
Nightshade, black	*Solanum nigrum*	Solanine
Nightshade, deadly	*Atropa belladonna*	Anticholinergic
Nightshade, deadly	*Solanum* sp	Solanine
Nightshade, poisonous	*Solanum dulcamara*	Solanine
Nightshade, yellow	*Urechites* sp	Cardiac glycosides
Noah's ark	*Cypripedium* sp	Dermatitis
Norfolk island pine	*Araucaria heterophylla*	Dermatitis
Norfolk pine	*Araucaria heterophylla*	Dermatitis
Nosebleed	*Achillea millefolium*	GI/dermatitis
Nutmeg	*Myristica fragrans*	Hallucinogen/anticholinergic
Nutmeg flower	*Nigella sativa*	Protoanemonin
Nux vomica	*Strychnos nux-vomica*	Strychnine
Oak	*Quercus* sp	Tannic acid/dermatitis
Oleander, common	*Nerium oleander*	Cardiac glycosides

(*continued*)

TABLE 62.1 Toxic Plants (*Continued*)

Common Name	Botanical Name	Toxins/Effects
Oleander, yellow	*Thevetia peruviana*	Cardiac glycosides
Olive, common	*Olea europaea*	Dermatitis/allergen
Onion (large quantities)	*Allium cepa*	GI/dermatitis/hypoglycemia
Orange (peels and thorns)	*Citrus sinensis*	Photodermatitis
Oriental poppy	*Papaver orientale*	Opioids
Ornamental cherry	*Prunus* sp	Cyanogenic glycosides
Ornamental pepper	*Capsicum annuum*	Capsaicin
Ornamental pepper	*Solanum pseudocapsicum*	Solanine
Ornamental plum	*Prunus* sp	Cyanogenic glycosides
Oxalis	*Oxalis* sp	Soluble oxalates
Pagoda tree, Japanese	*Sophora japonica*	Cytisine
Pagoda tree, weeping	*Sophora japonica*	Cytisine
Painted leaf	*Euphorbia cyathophora*	GI/dermatitis
Palm (thorns)	*Various*	Wound injury/dermatitis
Pansy (seeds only)	*Viola tricolor*	GI
Paper white narcissus	*Narcissus tazetta*	GI/dermatitis
Papyrus	*Cyperus* sp	Acute: GI
		Chronic: nephrotoxicity/CNS changes
Paradise plant	*Daphne mezereum*	Daphne
Paradise tree	*Melia azedarach*	Chinaberry
Parsley, false	*Cicuta maculata*	Stimulants
Parsley, spotted	*Cicuta maculata*	Stimulants
Parsley, wild	*Cicuta maculata*	Stimulants
Parsley, wild	*Heracleum mantegazzianum*	Photodermatitis
Parsnip (leaves)	*Pastinaca sativa*	Photosensitivity
Parsnip, poison	*Cicuta maculata*	Stimulants
Parsnip, wild	*Cicuta maculata*	Stimulants
Parsnip, wild	*Heracleum mantegazzianum*	Photodermatitis
Pasque flower	*Anemone* sp	Protoanemonin
Passion flower or vine	*Passiflora* sp	Cardiac glycosides/depressants
Peace lily	*Spathiphyllum floribundum*	Calcium oxalates
Peach (chewed pits)	*Prunus persica*	Cyanogenic glycosides
Peacock flower	*Caesalpinia pulcherrima*	Tannins/gastrointestinal
Pear (chewed seeds)	*Pyrus* sp	Cyanogenic glycosides
Pearly gates	*Ipomoea* sp	Lysergic acid alkaloids
Pelargonium	*Pelargonium* sp	Mild dermatitis may occur
Pencil cactus	*Opuntia* sp	Thorn injury
Pennyroyal	*Mentha pulegium*	Multiorgan failure/DIC
Peony	*Paeonia officinalis*	Juice from roots can cause paralysis, dermatitis
Pepper rod or Pepper bush	*Croton humilis*	Dermatitis
Pepper tree	*Schinus molle*	GI/dermatitis
Peppers	*Capsicum* sp	Capsaicin
Periwinkle	*Vinca rosea*	Vincristine/vinblastine

TABLE 62.1   Toxic Plants (*Continued*)

Common Name	Botanical Name	Toxins/Effects
Persian lilac	*Melia azedarach*	Chinaberry
Peruvian lily	*Alstroemeria* sp	GI/dermatitis
Peruvian lily	*Hymenocallis* sp	GI
Peyote; mescal	*Lophophora williamsii*	Hallucinogen
Philodendron	*Philodendron* sp	Calcium oxalates
Photinia	*Photinia arbutifolia*	Cyanogenic glycosides
Physic nut	*Jatropha curcas*	Toxalbumins
Pigeon berry	*Cornus canadensis*	Dermatitis
Pigeon berry or weed	*Phytolacca americana*	GI/headache
Pigeonberry	*Rivina humilis*	GI
Pikake	*Jasminum sambac*	Dermatitis
Pinks	*Dianthus* sp	Dermatitis
Plant of life	*Aloe* sp	Anthraquinones
Pleurisy root	*Asclepias* sp	Cardiac glycosides
Plum (chewed seeds)	*Prunus domestica*	Cyanogenic glycosides
Plumbago, blue	*Plumbago capensis*	Dermatitis
Podocarpus	*Podocarpus macrophylla*	GI
Poet's jessamine or jasmine	*Jasminum officinale*	Dermatitis
Poinciana	*Caesalpinia pulcherrima*	Tannins/GI
Poison bush or tree	*Acokanthera oppositifolia*	Cardiac glycosides
Poison daisy	*Anthemis cotula*	Dermatitis/allergen
Poison hemlock	*Conium maculatum*	Coniine
Poison ivy, oak, sumac	*Toxicodendron* sp	Allergic contact dermatitis
Poison nut	*Strychnos nux-vomica*	Strychnine
Poison parsley	*Conium maculatum*	Coniine
Poison tobacco	*Hyoscyamus niger*	Anticholinergic
Poison vine	*Toxicodendron radicans*	Allergic contact dermatitis
Poison water hemlock	*Cicuta douglasii*	Stimulants
Poke, Indian	*Phytolacca acinosa*	GI/headache
Poke, Indian	*Veratrum viride*	Veratrum alkaloids
Pokesalad plant	*Phytolacca* sp	GI/headache
Poplar	*Populus* sp	Dermatitis
Poppy, common	*Papaver somniferum*	Opioids
Potato (unripe, leaves)	*Solanum tuberosum*	Solanine
Potato vine	*Solanum jasminoides*	Solanine
Pothos	*Scindapsus aureus*	Calcium oxalates
Pothos or Pothos vine	*Epipremnum aureum*	Calcium oxalates
Prairie crocus	*Anemone* sp	Protoanemonin
Prayer bead or bean	*Abrus precatorius*	Toxalbumins
Precatory bean or pea	*Arbus precatorius*	Toxalbumins
Pregnant onion	*Ornithogalum caudatum*	Cardiac glycosides
Prickly pear	*Opuntia* sp	Contact dermatitis/wound injury from thorns
Prickly poppy	*Argemone mexicana*	Berberine
Pride of China	*Melia azedarach*	Chinaberry
Pride of India	*Melia azedarach*	Chinaberry
Pride of Madeira	*Echium* sp	Pyrrolizidine alkaloids
Primrose	*Primula* sp	Dermatitis

(continued)

TABLE 62.1 Toxic Plants (*Continued*)

Common Name	Botanical Name	Toxins/Effects
Primula	*Primula sp*	Dermatitis
Privet, California	*Ligustrum ovalifolium*	GI
Puke weed	*Lobelia inflata*	Lobeline/dermatitis
Purge nut	*Jatropha curcas*	Toxalbumins
Qat or Quat	*Catha edulis*	Stimulants
Quaker buttons	*Strychnos nux-vomica*	Strychnine
Quaking aspen	*Populus sp*	Dermatitis
Queen Anne's lace	*Daucus carota*	Dermatitis
Queen's delight	*Stillingia sp*	Dermatitis
Queen's lace	*Daucus carota*	Dermatitis
Queen's root	*Stillingia sylvatica*	Dermatitis
Ragweed	*Ambrosia artemisiifolia*	Dermatitis/allergen
Ragwort	*Senecio sp*	Pyrrolizidine alkaloids
Ranunculus	*Ranunculus sp*	Protoanemonin
Rattlebox	*Crotolaria sp*	Pyrrolizidine alkaloids
Rattlebox	*Sesbania sp*	Pyrrolizidine alkaloids
Rattlebox, purple	*Daubentonia sp*	Pyrrolizidine alkaloids
Rattlebush or Rattleweed	*Baptisia sp*	Cytisine
Rattlebush or weed	*Sophora tinctoria*	Cytisine
Red root	*Sanguinaria canadensis*	GI/depressant
Redberry	*Arctostaphylos uva-ursi*	Hydroquinones
Rhododendron	*Rhododendron genus*	Grayanotoxins
Rhubarb (leaves)	*Rheum sp*	Soluble oxalates/dermatitis
Rhubarb, wild	*Heracleum mantegazzianum*	Photodermatitis
Rock poppy	*Chelidonium majus*	GI/hepatotoxicity/dermatitis
Rock rose	*Cistus creticus*	Dermatitis
Rosary beads	*Senecio sp*	Pyrrolizidine alkaloids
Rosary bean or bead	*Senecio sp*	Pyrrolizidine alkaloids
Rosary bean or pea	*Abrus precatorius*	Toxalbumins
Rosary pearls	*Senecio sp*	Pyrrolizidine alkaloids
Rose periwinkle	*Catharanthus roseus*	Vincristine/vinblastine
Rubber tree	*Hevea brasiliensis*	Dermatitis/allergen
Rubber vine	*Cryptostegia grandiflora*	Cardiac glycosides
Rue	*Ruta graveolens*	Dermatitis/photosensitivity/abortion
Sacred Datura	*Datura inoxia*	Anticholinergic
Sacred lily of India	*Amorphophallus rivieri*	Calcium oxalates/dermatitis
Saffron	*Crocus sativus*	Bradycardia/hemorrhage/vasodilation/vertigo
Saffron crocus	*Crocus sativus*	Bradycardia/hemorrhage/vasodilation/vertigo
Sagebrush	*Artemisia sp*	Stimulants/depressants
Sago cycas	*Zamia sp*	Cyanogenic glycosides
Sago cycas/palm	*Cycas sp*	Cyanogenic glycosides
Salvia	*Salvia divinorum*	Hallucinogen
Sambucus (green parts)	*Sambucus caerulea*	GI
Sandberry	*Arctostaphylos uva-ursi*	Hydroquinones

TABLE 62.1   Toxic Plants (*Continued*)

Common Name	Botanical Name	Toxins/Effects
Sassafras	*Sassafras* sp	GI/depressant/hypersensitivity to touch
Scotch broom	*Cytisus scoparius*	Cytisine
Scotch broom	*Spartium scoparium*	Cytisine
Scotch heather	*Calluna vulgaris*	Grayanotoxin
Sea onion	*Scilla verna*	Cardiac glycosides
Sesbania	*Sesbania* sp	Pyrrolizidine alkaloids
Shamrock	*Oxalis* sp	Soluble oxalates
Shasta daisy	*Chrysanthemum* sp	Pyrethrums
Shell flower	*Alpinia zerumbet*	Dermatitis
Silybinin	*Silybum marianum*	GI/diaphoresis after chronic use
Silymarin	*Silybum marianum*	GI/diaphoresis after chronic use
Skunk cabbage	*Symplocarpus foetidus*	Calcium oxalates
Skunk cabbage	*Veratrum* sp	Veratrum alkaloids
Skunkweed	*Symplocarpus foetidus*	Calcium oxalates
Slipper flower or plant	*Pedilanthus tithymaloides*	GI
Slipper plant or flower	*Euphorbia tithymaloides*	GI
Slippery root	*Symphytum officinale*	Pyrrolizidine alkaloids
Snake flower	*Echium vulgare*	Pyrrolizidine alkaloids
Snakeroot	*Aristolochia* sp	Aristolochic acid
Snakeroot	*Asarum* sp	Aristolochic acid
Snakeroot	*Cicuta maculata*	Stimulants
Snakeroot	*Eupatorium* sp	Pyrrolizidine alkaloids
Snakeroot, black	*Zygadenus venenosus*	Veratrum alkaloids
Snakeroot, black	*Cimicifuga racemosa*	Cimicifuga
Snow on the mountain	*Euphorbia marginata*	GI/dermatitis
Snowberry	*Symphoricarpos* sp	GI/depressant
Snowdrop	*Galanthus* sp	GI
Snowflake	*Leucojum vernum*	GI
Snowflower	*Spathiphyllum floribundum*	Calcium oxalates
Soapberry	*Sapindus* sp	GI/dermatitis
Solandra	*Solandra* sp	Solanine/anticholinergic
Solomon's lily	*Arum palestinum*	Calcium oxalates
Son-before-the-father	*Colchicum autumnale*	Colchicine
Sorrel	*Oxalis* sp	Soluble oxalates
Sorrel	*Rumex* sp	Soluble oxalates
Spanish bayonet	*Yucca aloifolia*	GI/wound injury from thorns
Spanish broom	*Spartium junceum*	Cytisine
Spathe flower	*Spathiphyllum* sp	Calcium oxalates
Spathiphyllum	*Spathiphyllum* sp	Calcium oxalates
Spider flower or lily	*Hymenocallis americana*	GI
Spindle tree, Japanese	*Euonymus japonica*	GI
Spineless cactus	*Opuntia* sp	Contact dermatitis/wound injury from thorns
Split leaf philodendron	*Monstera deliciosa*	Calcium oxalates
Spotted cowbane	*Cicuta maculata*	Stimulants

(*continued*)

TABLE 62.1   Toxic Plants (*Continued*)

Common Name	Botanical Name	Toxins/Effects
Spotted hemlock	*Cicuta maculata*	Stimulants
Spotted hemlock	*Conium maculatum*	Coniine
Spotted parsley	*Cicuta maculata*	Stimulants
Spurge	*Euphorbia myrsinites*	GI/dermatitis
Spurge flax	*Daphne mezereum*	Daphne
Spurge nettle	*Cnidoscolus stimulosus*	Dermatitis
Spurge olive	*Daphne mezereum*	Daphne
Squill	*Urginea maritima*	Cardiac glycosides
St. John's wort	*Hypericum perforatum*	Photodermatitis/GI/depressant/ serotonin syndrome
St. Joseph lily	*Amaryllis* sp	GI
Star fruit	*Averrhoa carambola*	Soluble oxalates (in renal failure patients)
Star hyacinth	*Scilla amoena*	Cardiac glycosides
Star thistle, yellow	*Centaurea solstitialis*	Mucous membrane irritant/ allergen
Star-glory	*Ipomoea quamoclit*	Lysergic acid alkaloids
Star-of-Bethlehem	*Hippobroma longiflora*	Lobeline
Star-of-Bethlehem	*Laurentia longiflora*	Lobeline
Star-of-Bethlehem	*Ornithogalum* sp	Cardiac glycosides
Stinging spurge	*Cnidoscolus stimulosus*	Dermatitis
Stinking hellebore	*Helleborus foetidus*	Hellebore
Stinking rose	*Allium sativum*	GI/dermatitis/hypoglycemia
Stinkweed	*Datura stramonium*	Anticholinergic
String of beads	*Senecio* sp	Pyrrolizidine alkaloids
String of pearls	*Senecio* sp	Pyrrolizidine alkaloids
Strychnine tree	*Strychnos nux-vomica*	Strychnine
Sumac, poison	*Toxicodendron* sp	Allergic contact dermatitis
Summer skies	*Ipomoea tricolor*	Lysergic acid amides
Swamp sumac	*Toxicodendron* sp	Allergic contact dermatitis
Sweet clover	*Melilotus alba*	Warfarin
Sweet flag	*Acorus calamus*	Dermatitis
Sweet pea	*Lathyrus odoratus*	Large ingestions: late onset paralysis
Sweet William	*Dianthus* sp	Dermatitis
Swiss cheese plant	*Monstera deliciosa*	Calcium oxalates
Tansy	*Chrysanthemum* sp	Pyrethrums
Tansy	*Tanacetum vulgare*	Dermatitis
Taro	*Alocasia macrorrhiza*	Calcium oxalates
Taro	*Colocasia esculenta*	Calcium oxalates
Taro vine	*Epipremnum aureum*	Calcium oxalates
Texas snake root	*Aristolochia* sp	Aristolochic acid
Texas umbrella tree	*Melia azedarach*	Chinaberry
Thornapple	*Argemone mexicana*	Berberine
Thornapple	*Datura stramonium*	Anticholinergic
Tobacco	*Nicotiana* sp	Nicotine
Tobacco, Indian	*Lobelia inflata*	Lobeline/dermatitis
Tobacco, wild	*Lobelia inflata*	Lobeline/dermatitis
Tobacco, wild	*Nicotiana* sp	Nicotine

TABLE 62.1 Toxic Plants (*Continued*)

Common Name	Botanical Name	Toxins/Effects
Tomatillo (leaves, stems, unripe fruit)	*Physalis* sp	Solanine
Tomato (leaves, stems)	*Lycopersicon* sp	Solanine
Tomato (leaves, stems)	*Physalis* sp	Solanine
Tonka bean	*Dipteryx odorata*	Coumarin
Toyon (leaves)	*Photinia arbutifolia*	Cyanogenic glycosides
Tree tobacco	*Nicotiana glauca*	Nicotine
Trumpet bush or tree	*Tabebuia* sp	GI/dermatitis
Trumpet creeper or vine	*Campsis radicans*	Dermatitis
Trumpet flower	*Solandra longiflora*	Solanine/anticholinergic
Trumpet lily	*Datura stramonium*	Anticholinergic
Trumpet lily	*Zantedeschia aethiopica*	Calcium oxalates
Tuberose	*Polianthes tuberose*	GI
Tulip (bulb)	*Tulipa* sp	GI/dermatitis
Tung nut	*Aleurites fordii*	GI/dermatitis
Tung oil tree	*Aleurites fordii*	GI/dermatitis
Umbrella leaf	*Podophyllum peltatum*	Severe dermatitis/GI/depressant/alopecia
Umbrella plant	*Cyperus* sp	Acute: GI Chronic: nephrotoxicity/CNS changes
Uva-ursi	*Arctostaphylos uva-ursi*	Hydroquinones
Valerian	*Valeriana officinales*	Depressants
Valerian, American	*Cypripedium calceolus*	Dermatitis
Venus's shoe	*Cypripedium calceolus*	Dermatitis
Veratum	*Veratum* sp	Veratrum alkaloids
Vetch, yellow	*Lathyrus pratensis*	Large ingestions: Late-onset paralysis
Vinca minor or major	*Vinca rosea*	Vincristine/vinblastine
Vinca rosea	*Vinca rosea*	Vincristine/vinblastine
Viola (seeds only)	*Viola odorata*	GI
Violet (seeds only)	*Viola odorata*	GI
Virginia creeper	*Parthenocissus* sp	Soluble oxalates/calcium oxalates
Vomit nut	*Strychnos nux-vomica*	Strychnine
Voodoo lily	*Amorphophallus rivieri*	Calcium oxalates/dermatitis
Walnut, black (green shells)	*Juglans nigra*	Dermatitis
Wandering Jew	*Tradescantia* sp	Dermatitis
Water hemlock	*Cicuta* sp	Stimulants
Wax berry	*Symphoricarpos* sp	GI/depressant
Wax vine	*Senecio macroglossus*	Pyrrolizidine alkaloids
Waxberry	*Myrica cerifera*	Dermatitis
Weeping fig	*Ficus benjamina*	Dermatitis
Weeping tea tree	*Melaleuca leucadendron*	Dermatitis
Weeping willow	*Salix* sp	Dermatitis
Whippoorwill-shoe	*Cypripedium calceolus*	Dermatitis
Wild calla	*Calla palustris*	Calcium oxalates
Wild carrot	*Cicuta maculata*	Stimulants

(continued)

TABLE 62.1 Toxic Plants (*Continued*)

Common Name	Botanical Name	Toxins/Effects
Wild carrot	*Daucus carota*	Dermatitis
Wild cherry	*Prunus* sp	Cyanogenic glycosides
Wild coffee	*Polyscias guilfoyei*	Dermatitis/GI/depressant
Wild crocus	*Anemone* sp	Protoanemonin
Wild garlic	*Allium* sp	GI/dermatitis/hypoglycemia
Wild ginger	*Asarum* sp	Aristolochic acid
Wild indigo	*Baptisia tinctoria*	Cytisine
Wild indigo	*Sophora tinctoria*	Cytisine
Wild iris	*Iris versicolor*	GI/dermatitis
Wild lemon	*Podophyllum peltatum*	Severe dermatitis/GI/depressant/alopecia
Wild licorice	*Abrus precatorius*	Toxalbumins
Wild onion	*Allium* sp	GI/dermatitis/hypoglycemia
Wild parsnip	*Angelica archangelica*	Photodermatitis
Wild parsnip	*Cicuta maculata*	Stimulants
Wild parsnip	*Pastinaca sativa*	Photosensitivity
Wild pepper	*Daphne mezereum*	Daphne
Wild saffron	*Colchicum autumnale*	Colchicine
Wild tobacco	*Nicotiana* sp	Nicotine
Wild turnip	*Arisaema triphyllum*	Calcium oxalates/dermatitis
Windflower	*Anemone* sp	Protoanemonin
Winterberry	*Ilex* sp	GI
Wisteria	*Wisteria* sp	GI
Wolf's bane	*Arnica* sp	Arnica
Wolf's milk	*Euphorbia esula*	GI/dermatitis
Wolfsbane	*Aconitum napellus*	Aconitum
Wonder bulb	*Colchicum autumnale*	Colchicine
Wonderflower	*Ornithogalum thyrsoides*	Cardiac glycosides
Wood rose (seeds)	*Merremia tuberosa*	Lysergic acid amides
Wood rose, Hawaiian (seeds)	*Merremia tuberosa*	Lysergic acid amides
Wood rose, Hawaiian baby (seeds)	*Argyreia nervosa*	Lysergic acid alkaloids
Wood vine	*Gelsemium sempervirens*	Gelsemium
Woodbine	*Parthenocissus* sp	Soluble oxalates/calcium oxalates
Woodrose, Hawaiian baby (seeds)	*Merremia tuberosa*	Lysergic acid amides
Wormseed	*Chenopodium ambrosioides*	GI
Wormseed or Wormwood	*Artemisia* sp	Stimulants/depressants
Xanthosoma	*Xanthosoma* sp	Calcium oxalates
Yarrow	*Achillea millefolium*	GI/dermatitis
Yellow false jasmine	*Gelsemium sempervirens*	Gelsemium
Yellow jasmine or jessamine	*Gelsemium sempervirens*	Gelsemium
Yellow locust	*Robinia pseudoacacia*	Toxalbumins
Yellow oleander	*Thevetia peruviana*	Cardiac glycoside
Yerba mate	*Ilex paraguariensis*	Caffeine

TABLE 62.1	Toxic Plants *(Continued)*

Common Name	Botanical Name	Toxins/Effects
Yesterday-and-today	*Brunfelsia* sp	Stimulants
Yesterday-today-and-tomorrow	*Brunfelsia* sp	Stimulants
Ye w	*Taxus* sp	Cardiac glycosides
Yew, Japanese (do not confuse with *Taxus*)	*Podocarpus macrophylla*	GI
Yohimbine	*Corynanthe yohimbe*	α-2-Adrenoreceptor antagonist/ mild hallucinogen
Yucca	*Yucca aloifolia*	GI/thorn injury

CNS, central nervous system; GI, gastrointestinal.

Central nervous system (CNS) stimulation may be caused by a variety of plants with various mechanisms of action. Cicutoxin, found in water hemlock, is thought to cause status epilepticus from overstimulation of the cholinergic pathways. Seizures may occur as suddenly as 5 minutes after ingestion but may be delayed up to 1 to 2 hours. Postictal states following seizures may mislead the clinician into thinking that a depressant drug has been ingested (6,8).

Sudden onset of unconsciousness is seen after ingestion of monkshood, hellebore, or death camas. Ingestion of nicotiana, lantana, and large quantities of mescal beans may cause delayed CNS depression. Anticholinergic plants such as jimson weed or belladonna may cause hallucinations and delirium, along with CNS stimulation or depression (1,6,8).

Well-known hallucinogenic or perception-altering plants include marijuana and peyote. Other hallucinogenic plants include the morning glory, Hawaiian wood rose, four o'clock, and nutmeg (see Chapter 51). Usually, large amounts are required to result in any effect. Anticholinergic plants, such as jimsonweed and belladonna, also produce hallucinations (1,5,6,8). It should be noted that *Amanita muscaria* and *Amanita psilocybe* mushrooms are also used intentionally for their psychoactive properties (see Chapter 61).

Dermal exposure can cause skin irritation as a result of mechanical, chemical, or allergic reactions; photodermatitis; or a combination of these. Severity of symptoms depends on the amount of exposure, the individual sensitivity, and the part of the body exposed. Most cases are self-limiting and resolve within 14 to 21 days (6,8).

An allergic reaction is a true sensitization of an individual to the allergen contained in the plant. After the first exposure, the patient's next exposure has a 5- to 7-day latency period before the immunological response develops. Allergic contact dermatitis presents with pruritus and vesiculation. The affected area may be erythematous and edematous and may develop large bullae. Weeping and crusting of the affected areas may occur (6,8).

TABLE 62.2 Nontoxic Plants

Common Name	Botanical Name	Common Name	Botanical Name
Abelia	*Abelia* sp	Bigleaf palm	*Fatsia japonica*
Acanthus	*Acanthus* sp	Billbergia	*Quesnella* sp
Adobe lily	*Fritillaria pluriflora*	Birch tree	*Betula* sp
African daisy	*Gerbera jamesonii*	Bird cherry	*Osmaronia* sp
African daisy	*Dimorphotheca pluvialis*	Bird's nest fern	*Asplenium* sp
		Bishop's cap or hood	*Astrophytum myriostigma*
African violet	*Saintpaulia ionantha*	Bishop's elder or weed	*Aegopodium podagraria*
Aglaonema	*Aglaonema* sp	Black haw	*Crataegus* sp
Air plant	*Kalanchoe pinnata*	Black haw	*Viburnum lentago*
Ajuga	*Ajuga* sp	Black thorn	*Crataegus* sp
Albizia	*Albizia* sp	Blazing star	*Liatris* sp
Aluminum plant	*Pilea cadierei*	Bleeding glory bower	*Clerodendrum* sp
Alyssum	*Alyssum* sp		
Angel's tears	*Soleirolia soleirolii*	Bleeding heart	*Clerodendrum* sp
Arbutus	*Arbutus unedo*	Bluebell, English, Spanish, or Texas	*Endymion* sp
Areca palm	*Areca lutescens*		
Arrowroot	*Maranta* sp		
Artillery plant	*Pilea* sp		
Asparagus fern	*Asparagus sprengeri*	Blue spruce	*Picea pungens*
Aspidistra	*Aspidistra* sp	Boston fern	*Nephrolepsis exalta*
Aster, Chinese	*Callistephus chinensis*	Bottlebrush	*Callistemon* sp
		Brain plant	*Calathea makoyana*
Astilbe	*Astilbe japonica*	Brazilian firecracker	*Manettia bicolor*
Australian umbrella tree	*Brassala actinophylla*		
Baby's breath	*Gypsophila* sp	Breath of heaven	*Diosma ericoides*
Baby's tears	*Soleirolia soleirolii*	Breath of heaven	*Coleonema ericoides*
Baby's tears	*Hypoestes phyllostachya*	Bride's bonnet	*Clintonia uniflora*
Bachelor buttons	*Centaurea cyanus*	Bride's flower	*Stephanotis floribunda*
Balloon flower	*Platycodon grandiflorus*	Brodiaea	*Dichelostemma pulchellum*
Bamboo, common	*Phyllostachys aurea*		
Bamboo palm	*Chamaedorea erumpens*	Bromeliad king	*Vriesea hieroglyphica*
Basket plant or vine	*Aeschynanthus* sp	Bromeliad, blushing	*Neoregelia carolinae*
Bayberry	*Aeschynanthus* sp	Buchu	*Diosma ericoides*
Bear's breech	*Acanthus* sp	Buddleia	*Buddleia davidii*
Beauty berry	*Callicarpa* sp	Burro's tail	*Sedum morganianum*
Bee balm	*Monarda didyma*		
Bee balm	*Melissa officinalis*	Busy Lizzie	*Impatients wallerna*
Beech tree	*Fagus* sp	Butterfly bush	*Buddleia davidii*
		Butterfly lily	*Hedychium coronarium*
Bell flower	*Platycodon grandiflorus*		
Bell flower	*Campanula* sp	Butterfly palm	*Chrysalidocarpus lutescens*
Bells of Ireland	*Moluccella* sp		

TABLE 62.2   Nontoxic Plants (*Continued*)

Common Name	Botanical Name	Common Name	Botanical Name
Buttonball	*Platanus occidentali*	Christmas kalanchoe	*Kalanchoe blossfeldiana*
Button fern	*Pellaea rotundifolia*	Cigar flower	*Cuphea* sp
Buttons on a string	*Crassula rupestris*	Cinderella slippers	*Sinningia pusilla*
Cabbage kale	*Brassica oleracea*	Cinquefoil	*Potentilla* sp
Calathea	*Calathea* sp	Clarkia	*Clarkia* sp
Calendula	*Calendula officinalis*	Clianthus	*Clianthus* sp
California poppy	*Eschscholzia californica*	Cobra lily, orchid or plant	*Darlingtonia californica*
Camellia	*Camellia* sp	Cockscomb	*Celosia* sp
Canary date palm	*Phoenix canariensis*	Coleus	*Coleus* sp
Candle plant	*Plectranthus oetendahlii*	Columbine	*Aquilegia* sp
Candy corn plant	*Hypocyrta* sp	Coneflower	*Echinacea angustifolia*
Canna lily	*Canna* sp	Coral bells	*Kalanchoe uniflora*
Canterbury-bell gloxinia	*Gloxinia perennis*	Coral bells	*Heuchera sanguinea*
Cardinal flower	*Rechsteineria cardinalis*	Coral berry	*Ardisia crenata*
		Cordyline	*Cordyline australis*
Cardinal flower	*Sinningia cardinalis*	Coreopsis	*Coreopsis* spp
Carolina hemlock	*Tsuga* sp	Corn plant	*Dracaena fragrans*
Carpet bugle	*Ajuga* sp	Cornflower	*Centaurea cyanus*
Cast iron plant	*Aspidistra elatior*	Cornstalk plant	*Dracaena fragrans*
Catalpa	*Catalpa* sp	Cosmos	*Cosmos* sp
Cat ear	*Calochortus* sp	Cotton gum tree	*Nyssa aquatica*
Cathedral bells	*Cobaeae scandens*	Cotyledon	*Cotyledon* sp
Cathedral windows	*Calethea makoyana*	Cranberry tree	*Viburnum* sp
		Crape myrtle	*Lagerstroemia indica*
Cat tail	*Typha latifolia*	Crassula	*Crassula* sp
Cattleya orchid	*Cattleya* sp	Crataegus	*Crataegus* sp
Cedar of Lebanon	*Cedrus libani*	Creeping Charlie	*Plectranthus australis*
Celosia	*Celosia* sp		
Chain of love	*Antigonon leptopus*	Creeping Charlie	*Pilea nummulari-ifolia*
Chandelier plant	*Kalanchoe tubiforum*	Creeping Jenny	*Lysimachia nummularia*
Checker lily	*Fritillaria* sp		
Chenille plant, maroon	*Echeveria derenbergii*	Crocus, spring blooming	*Crocus* sp
Chicken and hens	*Echeveria elegans*	Crossandra	*Crossandra* sp
China doll	*Leea* sp	Crotolaria	*Crotolaria ramosissima*
China doll	*Radermachera* sp		
China rose	*Hibiscus* sp	Cup-and-saucer plant	*Gilla* sp
Chinese evergreen	*Aglaonema modestum*	Cup-and-saucer vine	*Cobaeae scandens*
Chocolate soldier	*Episcia cupreata*		
Christmas cactus	*Schlumbergera bridgesii*	Cupid's bower	*Achimenes erecta*
Christmas cheer	*Sedum* sp		

(continued)

TABLE 62.2 Nontoxic Plants (*Continued*)

Common Name	Botanical Name	Common Name	Botanical Name
Cupid's dart	*Catananche caerulea*	Evening primrose	*Oenothera caespitosa*
Curiosity plant	*Tolmiea menziesii*	Evergreen plant	*Radermachera sp*
Curtain plant	*Kalanchoe sp*	Evergreen thorn	*Pyracantha sp*
Cushionbush	*Calocephalus brownii*	Exacum	*Exacum affine*
		Fairwell-to-spring	*Clarkia amoena*
Cushion pink	*Silene acualis*	Fairy duster	*Calliandra eriophylla*
Dagger plant	*Yucca sp*	Fairy fountain	*Celosia sp*
Dahlia	*Dahlia sp*	False aralia	*Dizygotheca elegantissima*
Dandelion	*Taraxacum officinale*		
Day lily	*Hermocallis sp*	False heather	*Cuphea hyssopifolla*
Decorative kale	*Brassica oleracea*	False lily of the	*Maianthemum*
Deer's foot fern	*Davallia canariensis*	valley	*kamtschaticum*
Deer's tongue	*Liatris sp*	Farewell to	*Clarkia ameona*
Dipper gourd	*Lagenaria siceraria*	spring	
Dogwood, flowering	*Cornus florida*	Fatsia	*Fatsia japonica*
		Feathered	*Celosia sp*
Donkey tail	*Sedum morganianum*	amaranth	
		Feather fern	*Nephrolepis sp*
Double rose of China	*Hibiscus sp*	Fescue	*Festuca sp*
		Fever grass	*Cymbopogon citratus*
Douglas fir	*Pseudotsuga menziesii*		
		Ficus	*Ficus benjamina*
Dracaena	*Cordyline sp*	Fiery spike	*Aphelandra sp*
Dracaena	*Dracaena sp*	Fir tree	*Abies sp*
Dragon tree	*Dracaena draco*	Fir tree	*Pseudotsuga sp*
Dusty miller	*Lynchnis coronaria*	Fire ball plant	*Kalanchoe sp*
Earth star, green or brown	*Cryptanthus acaulis*	Firebird	*Heliconia bihai*
		Firecracker	*Gesneria cuneifolia*
Easter lily	*Lilium longiflorum*	Firecracker flower	*Crossandra spp*
Echeveria	*Echeveria sp*		
Echinacea	*Echinacea sp*	Firecracker plant	*Manettia bicolor*
Elephant's ear	*Enterolobium cyclocarpum*	Firecracker plant	*Cuphea sp*
		Fire lily	*Cyrtanthus sp*
Elephant's ear	*Bergenia cordifolia*	Firethorn	*Pyracantha sp*
Elephant's ear fern	*Platycerium angolense*	Fishpole bamboo	*Phyllostachys aurea*
		Fishtail fern	*Cyrtomium falcatum*
Elephant's foot	*Dioscorea elephantipes*	Fittonia	*Fittonia sp*
		Flame of the forest	*Spathodea campanulata*
Emerald feather or fern	*Asparagus densi-florus sprengeri*		
		Flaming sword	*Vriesea splendens*
Emerald ripple peperomia	*Peperomia caperata*	Flaming violet	*Episcia reptans*
		Flamingo plant	*Hypoestes phyl-lostachya*
Epidendrum orchid	*Epidendrum sp*		
		Floppers	*Kalanchoe sp*
Escallonia	*Escallonia sp*	Flowering kale	*Brassica oleracea*
Euryops	*Euryops sp*	Flowering quince	*Chaenomeles sp*

TABLE 62.2	Nontoxic Plants (*Continued*)

Common Name	Botanical Name	Common Name	Botanical Name
Flower of the Nativity	*Euphorbia pulcherrima*	Gold dust plant	*Alyssum* spp
Flox or Flocks	*Phlox* sp	Gold dust plant	*Aucuba japonica*
Fluted urn	*Billbergia* sp	Golden bells	*Forsythia* spp
Fool proof plant	*Billbergia* sp	Golden globe *or* glow	*Rudbeckia laciniata*
Forget-me-not	*Myosotis* sp		
Forsythia	*Forsythia* sp	Golden stars	*Mammillaria compressa*
Fort knight lily	*Dietes* sp		
Fox's brush	*Centranthus rubber*	Goldfish plant	*Hypocyrta* sp
Fragrant olive	*Osmanthus fragrans*	Goldins gold	*Calendula officinalis*
Freesia	*Freesia* sp	Good luck leaf	*Kalanchoe* sp
French mulberry	*Callicarpa Americana*	Good luck palm	*Chamaedorea elegans*
Friendship plant	*Pilea involucrate*	Good luck plant	*Cordyline terminalis*
Friendship plant	*Billbergia nutans*	Good luck plant	*Kalanchoe daigremontiana*
Fritillaria	*Fritillaria* sp		
Fruitless mulberry	*Morus* sp	Gourd	*Cucurbitaceae* sp
Fuchsia	*Fuchsia* sp	Granddaddy	*Chionanthus virginicus*
Fuzzy ears	*Cyanotis somaliensis*		
		Granny's bonnet	*Aquilegia vulgaris*
Garden canna	*Canna generalis*	Grape hyacinth	*Muscari* sp
Gardenia	*Gardenia* sp	Graybeard	*Tillandsia usneoides*
Garden lavender	*Lavandula officinalis*	Grecian vase	*Quesnelia* sp
Garland flower	*Hedychium coronarium*	Green ripple peperomia	*Peperomia caperata*
		Hackberry	*Celtis* sp
Gazania	*Gazania* sp	Hackberry, Japanese or Chinese	*Celtis* sp
Gerbera daisy	*Gerbera jamesonii*		
German violet	*Exacum* sp		
Ghost plant	*Graptopetalum paraguayense*	Hairy toad plant	*Stapelia* sp
		Harebell	*Endymion* sp
Ghost plant	*Sedum weinbergii*	Hare fern	*Davallia fejeensis*
Giant protea	*Protea cynaroides*	Hawaiian good luck plant	*Cordyline terminalis*
Ginger lily	*Hedychium coronarium*		
		Haws	*Crataegus* sp
Globe thistle	*Echinops* sp	Hawthorne	*Crataegus* sp
Glory of the snow	*Chionodoxa luciliae*	Heart of flame	*Bromelia balansae*
Glory pea	*Clianthus* sp	Heartsease	*Viola tricolor*
Glory tree	*Clerodendrum thomsoniae*	Hearts entangled	*Ceropegia woodii*
		Hearts-on-a-string	*Ceropegia woodii*
Glossy-leaved paper plant	*Fatsia japonica*		
		Heart vine	*Ceropegia woodii*
Glossy privet	*Ligustrum lucidium*	Heather, false	*Cuphea hyssopifolia*
Gloxinia	*Sinningia speciosa*	Heavenly bamboo	*Nandina domestica*
Gloxinia	*Gloxinia perennis*	Helmet flower	*Sinningia cardinalis*
Godetia	*Godetia* spp	Hemlock tree	*Tsuga* sp
Godetia	*Clarkia amoena*	Hen and chickens fern	*Asplenium bulbiferum*
Gold dust dracaena	*Dracaena* spp		
		Hen and chicks	*Echeveria* sp

(*continued*)

TABLE 62.2 Nontoxic Plants (*Continued*)

Common Name	Botanical Name	Common Name	Botanical Name
Hibiscus	*Hibiscus* sp	Japanese snowbell	*Styrax japonica*
Hickory tree	*Carya* sp		
Hollyhock	*Althaea rosea*	Jasmine	*Jasminum rex*
Honesty plant	*Lunaria annua*	Java glory bean	*Clerodendrum speciosum*
Honey flower *or* protea	*Protea mellifera*		
		Jelly beans	*Sedum pachyphyllum*
Honey locust	*Gleditsia triacanthos*		
		Job's tears	*Coix lacrymajobii*
Honey plant	*Hoya carnosa*	Jodetia	*Clarkia* sp
Horn of plenty	*Fedia cornucopiae*	Johnny jump up (except for seeds)	*Viola cornuta*
Horse mint	*Monardia didyma*		
Horse's tail	*Sedum morganianum*		
		Joshua tree	*Yucca brevifolia*
Hoya plant	*Hoya carnosa*	Joshua tree	*Sedum multiceps*
Ice plant	*Lampranthus* sp	Jupiter's beard	*Centranthus ruber*
Ice plant	*Aptenia cordifolia*	Kalanchoe	*Kalanchoe* sp
Ice plant	*Mesembryanthemum cordifolium*	Kale	*Brassica oleracea*
		Kangaroo vine	*Cissus antartica*
Impatiens *or* Impatients	*Impatiens* sp	Kentucky blue grass	*Poa pratensis*
Inch plant	*Zebrina pendula*		
Inch plant	*Callisia* sp	Kenya violet	*Saint Paulia* sp
Indian bean	*Catalpa* sp	King and queen fern	*Asplenium* sp
Indian hawthorn	*Raphiolepsis indica*		
Indian kale	*Zanthosoma lindeni*	Kingfisher daisy	*Felicia bergerana*
Indian paint brush	*Castilleja* sp	King of bromeliads	*Vriesea hieroglyphica*
		King of the forest	*Anoectochilus setaceus*
Indian strawberry	*Duchesnea indica*		
Indian tobacco	*Eriogonum umbellatum*	King protea	*Protea cynaroides*
		Knot root	*Stachys affinis*
India rubber plant	*Ficus elastica*	Kohleria	*Kohleria lindeniana*
Iron fern	*Rumohra adiantiformis*	Lace flower vine	*Episcia dianthiflora*
		Lady palm	*Rhapis* sp
Iron plant	*Aspidistra* sp	Lady's ear drops	*Fuchsia* sp
Italian cypress	*Cupressus sempervirens*	Lady's pocketbook	*Calceolaria crenatiflora*
Jacaranda tree	*Jacaranda* sp	Lamb's ears	*Stachys byzantina*
Jack jump about	*Aegopodium podagraria*	Lamb's tail	*Sedum morganianum*
Jade plant *or* tree	*Crassula* sp	Lasiandra	*Tibouchina* sp
Jade vine	*Strongylodon macrobotrys*	Lavender	*Lavandula officinalis*
		Lead plant	*Amorpha canescens*
Japanese aralia	*Fatsia japonica*	Leather fern	*Rumohra adiantiformis*
Japanese lantern	*Hibiscus* sp		
Japanese lily	*Lilium* sp	Lemon balm	*Melissa offinalis*
Japanese mahonia	*Mahonia japonica*	Lemon grass	*Cymbopogon citratus*
Japanese maple	*Acer palmatum*		

TABLE 62.2 Nontoxic Plants (*Continued*)

Common Name	Botanical Name	Common Name	Botanical Name
Leopard flower	*Belamcanda chinensis*	Maid fern *or* Maidenhair fern	*Adiantum decorum*
Leopard lily	*Lachenalia lilacina*		
Liatris	*Liatris* sp	Maidenhair vine	*Muehlenbeckia complexa*
Life plant	*Kalanchoe* sp		
Lilac	*Syringa* sp	Maltese cross	*Lychis chalcedonica*
Lipstick plant *or* vine	*Aeschynanthus* sp	Mandevilla vine	*Mandevilla* sp
		Manzanita	*Arbutus* sp
Liquidamber	*Liquidamber orientalis*	Manzanita, wooly	*Arctostaphylos tomentosa*
Linden tree	*Tilia americana*	Maple tree	*Acer* sp
Live forever	*Sedum telephium*	Maranta	*Calathea* sp
Living rock *or* stone	*Pleiospilos* sp	Maranta	*Maranta* sp
		Marbled spoon	*Cryptanthus* sp
Living rock	*Ariocarpus fissuratus*	Marble plant	*Lithops* sp
		Marbled spoon	*Cryptanthus* sp
Living stone	*Lithops karasmontana*	Marigold	*Calendula* sp
		Marine ivy or vine	*Cissus incisa*
Living stone	*Dinteranthus vanzylii*	Mariposa lily	*Calochortus* sp
Lobster claws	*Vriesea hieroglyphica*	Maternity plant	*Kalanchoe* sp
		Matilija poppy	*Romneya coulteri*
Lobster plant	*Euphorbia pulcherrima*	Merry Christmas	*Begonia rex*
		Mesquitilla	*Calliandra eriophylla*
Locust pods	*Ceratonia siliqua*	Mexican evening primrose	*Oenothera caespitosa*
Loosestrife	*Lysimachia* sp		
Lote tree	*Celtis australis*	Mexican firecracker	*Echeveria* sp
Love charm	*Clytostoma callistegioides*	Mexican flameleaf *or* flametree	*Euphorbia pulcherrima*
Love tree	*Cercis siliquastrum*		
Love vine	*Antigonon leptopus*	Mexican hat	*Ratibida columnaris*
Lucky bamboo	*Dracaena sanderiana*	Mexican heather	*Cuphea hyssopifolia*
		Mexican love plant	*Kalanchoe* sp
Madagascar dragon tree	*Dracaena marginata*		
Madagascar jasmine	*Stephanotis floribunda*	Mexican rose	*Oenothera caespitosa*
Madagascar lace plant	*Aponogeton senetralis*	Mexican shrimp plant	*Justicia brandegeana*
Madeira vine	*Anredera cordifolia*	Mexican snowball	*Echeveria* sp
Madrone	*Arbutus menziesil*		
Magic flower	*Cantua buxifolia*	Mimicry plant	*Pleiospilos* sp
Magic flower	*Achimenes* sp	Mimosa	*Albizia julibrissin*
Magnolia	*Magnolia* sp	Mind your own business	*Soleirolia soleirolii*
Mahonia	*Mahonia* sp		
Maiden's tears	*Silene acaulis*	Miner's candle	*Verbascum thapsus*
		Ming aralia	*Polyscias fruticosa*
		Miracle leaf	*Kalanchoe* sp

(*continued*)

TABLE 62.2 Nontoxic Plants (*Continued*)

Common Name	Botanical Name	Common Name	Botanical Name
Mirror plant	*Coprosma* sp	Nanny berry *or* plum	*Viburnum* sp
Mock orange	*Pittosporum tobira*		
Mock orange	*Philadelphus* sp	Nasturtium	*Tropaeolum* sp
Mock plane	*Acer pseudoplan-tanas*	Necklace vine	*Crassula rupestris*
		Necklace vine	*Muehlenbeckia complexa*
Mock strawberry	*Duchesnea indica*		
Monastery bells	*Cobaeae scandens*	Nerve plant	*Fittonia* sp
Money plant	*Lunaria annua*	Night-blooming cereus	*Hylocereus undatus*
Monkey bread plant	*Adansonia digitata*		
		Night jasmine	*Nyctanthes arbortristis*
Monkey plant	*Ruellia makoyana*		
Morning primrose	*Oenothera caespitosa*	Noble fir	*Abies procera*
		Norway spruce	*Picea abies*
Mosaic plant	*Fittonia argyroneura*	Oak leaf acanthus	*Acanthus* sp
Mosquito plant	*Cyananchum* sp		
Mosquito plant	*Azolla caroliniana*	Octopus tree	*Brassaia actinophylla*
Mother fern	*Aspelenium* sp		
Mother of hundreds	*Mammillaria compressa*	Old man of the mountains	*Hymenoxys grandiflora*
Mother of millions	*Kalanchoe pinnata*	Old man of the mountains	*Rudbergia grandiflora*
Mother of pearl plant	*Graptopetalum paraguayense*	Old man's beard	*Chionanthus virginicus*
Mother of pearl plant	*Sedum weinbergii*	Orchid	*Cattleya* sp
		Orchid	*Oncidium* sp
Mother of thousands	*Saxifraga stolonifera*	Orchid	*Epidendrum* sp
		Orchid	*Bulbophyllum* sp
Mother of thousands	*Kalanchoe pinnata*	Orchid	*Cymbidium* sp
		Orchid ginger	*Alpinia mutica*
Mother of thousands	*Tolmiea menziesii*	Oregon grape	*Mahonia aquifolium*
		Ox tongue	*Gasteria hybrida*
Mountain acanthus	*Acanthus* sp	Pagoda flower	*Clerodendrum* sp
		Paint brush	*Castilleja* sp
Mountain grape	*Mahonia* sp	Painted cup	*Castilleja* sp
Mountain rose	*Antigonon leptopus*	Painted dragon lily	*Dracaena fragrans*
Mountain tea	*Gaultheria procum-bens*	Painted feather	*Vriesea hiero-glyphica*
Mount Etna broom	*Genista aetnensis*	Painted lady	*Echeveria* sp
Mulberry	*Morus* sp	Painted leaf	*Euphorbia pulcherrima*
Mulberry, fruitless	*Morus* sp	Palm lily	*Cordyline australis*
Mullein	*Verbascum* sp	Palo verde	*Cercidium micro-phyllum*
Multiplication plant	*Kalanchoe* sp		
Muscari	*Muscari* sp	Pampas grass	*Cortaderia selloana*
Nandina	*Nandina domestica*	Panda plant	*Kalanchoe tomentosa*

TABLE 62.2 Nontoxic Plants (*Continued*)

Common Name	Botanical Name	Common Name	Botanical Name
Panda bear plant	Kalanchoe tomentosa	Poinsettia	Euphorbia pulcherrima
Pansy (except for seeds)	Viola tricolor	Polka dot plant	Hypoestes phyllostachya
Paper plant	Fatsia japonica	Poker plant	Kniphofia sp
Parlor palm	Chamaedorea elegans	Pond lily	Numphaea odorata
Parrot's beak or bill	Clianthus sp	Pony tail plant	Beaucarnea recurvata
Passion vine, purple	Gynura aurantiaca	Portulaca	Portulaca oleracea
Patience plant	Impatiens sp	Potentilla	Potentilla sp
Patient Lucy	Impatients sp	Prairie rocket	Cheirinia aspera
Peacock plant	Calathea makoyana	Prairie rocket	Erysimum sp
Peacock plant	Kaempferia roscoeana	Prairie snowball	Abronia sp
Pea shrub or tree	Caragana arborescens	Prayer plant	Maranta leuconeura
		Pregnant plant	Kalanchoe pinnata
Peperomia	Peperomia sp	Prince Albert's yew	Saxegothaea conspicua
Pepper vine	Ampelopsis arborea	Princess flower	Tibouchina sp
Persian violet	Exacum affine	Princess tree	Paulownia sp
Petunia	Petunia sp	Privet, wax-leaf	Ligustrum sp
Pheasant plant	Cryptanthus zonatus	Propeller plant	Crassula cultrate
Phlox	Phlox sp	Protea	Protea sp
Photinia	Photinia fraseri	Purple beard tongue	Penstemon pachyphyllus
Pick-a-back plant	Tolmiea menziesii	Purple beauty berry	Callicarpa sp
Piggyback plant	Tolmiea menziesii	Purple fringe	Phacelia sp
Pilea	Pilea sp	Purple passion vine	Gynura aurantiaca
Pincushion flower	Scabiosa sp		
Pine tree	Pinus sp	Purslane	Portulaca oleracea
Pink dot	Hypoestes phyllostachya	Pussy ears	Kalanchoe tomentosa
Pink fritillaria	Fritillaria pluriflora	Pussy ears	Cyanotis somaliensis
Pink polka dot	Hypoestes phyllostachya	Pyracantha	Pyracantha sp
Pink splash plant	Hypoestes phyllostachya	Queen cup	Clintonia uniflora
		Queen elkhorn	Platycerium sp
Pipe plant	Aeschnanthus sp	Queen of dracaenas	Dracaena goldieana
Pitcher plant	Darlingtonia californica	Queen of the night	Epiphyllum oxypetalum
Pittosporum	Pittosporum sp	Queen's jewels	Antigonon leptopus
Plane tree	Platanus occidentalis	Queen's tears	Billbergia nutans
Plumbago, Chinese	Ceratostigma willmottianum	Queen's umbrella tree	Brassaia actionophylla
Plush vine	Mikania apiifolia	Queen's wreath	Antigonon leptopus
Pocket plant	Calceolaria sp	Queensland arrowroot	Canna edulis
Pocketbook plant	Calceolaria sp		

(continued)

TABLE 62.2 Nontoxic Plants (*Continued*)

Common Name	Botanical Name	Common Name	Botanical Name
Queensland tree	*Aceratium megalospermum*	Sage tree	*Vitex* sp
		Salmon berry	*Rubus spectabilis*
Queensland umbrella tree	*Brassaia actinophylla*	Sand dollar cactus	*Astrophytum asterias*
Quince, common	*Cydonia oblonga*	Sand lily	*Leucocrinum montanum*
Quince, flowering	*Chaenomeles* sp		
Quince, Japanese	*Chaenomeles* sp	Sand lily	*Oenothera caespitosa*
Rabbit's foot	*Maranta leuconeura*		
Rabbit's foot fern	*Davallia fejeensis*	Sand verbena	*Abronia* sp
Rainbow plant	*Billbergia* sp	Santolina	*Santolina* sp
Rattlesnake plant	*Calathea insignis*	Satin flower	*Clarkia* sp
Red bud	*Cercis Canadensis*	Scarlet fritillaria	*Fritillaria* sp
Red gum	*Liquidamber* sp	Scarlet sumac	*Rhus glabra*
Red hot poker	*Kniphofia* sp	Schefflera	*Brassaia actinophylla*
Red-white-and-blue flower	*Cuphea* sp		
		Schefflera	*Schefflera* sp
Resurrection lily	*Kaempferia* sp	Scotch thistle	*Onopordum acanthium*
Resurrection plant	*Selaginella lepidophylla*		
		Sedum	*Sedum* sp
Ribbon plant	*Dracaena sanderiana*	Sego lily	*Calochortus* sp
		Sensitive fern	*Onoclea sensibilis*
Ribbon plant	*Chlorophytum comosum*	Sensitive plant	*Mimosa pudica*
		Sentry palm	*Howea forsterana*
Rock rose	*Cistus* sp	Serpentaria	*Lysimachia nummularia*
Rock rose	*Oenothera caespitosa*		
		Shell flower	*Alpinia nutans*
Rosary bead plant	*Ceropegia woodii*	Shell flower	*Molucella* sp
		Shell ginger	*Alpinia nutans*
Rosary plant	*Crassula rupestris*	Shoelace plant	*Crassula* sp
Rosary vine	*Crassula rupestris*	Shooting star	*Dodecatheon* sp
Rosary vine	*Ceropegia woodii*	Shrimp plant	*Beloperone guttata*
Rose	*Rosa* sp (except for *Rosa rugose*)	Shrimp plant *or* bush	*Justicia brandegeana*
Rose moss	*Portulaca grandiflora*	Siberian pea shrub *or* tree	*Caragana arborescens*
Rose of China	*Hibiscus senensis*	Silk tree	*Albizia julibrissin*
Rose of heaven	*Lychnis coeli-rosa*	Silver bell	*Halesia carolina*
Rose of Mexico	*Oenothera speciosa*	Silver berry	*Elaeagnus* sp
Rose of Sharon	*Hibiscus syriacus*	Silver calathea	*Calathea argyraea*
Rose verbena	*Verbena canadensis*	Silver crown	*Cotyledon undulata*
Rubber plant	*Ficus elastica*	Silver dollar	*Astrophytum asterias*
Rubber tree plant	*Ficus elastica*		
Russian olive	*Elaegans* sp	Silver dollar	*Crassula arborscens*
Sacred bamboo	*Nandina domestica*	Silver evergreen	*Aglaonema* sp
Sacred flower of Peru	*Cantua buxifolia*	Silver fittonia	*Fittonia argyroneura*
		Silver gum	*Eucalyptus cordata*
Sacred flower of the Incas	*Cantua buxifolia*	Silver king	*Aglaonema* sp
		Silver maple	*Acer saccharinum*

TABLE 62.2 Nontoxic Plants (*Continued*)

Common Name	Botanical Name	Common Name	Botanical Name
Silver nerve plant	*Fittonia argyroneura*	Strawberry begonia	*Saxifraga* sp
Silver net plant	*Fittonia argyroneura*		
Silver queen	*Aglaonema* sp	Strawberry geranium	*Saxifraga* sp
Silver ruffles	*Cotyledon undulata*		
Silver star	*Cryptanthus lacerdae*	Strawberry tree	*Arbutus unedo*
		Strawflower	*Helichrysum bracteatum*
Silver threads	*Fittonia argyroneura*		
Silver weed	*Potentilla* sp	String of buttons	*Crassula rupestris*
Slipper plant	*Calceolaria* spp	String of hearts	*Ceropegia woodii*
Slipper plant	*Sinningia pusilla*	Striped inch plant	*Callisia* sp
Skunk bush *or* plant	*Osmaronia* sp	Sugar bush	*Protea mellifera*
		Sugar pods	*Ceratonia siliqua*
Snapdragon	*Antirrhinum majus*	Sulfur flower	*Eriogonum umbellatum*
Snowball bush	*Viburnum* sp		
Snowbell tree	*Halesia carolina*	Sultana	*Impatients* sp
Snowbush	*Breynia disticha*	Sundrops	*Oenothera* sp
Soap berry	*Shepherdia* sp	Sunflower	*Helianthus annuus*
Soap weed	*Yucca* sp	Sun god	*Hymenoxys grandiflora*
Society garlic	*Tulbaghia violacea*		
Song of India	*Pleomele reflexa*	Sun god	*Rudbergia grandiflora*
Sonoran palo verde	*Cercidium praecox*		
		Swedish ivy	*Plectranthus australis*
Southern magnolia	*Magnolia grandiflora*		
		Sweet alyssum	*Lobularia maritime*
Spanish bayonet	*Yucca* sp	Sweet alyssum	*Alyssum* sp
Spanish moss	*Tillandsia usneoides*	Sweetberry	*Viburnum lentago*
Sparaxis	*Sparaxis* sp	Sweet flag	*Acorus* sp
Spider aralia	*Dizygotheca elegantissima*	Sweet gum	*Liquidambar* sp
		Sweet olive	*Osmanthus fragrans*
Spider plant	*Chlorophytum comosum*	Sweet viburnum	*Viburnum* sp
		Sweet William phlox	*Phlox diuaricata*
Spiraea	*Astilbe japonica*		
Spirea	*Spirea* sp	Sweet woodruff	*Asperula odorata*
Spruce tree	*Picea* sp	Sword fern	*Nephrolepsis* spp
Staghorn fern	*Platycerium* sp	Sword fern	*Polystichum munitum*
Starfish flower	*Stapelia* sp		
Star jasmine	*Trachelospermum jasminoides*	Sword grass	*Scirpus pungens*
		Sycamore tree	*Acer pseudoplatanus*
Starfish flower	*Stapelia* sp		
Stargazer lily	*Lilium* sp	Tahitian bridal veil	*Tradescantia multiflora*
Star lily	*Lilium* sp		
Star of Bethlehem	*Euphorbia pulcherrima*	Teaberry	*Gaultheria* sp
		Tea olive	*Osmanthus fragrans*
Statice	*Limonium* sp	Tea plant	*Viburnum* sp
Stephanotis	*Stephanotis floribunda*	Teddy bear vine *or* plant	*Cyanotis kewensis*
Stock	*Matthiola incana*	Temple bells	*Smithiantha cinnabarina*

(*continued*)

TABLE 62.2 Nontoxic Plants (*Continued*)

Common Name	Botanical Name	Common Name	Botanical Name
Ten command-ments plant	*Maranta* sp	Viburnum	*Viburnum* sp
		Vinegar tree	*Rhus glabra*
Texas bluebell	*Eustoma lisianthus*	Violas (except for seeds)	*Viola* sp
Thatch palm	*Coccothrinax crinita*		
Thorn apple *or* plum	*Crataegus* sp	Violets (except for seeds)	*Viola odorata*
Thrift	*Armeria maritime*	Viper's grass	*Scorzonera hispanica*
Ti plant	*Cordyline terminalis*		
Tickseed	*Coreopsis californica*	Wandering Jenny	*Lysimachia nummularia*
Tiger lily	*Lilium* sp	Wandering Jew	*Zebrina pendula*
Tomato tree	*Cyphomandra betacea*	Wandering sailor	*Lysimachia nummularia*
Torch lily	*Kniphofia* sp	Wandering tailor	*Lysimachia nummularia*
Touch-me-not	*Impatiens* spp		
Touch-me-not	*Mimosa pudica*	Wand flower	*Sparaxis* sp
Transvaal daisy	*Gerbera jamesoni*	Water hyacinth	*Eichhornia crassipes*
Tree of kings	*Cordyline terminalis*	Water lily	*Nymphaea* sp
Tree of life	*Mauritia flexuosa*	Watermelon pilea	*Pilea cadierei*
Tree of sadness	*Nyctanthes arbortritis*	Watsonia	*Watsonia* sp
Tree privet	*Ligustrum licidium*	Wax flower	*Stephanotis floribunda*
Trumpet vine	*Distictis* sp		
Tubeflower	*Clerodendrum indicum*	Wax leaf privet	*Ligustrum japonicum*
Tulip poplar *or* tree	*Liriodendron tulipifera*	Wax plant	*Hoya carnosa*
		Wax rosette	*Echeveria* sp
Tulip tree	*Spathodea campanulata*	Weeping fig	*Ficus benjamina*
		Weigela	*Weigela* sp
Tupelo gum tree	*Nyssa aquatica*	Western wallflower	*Cheirinia aspera*
Twistwood	*Viburnum* sp		
Umbrella plant	*Eriogonum umbellatum*	Western wallflower	*Erysimum* sp
Umbrella tree	*Brassaia actinophylla*	West Indian holly	*Leea* sp
		Whirling butterflies	*Gaura* sp
Upland sumac	*Rhus glabra*		
Urn plant	*Aechmea fasciata*	White ginger	*Hedychium coronarium*
Valor plant	*Crassula argentea*		
Vanilla plant	*Liatris* sp	Whitewood	*Liriodendron tulipifera*
Veldt daisy	*Gerbera jamesonii*		
Velvet leaf	*Abutilon theophrasti*	Whitewood	*Tilia americana*
Velvet leaf	*Kalanchoe beharensis*	Wild olive	*Halesia Carolina*
		Wild olive	*Nyssa aquatica*
Velvet plant	*Gynura* sp	Wild olive	*Osmanthus americanus*
Verbena	*Verbena* sp (except *Verbena hastata*)		
		Wild strawberry	*Fragaria* sp
Veronica	*Veronica* sp	Winter cherry	*Cardiospermum halicacabum*
Veronica	*Hebe* sp		

TABLE 62.2	Nontoxic Plants (*Continued*)		
Common Name	**Botanical Name**	**Common Name**	**Botanical Name**
Wolfberry	*Symphoricarpos* sp	Zebra plant	*Aphelandra squarrosa*
Woolflower	*Celosia* sp		
Xylosma	*Xylosma* sp	Zebra plant	*Calathea zebrine*
Yellow wood	*Cladrastis lutea*	Zebra plant	*Cryptanthus zonatus*
Yellow wood	*Rhodosphaera rhodanthema*	Zinnia	*Zinnia* sp
		Zulu giant	*Stapelia gigantea*
Yucca	*Yucca* sp	Zygocactus	*Schlumbergera bridgesii*

Capsaicin alkaloids are thought to deplete nerve terminals of substance P that stimulates sensory nerve endings resulting in pain and burning. Nettle plants have "hairs" that inject the skin with histamine, acetylcholine, and serotonin, resulting in wheals, pruritus, and burning at the sting (6,8).

Photodermatitis may result after exposure to plants containing oils that intensify the skin's sensitivity to sunlight. Onset occurs within hours but can be delayed for up to 48 hours. A rash similar to sunburn occurs, but only skin that has both been in contact with the plant and exposed to the sun is affected (1,6,8).

Mechanical trauma after exposure to the thorns, spines, and barbs of any plant species can occur. Spines or thorns breaking off in the skin may cause secondary infections and wound ulceration (4).

ED EVALUATION

A history of exposure is critical in alerting the clinician to the possibility of plant toxicity. Questions concerning the use of or contact with plants should be asked when a patient presents with an illness of uncertain cause. Additionally, patients should be asked about the ingestion of homemade tea used to treat themselves or their sick children.

In children, even if ingestion was not witnessed, questions should be asked about plant availability. Evidence of plant exposure may include plant material on a child, missing parts on a plant, or plant material in the stool or vomitus. If possible, any suspect plant (or a sample) should be brought with the patient to the ED (1,8).

Many plants have multiple common and scientific names. Some plants sharing common names may include both toxic and nontoxic species. If the patient provides a common name of a plant, the correct identity should be confirmed by the scientific Latin name, as well as a botanic description (2). Plant nurseries, botanic gardens, park rangers, university agricultural departments, garden clubs, and floral or garden shops may be of value in identifying unknown plants (1). Poison control centers may also help with information on plant toxicity and treatment options.

Depending on the patient's signs and symptoms, a complete physical examination is appropriate. All patients should have a complete set of vital signs, including temperature. Depending on the history and physical findings, a rhythm strip or electrocardiogram interpretation may be indicated (1,6,8). Laboratory testing may be necessary for the assessment of fluid and electrolyte, hematologic, liver, or renal function abnormalities. With few exceptions (e.g., cardiac glycoside plants), specific toxicology testing is unlikely to be helpful. Digoxin radioimmunoassays can be used to detect digitalis glycosides. Interpretation of quantitative results for plant cardiac glycosides is limited, and the results should only be used as a qualitative marker (1,8).

Finally, the possibility should be kept in mind that the plant may have been treated with a pesticide or herbicide that may be causing the symptoms rather than the plant itself (see Chapters 21, 23, and 24).

ED MANAGEMENT

Supportive care and GI and skin decontamination are the primary treatment modalities. Although rarely necessary, advanced life-support measures should be instituted when appropriate. Supportive therapy includes replacement of volume deficits with intravenous (IV) crystalloids and correction of electrolyte abnormalities. Patients with CNS depression may require airway protection and ventilatory support. Patients manifesting seizures and CNS stimulation usually respond to treatment with benzodiazepines. Refractory seizures can be treated with benzodiazepines and phenobarbital. Allergic reactions and hematologic, liver, and renal toxicity are treated with standard measures (1,6,8).

Local pain and irritation from the ingestion of plants containing insoluble oxalate crystals can be treated with age-appropriate cold foods or liquids such as juice bars, ice cream, yogurt, milk, or ice cubes, which decrease mouth pain and help alleviate any localized oral swelling. The pain usually lasts 15 to 30 minutes, and other treatment is usually not needed (1,3,6).

Decontamination varies with the nature of the exposure. Dilution with small amounts of clear liquids is usually sufficient for the ingestion of plants that only cause gastroenteritis. Because many plant toxins are large molecules, activated charcoal should be effective and is the preferred method of GI decontamination for recent ingestions of agents with potential systemic toxicity (1,6,8).

Skin and eye exposures are treated with thorough irrigation. Some cactus spines can be removed with tweezers or forceps (4,6). Fine spines have been removed with tape, facial masks, glue mixtures, warm wax, and wood pastes applied to the skin and then peeled off. Oily materials, such as the toxicodendrol oils from poison ivy or poison oak, should be washed thoroughly with soap and water to prevent spread to other parts of the body, clothing, or to ED staff. Affected clothing may also need to be washed to prevent further contamination. Antihistamines, topical or oral systemic steroids, and analgesics for itching and pain may be required for some dermal exposures. Topical antiseptics and tetanus prophylaxis may be useful if there are puncture wounds (6,8).

There are few antidotes for plant poisonings. Those that are useful are generally similar in effectiveness and are given in the same dosage as when administered for a nonplant exposure to the same toxic substance. For example, cardiac glycoside poisoning may be treated with digoxin-specific Fab-fragment antibodies (see Chapter 30), although calculating a dose is challenging. Severe anticholinergic plant poisoning is potentially treatable with physostigmine (see Chapter 49). Patients with symptomatic cyanogenic glycoside poisoning should be treated with specific cyanide antidotes (see Chapter 34) (1,6–8).

CRITICAL INTERVENTIONS

- Obtain complete vital signs, including temperature, on all patients with suspected plant ingestions.
- Obtain an accurate name of the plant, including the common and scientific name.
- Evaluate patients with plant ingestions for possible upper airway obstruction.
- Provide supportive care as clinically necessary.

DISPOSITION

Although the vast majority of patients with plant exposures can be treated at home or discharged from the ED, patients with acute ingestions of a potentially toxic plant should be observed until symptoms have resolved. Patients who are symptomatic after ingesting plants containing cardiac glycoside and CNS toxins should be admitted for close observation, monitoring, and treatment. The level of care should be dictated by clinical severity. If severe, patients with fluid and electrolyte imbalance, allergic reactions, and hematologic, liver, or renal toxicity may also require admission (1,8).

COMMON PITFALLS

- Failure to appreciate that plant poisoning can affect virtually any organ system
- Failure to inquire about plant exposure and herbal use in patients with unexplained complaints, particularly GI and CNS symptoms and rashes
- Failure to appreciate that different plants may have the same common name, which may include both toxic and nontoxic plant species
- Failure to appreciate that some edible plants also have toxic components
- Failure to appreciate that specific antidotes are available for the treatment of anticholinergic, cardiac glycoside, and cyanogenic glycoside plant poisoning
- Failure to appreciate that plants may have been treated with pesticides, which may be the cause of the symptoms

ICD9

988.2 Toxic effects of berries and other plants eaten as food

REFERENCES

1. Alsop JA. Plants. In: Olson KR, ed. *Poisoning and drug overdose,* 5th ed. New York: Lange Medical Books/McGraw-Hill, 2007;309–321.
2. DiTomaso JM. Problems associated with the use of common names in the identification of poisonous plants. *Vet Hum Toxicol* 1993;35:465–466.
3. Franceschi VR, Nakata PA. Calicum oxalate in plants: formation and function. *Ann Rev Plant Biol* 2005;56:41–71.
4. Lindsey D, Lindsey WE. Cactus spine injuries. *Am J Emerg Med* 1988;6:362–369.
5. Mrvos R, Krenzelok EP. Toxidromes associated with the most common plant ingestions. *Vet Hum Toxicol* 2001;43:366–369.
6. *POISINDEX® system,* Klasco RK, ed. Greenwood Village, CO: Thomson Healthcare, 2008.
7. Rich SQ, Libera JM, Locke RJ. Treatment of foxglove extract poisoning with digoxin-specific fab-fragments. *Ann Emerg Med* 1993;22:1904–1907.
8. Smolinske SC, Daubert GP, Spoerke DG. Poisonous plants. In: Shannon MW, Borron SW, Burns MJ, eds. *Haddad and Winchester's clinical management of poisoning and drug overdose,* 4th ed. Saunders Elsevier, 2007;473–506.

Dietary Supplements and Herbal Medications

CLINICAL PRESENTATION

Dietary supplements form a category that is broadly unified in terms of intended use but not by any equivalence of biochemical composition or physiologic effect. Manifestations of toxicity are therefore varied. Acute effects may include allergy, any of the toxidromes, cardiac dysrhythmias, gastrointestinal distress, hepatitis, hepatic veno-occlusive disease, renal impairment, metabolic or electrolyte disturbance, hemorrhage, nervous system stimulation or depression (Table 63.1). Detailed information about specific agents and central potential interactions may be found at the National Center for Complementary and Alternative Medicine website (http://nccam.nih.gov). The Natural Medicines Comprehensive Database (http://www.naturaldatabase.com) is also a credible source of information.

DIFFERENTIAL DIAGNOSIS

The toxic effects of various herbal preparations are varied, and an appropriate differential diagnosis should be constructed with respect to these specific signs and symptoms. Conversely, because herbal preparations can affect every organ system, toxicity from dietary supplements should be considered in the differential diagnosis of any unexplained metabolic or organ failure.

ED EVALUATION

The initial evaluation of a patient with potential toxicity from dietary supplements should proceed as for any other emergency department patient, with immediate attention given to the stabilization of the ABCs (airway, breathing, and circulation) and vital signs. A history of exposure to dietary supplements is clearly helpful in evaluating the potential for adverse effects. Clinicians should be aware that many patients believe that dietary supplements are benign and may not include them on a list of "medications" unless explicitly prompted. Others may be hesitant to admit their use of herbals and supplements to a physician for fear of censure or judgment. Clinicians should also be aware that products may be contaminated or that labeling may be unclear or misleading. Ultimately, the best gauge of toxicity is

TABLE 63.1	Toxic Manifestations of Selected Dietary Supplements by Presenting Complaint

Anticholinergic toxidrome: bittersweet (*Celastrus scandens*); burdock (*Arctium lappa*); deadly nightshade (*Atropa belladonna*); henbane *(Hyocyamus niger)*; Jimsonweed (*Datura stramonium*); lobelia (*Lobelia inflata*); mandrake (*Mandragon officinarum*)

Bradycardia: cardiac glycosides: e.g., *Bufo* sp venom; dogbane (*Apocynum cannabimum*); foxglove (*Digitalis purpurea, D. Lanata*); lily-of-the-valley (*Convallaria majalis*); oleander (*Negrium oleanderi*); red squill (*Urginea maritima*)

Cardiac dysrhythmias (other): metals; monkshood (*Aconitum* species; "Caowu"), larkspur (*Delphinium sp.*) [Na$^+$ channel activation]; quinine (*Chinchona* species) [Na$^+$ channel blockade]; see also "Stimulants"

Coagulopathy: danshen (*Salvia miltiorrhiza*); dong quai (*Angelica polymorpha*); garlic (*Allium sativum*); ginko (*Ginkgo biloba*); tonka beans (*Dipteryx* sp)

Gastroenteritis: common: e.g., pokeweed (*Phytolacca americana*); senna (*Cassia angustifolia*); salmonella infection from rattlesnake meat; particularly concerning if due to metals

Hepatitis: borage (*Borago officinalis*); boron; chaparral (*Covillea tridentata, Larrea tridentata*); coltsfoot (*Tussilago farfara*); germander (*Teucrium chamaedrys*); kava kava (*Piper methysticum*)

Hepatic venoocclusive disease: comfrey (*Symphytum officinale*); gordolobo (*Senecio* sp); heliotrope (*Crotalaria specatabilli; Heliotropium europaeum*); T'u-san-chi (*Gynura segetum*)

Hypotension: black cohosh (*Cimicifuga racemosa*); false hellebore (*Veratrum* sp); Hawthorn (*Crataegus laevigata*); white cohosh (*Actea* sp)

Renal failure: aristolochic acid (*Aristolochia fangchi*); autumn crocus (*Colchicum autumnale*); colloidal silver; germanium (dioxide); juniper (*Juniper communis*), licorice (*Glycyrrhiza glabra*)

Peripheral neuropathy: clove oil (*Eugenia aromatic*); metals (arsenic, germanium, lead, mercury, thallium); podophyllum (*Podophyllum peltatum*); pyridoxine (B6); selenium

Sedative-hypnotic: hawthorn (*Crataegus oxyacantha*); hops (*Humulus lupulus*); kava kava (*Piper methysticum*); valerian (*Valeriana* sp)

Seizures: camphor (*Cinnamomum camphora*); Chinese cucumber (*Compound Q*); fennel oil (*Foeniculum vulgare*); wormwood (*Artemesia absinthium*); see "Anticholinergics" and "Stimulants"

Stimulants: betel (*Areca catechu*); methylxanthines (cocoa [*Theobromo cacao*], coffee [*Coffee arabica*], tea [*Camellia sinensis*], kola [*Cola nitida/acuminata*], maté [*Ilex paraguariensis*], guarana [*Paullinia cupana*]); ephedra (*Ephedra sinica;* ma huang; "herbal ecstasy"); khat (*Catha edulis*); bitter orange (*Citrus aurantium*); tobacco (*Nicotiana tobacum*); nutmeg (*Myristica fragrans*)

a focused history and physical examination in conjunction with selected ancillary tests of metabolic and organ-system dysfunction.

ED MANAGEMENT

The acute care of a patient with actual or potential toxicity from a dietary supplement is based on the nature and severity of illness. Gastrointestinal decontamination may be appropriate for patients who present early after a significant ingestion of a potentially toxic substance. Good supportive care is sufficient to treat most overdoses, but there are some notable exceptions. For example, poisoning with cardiac glycosides warrants therapy with multidose activated charcoal or digoxin-specific Fab fragments. Cyanide toxicity warrants specific therapy with sodium thiosulfate or hydroxocobalamin. Heavy-metal poisoning may require chelation therapy. Patients with anticholinergic toxicity may benefit from judicious use of physostigmine. All patients with possible toxicity from a dietary supplement should be advised to discontinue its use. All toxicity from herbals and dietary supplements should be reported to the regional poison center. This may help identify products that are contaminated, misrepresented, or pose significant public health risks in addition to serving as an informational resource for the clinician.

CRITICAL INTERVENTIONS

- Routinely ask about the use of dietary supplements while taking the medication history.
- Report all suspected drug interactions and adverse effects of dietary supplements by calling your regional poison center, or the FDA MedWatch program at 1-800-FDA-1088. (You may also report these online at http://www.fda.gov/Safety/MedWatch.)

DISPOSITION

Patient disposition depends on the presentation. Significant organ dysfunction demands admission to a higher level of care and a rigorous examination of all potential causes. Patients who take intentional overdoses should also have psychiatric evaluation prior to discharge.

COMMON PITFALLS

- Failure to recognize that most people regard herbals and dietary supplements as benign and may not alert the clinician to their use unless specifically prompted
- Failure to consider toxicity from herbals and dietary supplements in the differential diagnosis of unexplained organ dysfunction
- Failure to warn patients of potential interactions between medications and herbals and dietary supplements

CHAPTER 64

Seafood Toxins

CLINICAL PRESENTATION

Seafood toxin poisoning typically affects the gastrointestinal (GI) and neurologic systems.

Ciguatera poisoning typically occurs 2 to 30 hours after ingestion of ciguatoxic fish. Patients characteristically present with circumoral and/or extremity paresthesias, arthralgias, myalgias, diarrhea, vomiting, bradycardia, and pruritus. A classic, though uncommon, finding is hot-cold temperature sensation reversal in which a burning or painful sensation is associated with touching cold objects (1). Patients may present initially with only neurologic symptoms; these may be delayed up to 72 hours after ingestion or may occur without GI symptoms. Hypotension is common and may be due to fluid loss, bradycardia, peripheral vasodilatation, or myocardial depression. Symptoms vary among different patients and depend on where the fish were caught and what parts were eaten. More severe toxicity, especially hypotension and bradycardia, occurs in patients who were previously poisoned by ciguatera. Other common neurologic symptoms include asthenia, paresis, tremors, and pain affecting the joints, head, and abdomen. The paresthesias do not conform to dermatomal or peripheral nerve distribution. A sensation of looseness of the teeth is another unusual symptom. Insomnia, neurosis, depression, and hallucinations may occur. Other features include dyspnea, diaphoresis, salivation, tearing, chills, neck stiffness, pruritus, rashes, and tachycardia. In pregnant patients, violent fetal movements have been described. Less commonly, transient blindness, convulsions, rhabdomyolysis, polymyositis, or paralysis may occur. Death, although uncommon, may result from severe dehydration or cardiac or respiratory failure (1).

The onset of scombroid poisoning is normally within 1 hour of ingestion. The presentation is similar to, but generally less severe than, IgE-mediated allergic (anaphylactic) or anaphylactoid reactions. Patients experience intense flushing of the upper trunk and face, nausea, vomiting, hives, pruritus, tachycardia, bronchospasm, and occasionally hypotension. Severe reactions, such as bronchospasm, hypotension, and supraventricular tachyarrhythmias, are more likely to occur in patients with pre-existing cardiac or respiratory disease. Findings usually resolve within 6 to 12 hours from the time of ingestion (10).

Patients with tetrodotoxin poisoning usually present within 10 to 45 minutes after ingesting the toxic seafood. However, cases presentations delayed up to

20 hours are reported. Early symptoms include a feeling of exhilaration. Four stages of poisoning have been described. Initially, circumoral paresthesias, salivation, nausea, and vomiting occur, followed by peripheral paresthesias and numbness. Sensory symptoms then become more generalized, with ascending paralysis of the extremities, although deep-tendon reflexes remain intact. In the third stage, ataxia and paralysis of peripheral and bulbar muscles occur. Finally, respiratory muscles are affected, although patients may still be conscious (8). Patients may become unconscious and completely paralyzed, with dilated nonreactive pupils and loss of all brainstem reflexes. Owing to its effect on the sodium channel, cardiac arrhythmias, including A-V blocks, are also reported (5). Recovery occurs over a period of days and, unless complicated by anoxia, is complete. Death is usually due to paralysis of the respiratory muscles.

Paralytic shellfish poisoning occurs within minutes of ingestion and usually begins with neurologic symptoms including perioral, hand, and finger paresthesias, with associated nausea and abdominal pain. These are followed by paresthesias of the face and extremities and progressive muscle paralysis. Bulbar muscles are often affected, causing dysarthria, dysphagia, diplopia, and loss of the gag reflex. Other features include vertigo, ataxia, transient blindness, altered temperature perception, hypotension, headache, and low back pain. The paresthesias then become generalized, and a progressive paralysis including loss of deep-tendon reflexes and fixed-dilated pupils develops. Respiratory paralysis may be fatal without rapid intervention. Complete recovery typically occurs within 24 to 48 hours (4).

Neurotoxic shellfish poisoning causes a syndrome similar to ciguatera. Circumoral paresthesias that generalize, headache, tachycardia, and muscle cramps are common. Nausea, abdominal pain, vomiting, and diarrhea also occur. Seizures and coma have occurred with severe poisonings.

Amnestic shellfish poisoning also produces neurologic and GI findings, with onset of effects from minutes to 38 hours. Abdominal pain, nausea, and diarrhea, with loss of memory, severe headache, confusion, and disorientation commonly occur. Severe intoxication can result in seizures and coma. Improvement occurred 24 hours to 12 weeks after ingestion of mussels containing domoic acid (11).

The main symptoms from diarrheic shellfish poisoning and azaspiracid poisoning are gastrointestinal in origin. Onset occurs from 30 minutes to 10 hours after ingestion of seafood (3). Predominant effects include diarrhea, nausea, vomiting, abdominal cramps, and chills. Patients usually do not have a fever (3,6). Full recovery from this self-limited illness occurs within 3 to 4 days (12).

Ichthyoallyeinotoxism, hallucinatory fish poisoning, begins within minutes to 2 hours of ingestion of toxic fish. Initial symptoms resemble ethanol intoxication and include ataxia, incoordination, and general malaise/weakness. Within hours, patients report hallucinations (visual and/or auditory) and become delirious. Nightmares can occur. Less commonly, some patients experience vomiting and diarrhea. Symptoms usually resolve within 24 to 36 hours, although weakness can persist for days (2).

DIFFERENTIAL DIAGNOSIS

Patients who present with illness related to seafood toxins generally have a predominance of GI and neurologic signs and symptoms. The clinical presentation of ciguatera, neurotoxic shellfish, palytoxin, tetrodotoxin, and paralytic shellfish poisoning may be difficult to distinguish, as all may involve symptoms of paresthesias, weakness, and ataxia. Location, predominant symptoms, and the type of fish eaten are used to determine the specific etiology. A common shellfish origin has been found for toxins associated with tetrodotoxin and paralytic shellfish poisoning.

Infectious viral and bacterial gastroenteritis must be considered in any patient presenting with GI complaints. Common seafood pathogens include hepatitis A, Norwalk virus, *Vibrio spp.* (including *V. cholerae, V. parahaemolyticus,* and *V. vulnificus*).

Encephalitis, meningitis, Guillain-Barre, botulism, and transient ischemic attack, or stroke, should be considered in patients presenting with paralysis or other neurologic findings. In patients presenting with seizures, electrolyte and metabolic abnormalities, other toxins or an underlying seizure disorder should also be considered.

Anaphylaxis to seafood should be considered, especially in patients with signs and symptoms of scombroid poisoning. A metallic or strong peppery taste to the fish and the type of fish may distinguish scombroid from a true allergic reaction. Skin flushing can occur with scombroid poisoning but also with red man syndrome, niacin ingestion, monosodium glutamate ingestion, and ethanol-disulfiram interactions.

ED EVALUATION

One should obtain a history of foods ingested in patients with the combination of GI and neurologic symptoms. Special attention should be paid to the type of seafood ingested, locale, time of ingestion, and onset of symptoms. The origin of the seafood should be identified if possible, as this may help to differentiate poisonings specific to certain regions.

Public health officials may be able to assist in this process and provide information about similar cases or known quarantined fishing areas. Physical examination should focus on vital signs, respiratory function, and the neurologic examination, including deep-tendon reflexes and sensation. Patients with tachycardia or hypotension should be evaluated for hypovolemia. Patients with prominent neurologic findings should have objective measurement of the forced vital capacity and/or negative inspiratory force. The skin should be examined for rashes, hives, or flushing.

Laboratory evaluation should include fingerstick glucose in patients with altered mental status and a basic metabolic panel to evaluate for abnormal electrolytes, blood urea nitrogen, and serum creatinine. These tests are helpful to exclude nontoxin-related illnesses.

Assays for specific seafood toxins in the patient's blood are not readily available. However, if the seafood or seafood from the restaurant or home is available, testing may be available through public health authorities.

ED MANAGEMENT

Supportive care is the mainstay of therapy in all seafood toxin–related syndromes. Airway, breathing, and circulation (ABCs) should be addressed initially. Patients should have intravenous access and cardiac monitoring as appropriate. In patients with abnormal ventilation as demonstrated by decreased vital capacity, negative inspiratory force, or hypopnea or apnea, intubation and mechanical ventilation should be considered. Abnormal heart rhythms such as bradycardia should be addressed. Patients with tachycardia or hypotension should initially receive intravenous saline, but vasopressors such as dopamine, norepinephrine, or phenylephrine may be required if hypotension is unresponsive to saline.

In patients who may still have seafood in their stomach, activated charcoal (1 g/kg) should be considered. Antiemetics should be used for nausea and vomiting.

Specific therapy has been used in ciguatera poisoning. Mannitol, 1 g/kg, is often recommended for patients with severe neurologic toxicity such as coma, although there are conflicting data on its efficacy (7,9). Amitriptyline, which may act by blocking sodium channels, usually provides some relief from the chronic neurologic symptoms of ciguatera poisoning. Other agents used with varying degrees of success include fluoxetine, nifedipine, vitamins B_{12} and C, calcium gluconate (1–3 g intravenously over 24 hours), lidocaine, and tocainide. Two patients who were treated with gabapentin (400 mg orally three times daily) experienced a rapid improvement and recurrence of symptoms after therapy was discontinued. Other medications commonly used for neuropathic pain have been used for persistent paresthesias. Indomethacin and cyproheptadine are commonly used to relieve arthralgia and pruritus, respectively.

For scombroid poisoning, treatment includes H_1- and H_2-receptor antagonists. H_2 blockers such as cimetidine appear more effective than type 1 blockers such as diphenhydramine (4). Epinephrine may benefit the rare severely ill patient with hypotension who is not responsive to intravenous saline or with bronchospasm not responsive to albuterol. Corticosteroids are of little benefit, as this poisoning is due to histamine only (i.e., no secondary mediators such as leukotrienes are released). Once stabilized, patients with scombroid poisoning can be discharged on oral antihistamines for 48 hours.

Benzodiazepines are useful to manage the disturbing hallucinations and nightmares experienced by patients with hallucinatory fish poisoning. Edrophonium and neostigmine have been used to reverse motor paralysis due to tetrodotoxin poisoning but have not been studied in controlled trials.

Besides supportive care, prevention is the best treatment of all. Fish weighing >2 kg or of those types known to be frequently affected should be avoided to prevent ciguatera. Patients should also avoid eating specific organs in which the toxins accumulate, such as the liver and gonads for ciguatera and tetrodotoxin. The government aids in prevention by banning the sale of certain fish known to carry the toxin. In Miami, barracuda is banned from sale owing to the risk of ciguatera poisoning. The government also periodically tests shellfish for certain toxins and when red tides occur, and quarantines are instituted as appropriate.

CRITICAL INTERVENTIONS

- Assess ABCs and evaluate pulmonary function early with measurements of forced vital capacity and negative inspiratory force.
- Provide supportive care, including antiemetics for nausea and vomiting and intravenous saline for dehydration and hypotension.
- Treat scombroid poisoning with H_1- and H_2-receptor antagonists.
- Consult a regional poison center and/or public health officials for current treatment advice and to report outbreaks.

DISPOSITION

Most patients may be discharged home after evaluation and supportive treatment in the emergency department. Outpatient follow-up should be arranged. Patients with abnormal vital signs, neurologic symptoms, persistent vomiting, or inability to tolerate oral fluids should be admitted to the hospital. Patients with neurologic symptoms or those at risk for development of respiratory weakness or paralysis should be admitted to an intensive care unit for close monitoring. Local or state departments of health should be notified of all cases of suspected seafood poisoning, as timely intervention may prevent additional exposures.

COMMON PITFALLS

- Failure to consider seafood poisonings in patients with gastroenteritis and/or neurologic symptoms
- Failure to admit patients with neurologic findings for monitoring
- Failure to treat scombroid poisoning with anti-histamines

ICD9

988.0 Toxic effect of fish and shellfish eaten as food

REFERENCES

1. Bagnis R, Kuberski T, Laugier S. Clinical observations on 3,009 cases of ciguatera (fish poisonings) in the South Pacific. *Am J Trop Med Hyg* 1979;28:1067–1073.
2. de Haro L, Pommier P. Hallucinatory fish poisoning (ichthyoallyeinotoxism): two case reports from the western Mediterranean and literature review. *Clin Toxicol* 2006;44:185–188.
3. Economou V, Papadopoulou C, Brett M, et al. Diarrhetic shellfish poisoning due to toxic mussel consumption: the first recorded outbreak in Greece. *Food Addit Contam* 2007;24:297–305.
4. Gessner BD, Middaugh JP, Doucette GJ. Paralytic shellfish poisoning in Kodiak, Alaska. *West J Med* 1997;167:351–353.
5. How C, Chern C, Huang Y, et al. Tetrodotoxin poisoning. *Am J Emerg Med* 2003;21:51–54.
6. James KJ, Moroney C, Roden C, et al. Ubiquitous "benign" alga emerges as the cause of shellfish contamination responsible for the human toxic syndrome, azaspiracid poisoning. *Toxicon* 2003;41:145–151.
7. Palafox NA, Jain LG, Pinano AZ, et al. Successful treatment of ciguatera fish poisoning with intravenous mannitol. *JAMA* 1988;259:2740–2742.

8. Perl TM, Bedard L, Kosatsky T, et al. An outbreak of toxic encephalopathy caused by eating mussels contaminated with domoic acid. *N Engl J Med* 1990;322:1775–1780.
9. Schnorf H, Taurarii M, Cundy T, et al. Ciguatera fish poisoning: a double-blind randomized trial of mannitol therapy. *Neurology* 2002;58:873–880.
10. Smart DR. Scombroid poisoning. A report of seven cases involving the Western Australian salmon, *Arripis truttaceus*. *Med J Aust* 1992;157:748–751.
11. Teitelbaum JS, Zatorre RJ, Carpenter S, et al. Neurologic sequelae of domoic acid intoxication due to the ingestion of contaminated mussels. *N Engl J Med* 1990;322:1781–1787.
12. Whittle K, Gallacher S. Marine toxins. *Br Med Bull* 2000;56:236–253.

INDEX

Page numbers followed by "f" indicate figures; those followed by "t" indicate tables.

CCS0412